TOP TRAILS™
Yosemite

Written by
Jeffrey P. Schaffer

Series created by
Joseph Walowski

 WILDERNESS PRESS · BERKELEY, CALIFORNIA

Top Trails Yosemite

1st EDITION April 2007
  2nd Printing October 2007

All photos copyright by Jeffrey P. Schaffer, except where noted
Maps: Lohnes + Wright
Cover design: Frances Baca Design and Lisa Pletka
Interior design: Frances Baca Design
Book production: Pease Press
Book editor: Elaine Merrill

ISBN: 978-0-89997-425-5
UPC: 7-19609-97425-3

Manufactured in Canada

Published by: **Wilderness Press**
               1200 5th Street
               Berkeley, CA 94710
               (800) 443-7227; FAX (510) 558-1696
               info@wildernesspress.com
               www.wildernesspress.com
Visit our website for a complete listing of our books and for ordering information.

Cover photos: Four Mile Trail takes the hiker past spectacular views of Yosemite Falls, by John Elk III/Lonely Planet Images; Ground squirrel (inset), by Thomas Winnett

SAFETY NOTICE: Although Wilderness Press and the author have made every attempt to ensure that the information in this book is accurate at press time, they are not responsible for any loss, damage, injury, or inconvenience that may occur to anyone while using this book. You are responsible for your own safety and health while in the wilderness. The fact that a trail is described in this book does not mean that it will be safe for you. Be aware that trail conditions can change from day to day. Always check local conditions and know your own limitations.

The Top Trails™ Series

D0003084

Wilderness Press

When Wilderness Press published *Sierra North* in 1967, no other trail guide like it existed for the Sierra backcountry. The first run of 2800 copies sold out in less than two months and its success heralded the beginning of Wilderness Press. In the past 35 years, we have expanded our territories to cover California, Alaska, Hawaii, the U.S. Southwest, the Pacific Northwest, New England, Canada, and Baja California.

Wilderness Press continues to publish comprehensive, accurate, and readable outdoor books. Hikers, backpackers, kayakers, skiers, snowshoers, climbers, cyclists, and trail runners rely on Wilderness Press for accurate outdoor adventure information.

Top Trails

In its Top Trails guides, Wilderness Press has paid special attention to organization so that you can find the perfect hike each and every time. Whether you're looking for a steep trail to test yourself on or a walk in the park, a romantic waterfall or a city view, Top Trails will lead you there.

Each Top Trails guide contains trails for everyone. The trails selected provide a sampling of the best that the region has to offer. These are the "must-do" hikes, walks, runs and bike rides, with every feature of the area represented.

Every book in the Top Trails series offers:

- The Wilderness Press commitment to accuracy and reliability
- Ratings and rankings for each trail
- Distances and approximate times
- Easy-to-follow trail notes
- Maps & permit information

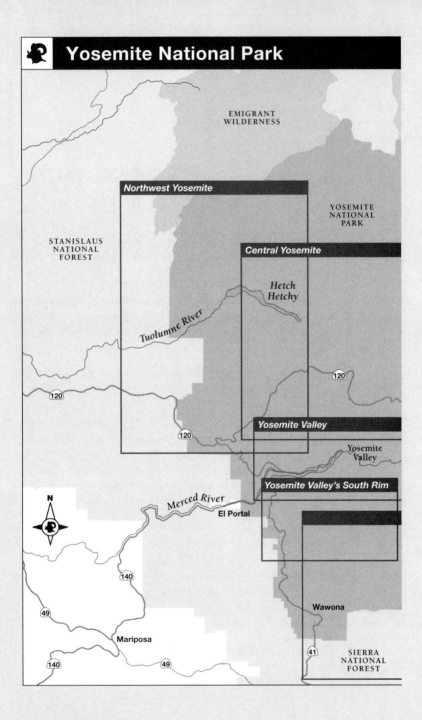

Yosemite National Park

EMIGRANT
WILDERNESS

Northwest Yosemite

YOSEMITE
NATIONAL
PARK

STANISLAUS
NATIONAL
FOREST

Central Yosemite

Hetch
Hetchy

Tuolumne River

120

120

120

Yosemite Valley

Yosemite
Valley

Yosemite Valley's South Rim

N

Merced River

El Portal

140

49

Mariposa

Wawona

41

140

49

SIERRA
NATIONAL
FOREST

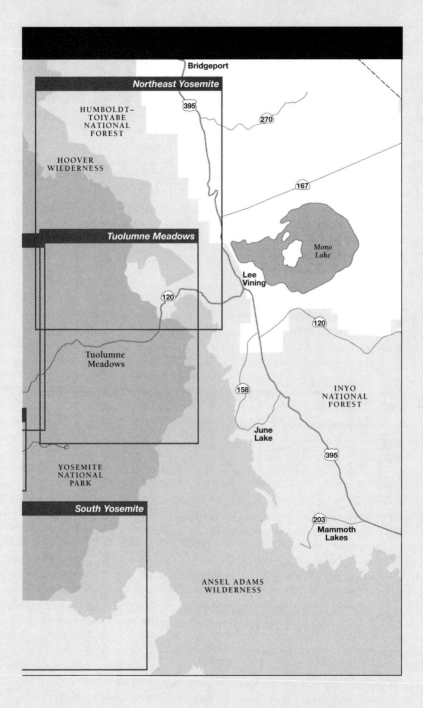

Yosemite Trails

Trail Number and Name	Page	Difficulty -12345+	Length in Miles	Type	Backpacking	Dayhiking	Horses	Running	Handicap Access	Child Friendly
1. Northeast Yosemite										
1 Barney Lake and Peeler Lake	31	3/4	16.4	Out & Back	✓	✓	✓	✓		
2 Green Creek Basin	37	2/3	6.2	Out & Back	✓	✓				
3 Virginia Lakes Basin to Green Creek	43	3	11.9	Point-to-Point	✓	✓	✓			
4 Twenty Lakes Basin	53	2	7.6	Loop		✓				
5 Mount Dana	59	3	5.8	Out & Back		✓				
6 Gaylor Lakes and Great Sierra Mine	65	2	4.0	Out & Back		✓				
2. Tuolumne Meadows										
7 Lembert Dome, Dog Dome, and Dog Lake	81	2/3	4.6	Out & Back		✓	✓			
8 Pothole Dome and the Tuolumne River	87	1	3.0	Out & Back		✓				✓
9 Young Lakes	93	4	16.4	Loop	✓	✓	✓			
10 Glen Aulin and Waterwheel Falls	101	3	12.0	Out & Back	✓	✓	✓	✓		
11 Vogelsang High Sierra Camp Lakes	109	4	15.4	Out & Back	✓	✓				
12 Elizabeth Lake	115	2	5.0	Out & Back	✓	✓				
13 Lower Cathedral Lake	119	2	7.6	Out & Back	✓	✓	✓			
14 High Sierra Camps Loop, northwest part	123	4	17.6	Point-to-Point	✓			✓		
15 High Sierra Camps Loop, southeast part	133	5	33.0	Point-to-Point	✓		✓			
3. Central Yosemite										
16 Sunrise Lakes and Sunrise High Sierra Camp	153	3	11.6	Out & Back	✓	✓				
17 Clouds Rest	159	4	14.0	Out & Back	✓	✓	✓			
18 May Lake and Mount Hoffmann	165	2/3	2.4	Out & Back	✓	✓	✓			✓
19 North Dome	169	3	9.2	Out & Back	✓	✓	✓			
20 Ten Lakes Basin	175	4	12.6	Out & Back	✓	✓	✓			
21 Lukens Lake	183	1	2.2	Out & Back		✓		✓		✓
22 Harden Lake	187	2	5.6	Out & Back	✓	✓	✓	✓		✓

Legend

USES & ACCESS
- Day Hiking
- Backpacking
- Horses
- Running
- Biking
- Handicap Access
- Child Friendly

TYPE
- Loop
- Out & Back
- Point-to-Point

DIFFICULTY
- 1 2 3 4 5 +
less ————— more

TERRAIN
- Canyon
- Mountain
- Summit
- Stream
- Waterfall
- Lake

FLORA & FAUNA
- Autumn Colors
- Wildflowers
- Giant Sequoias

FEATURES
- Great Views
- Camping
- Swimming
- Secluded
- Steep

	TERRAIN					FLORA & FAUNA				OTHER				
Canyon	Mountain	Summit	Lake	Stream	Waterfall	Autumn Colors	Wildflowers	Giant Sequoias	Great Views	Camping	Swimming	Secluded	Steep	
✓			✓	✓		✓	✓			✓	✓			
✓			✓	✓		✓	✓		✓	✓	✓			
✓			✓	✓		✓	✓		✓	✓	✓			
✓			✓				✓		✓					
	✓								✓			✓		
			✓				✓		✓					
		✓	✓						✓	✓	✓			
		✓		✓					✓	✓	✓			
			✓	✓			✓		✓	✓	✓			
✓				✓	✓				✓	✓	✓			
✓			✓	✓			✓			✓	✓			
			✓	✓			✓			✓				
			✓	✓						✓	✓			
✓			✓	✓	✓				✓	✓	✓			
✓			✓	✓			✓		✓	✓	✓			
			✓	✓			✓		✓	✓	✓			
	✓	✓		✓			✓		✓	✓				
	✓	✓		✓					✓	✓	✓			
		✓		✓			✓		✓	✓	✓			
✓			✓	✓			✓		✓	✓	✓	✓		
			✓				✓				✓			
			✓			✓	✓			✓	✓			

Yosemite Trails

TRAIL NUMBER AND NAME	Page	Difficulty ~12345+	Length in Miles	Type	Backpacking	Dayhiking	Horses	Running	Handicap Access	Child Friendly
4. Northwest Yosemite										
23 Kibbie Lake	199	2	8.0	↗	🎒	🚶	🐎			👪
24 Laurel Lake and Lake Vernon	205	5	24.8	↗	🎒		🐎			
25 Wapama Falls and Rancheria Falls Camp	213	3	12.8	↗	🎒	🚶	🐎	🏃		
26 Tuolumne Grove of Big Trees	219	2	2.4	↗		🚶				
27 El Capitan from Tamarack Flat	223	4	17.0	↗	🎒	🚶				
5. Yosemite Valley										
28 Bridalveil Fall	239	1	0.4	↗		🚶			♿	👪
29 Lower Yosemite Fall	243	1	1.1	↻		🚶			♿	👪
30 Upper Yosemite Fall and Eagle Peak	249	4	7.0	↗	🎒	🚶				
31 Mirror Lake	257	1	2.0	↗		🚶	🐎	🏃		👪 🚴
32 Vernal Fall Bridge	261	2	2.0	↗		🚶				
33 Vernal Fall–Nevada Fall Loop	265	3	6.5	↻		🚶				
34 Half Dome	273	5	15.5	↗	🎒	🚶	🐎			
35 Merced Lake	285	5	28.4	↗	🎒		🐎			
6. Yosemite Valley's South Rim										
36 Dewey Point	303	2	8.2	↗		🚶	🐎	🏃		👪
37 Taft Point	307	1/2	2.6	↗	🎒	🚶		🏃		
38 Sentinel Dome	311	1/2	2.4	↗		🚶		🏃		
39 Glacier Point	315	1	0.4	↗		🚶			♿	
40 Four Mile Trail	319	2	4.6	↘		🚶				
41 Glacier Point–Panorama Trail	323	3	9.2	↘		🚶				
7. South Yosemite										
42 Ostrander Lake	337	3	12.8	↗	🎒	🚶	🐎			
43 Buena Vista Loop	341	5	30.4	↻	🎒		🐎			
44 Mariposa Grove of Big Trees	349	2	6.2	↻		🚶				👪
45 Vanderberg–Lillian Lakes Loop	355	4	12.6	↻	🎒	🚶	🐎			👪

| | TERRAIN | | | | | | FLORA & FAUNA | | | | | OTHER | | | | | |
Canyon	Mountain	Summit	Lake	Stream	Waterfall	Autumn Colors	Wildflowers	Giant Sequoias	Birds	Wildlife	Great Views	Photo Opportunity	Camping	Swimming	Secluded	Steep
			●	●		●							●	●		
			●	●		●					●		●	●		
●			●	●	●	●					●		●	●		
								●							●	
		●		●		●					●		●		●	
				●	●											
				●	●											
		●		●	●						●		●		●	
●			●	●							●					
●				●	●						●		●		●	
●				●	●						●		●		●	
●	●	●		●	●						●		●		●	
●			●	●	●	●					●		●	●		
		●		●		●					●					
		●		●		●					●					
		●				●					●					
		●			●						●					
											●				●	
●				●	●	●					●					
			●	●							●		●	●		
			●	●		●					●		●	●		
						●		●								
			●	●		●							●	●	●	

Contents

CHAPTER 1

Northeast Yosemite 23

CHAPTER 2

Tuolumne Meadows .71

CHAPTER 3

Central Yosemite 145

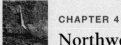
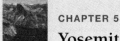
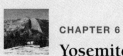

Map Legend

Trail		River	
Other Trail		Stream	
		Seasonal Stream	
Freeway		Body of Water	
Major Road			
Minor Road		Marsh/Swamp	
Tunnel		Dam	
Bridge	)(	Peak	▲
Building		Park/Forest	
		Boundary	
Trailhead Parking	P	Start/Finish	start & finish
Picnic	禾		
Camping	▲		
Gate	•—•	North Arrow	N

Using Top Trails™

Organization of Top Trails

Top Trails is designed to make identifying the perfect trail easy and enjoyable, and to make every outing a success and a pleasure. With this book you'll find it's a snap to find the right trail, whether you're planning a major hike or just a sociable stroll with friends.

The Region

Top Trails begins with the **Yosemite National Park map** (pages iv-v), displaying the entire region covered by the guide and providing a geographic overview. The map is clearly marked to show which area is covered by which chapter.

After the Regional Map comes the **Yosemite National Park Trails Table** (pages vi-ix), which lists every trail covered in the guide along with attributes for each one. A quick reading of the Regional Map and the Trail

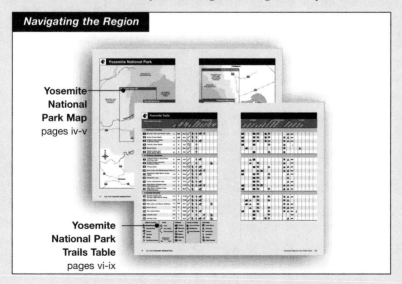

Navigating the Region

Yosemite National Park Map pages iv-v

Yosemite National Park Trails Table pages vi-ix

Table will give you a good overview of the entire region covered by this book.

The Areas

The region covered by this book is divided into Areas, with each chapter corresponding to one area in the region.

Each Area chapter starts with information to help you choose and enjoy a trail each time out. Use the table of contents or the Regional Map to identify an area of interest, then turn to the Area Chapter to find the following:

- An Overview of the Area, including permits and maps
- An Area Map with all trails clearly marked
- A Trail Feature Table providing Trail-by-Trail details
- Trail Summaries, written in a lively, accessible style

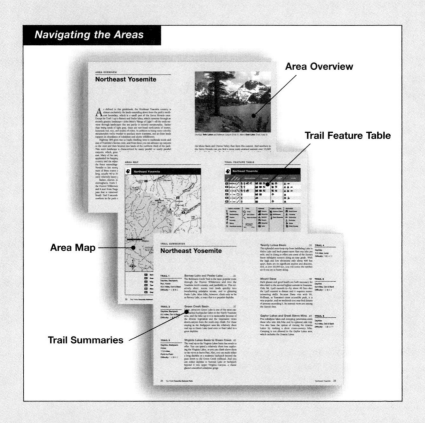

Navigating the Areas

Area Overview

Trail Feature Table

Area Map

Trail Summaries

The Trails

The basic building block of the Top Trails guide is the Trail Entry. Each one is arranged to make finding and following the trail as simple as possible, with all pertinent information presented in an easy-to-follow format:

- A Trail Map
- Trail Descriptors covering difficulty, length, and other essential data
- A written Trail Description
- Trail Milestones, providing easy-to-follow, turn-by-turn trail directions

Some Trail Descriptions offer additional information:

- An Elevation Profile
- Trail Options
- Trail Highlights

In the margins of the Trail Entries, look for icons that point out notable features at specific points along the trail.

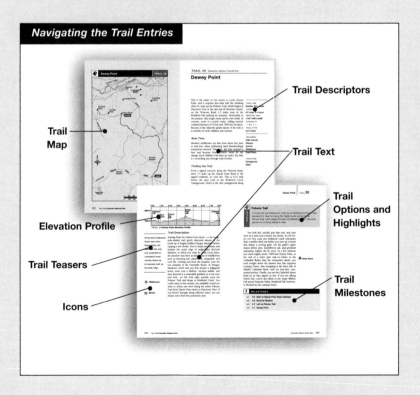

Navigating the Trail Entries

Trail Map

Elevation Profile

Trail Teasers

Icons

Trail Descriptors

Trail Text

Trail Options and Highlights

Trail Milestones

Choosing a Trail

Top Trails provides several different ways of choosing a trail, presented in easy-to-read tables, charts, and maps.

Location

If you know in general where you want to go, Top Trails makes it easy to find the right trail in the right place. Each chapter begins with a large-scale map showing the starting point of every trail in that area.

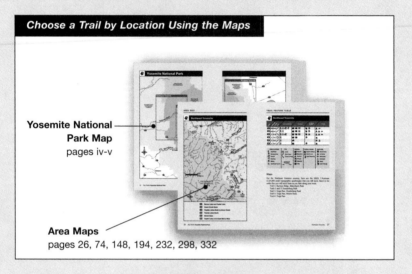

Choose a Trail by Location Using the Maps

Yosemite National Park Map
pages iv-v

Area Maps
pages 26, 74, 148, 194, 232, 298, 332

Features

This guide describes the Top Trails of Yosemite National Park, and each trail is chosen because it offers one or more features that make it appealing. Using the trail descriptors, summaries, and tables, you can quickly examine all the trails for the features they offer, or seek a particular feature among the list of trails.

Season and Condition

Time of year and current conditions can be important factors in selecting the best trail. For example, an exposed, low-elevation trail may be a riot of color in early spring, but an oven-baked taste of hell in midsummer. Wherever relevant, Top Trails identifies the best and worst conditions for the trails you plan to hike.

Difficulty

Each trail has an overall difficulty rating on a scale of 1 to 5, largely based on total length and total elevation change. Also taken into consideration is elevation, since above 8000 feet you are likely to hike slower with ever-increasing elevation. Generally, the longer the trail, the more elevation gain and loss. However, some relatively short trails have a lot of elevation change, such as Trail 30 to the top of Upper Yosemite Fall, in contrast to Trail 4 through Twenty Lakes Basin, which is slightly longer but has only about one-fourth of the elevation gain and loss. Then too, Trail 41 has much more descent than ascent, and so is relatively easy, if you don't mind all the braking downhill. Also, some hikes have more than one destination, and often these have two difficulty ratings, since a second destination may be significantly farther than the first. But then, some hikes just seem to straddle two difficulty ratings, so both are identified.

The ratings assume you are an able-bodied adult in reasonably good shape, using the trail for hiking. The ratings also assume normal weather conditions—clear and dry.

Readers should make an honest assessment of their own abilities and adjust time estimates accordingly. Also, rain, snow, heat, wind, and poor visibility can all affect the pace on even the easiest of trails.

Choose a Trail by Length, Difficulty, or Features Using the Tables

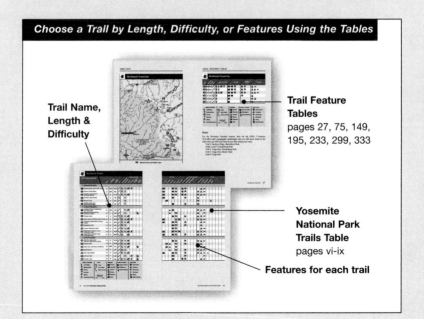

Trail Name, Length & Difficulty

Trail Feature Tables
pages 27, 75, 149, 195, 233, 299, 333

Yosemite National Park Trails Table
pages vi-ix

Features for each trail

Vertical Feet

Every trail description contains the approximate trail length and amount of elevation changes over the course of the trail. It's important to use all the figures when considering a hike: on average, plan one hour for every 2 miles, and add an hour for every 1000 feet you climb. (But if you are in great shape, you will complete the hike in half the time, as I did in my 20s and 30s. Indeed, back then I could have day-hiked every one of these trails, even Trail 15, at 33.7 miles, and I was no super athlete. If you can do this, you don't need a wilderness permit or a bear canister.) Elevation change is often underestimated by hikers when looking at a topographic map, since they notice the major ascents and tend to ignore the minor ups and downs, which can add up. For example, Trail 25 from O'Shaughnessy Dam east along Hetch Hetchy Reservoir to Rancheria Falls Camp has a net gain of about 700 feet, but because it roller coasters eastward to that camp, you do an extra 800 feet of ascending (and descending). No wonder a traversing trail that looks like a stroll on a map seems so hard in reality!

The calculation of Vertical Feet in this Top Trails guide is accomplished by measuring all ups and downs along each route as mapped by the author. For routes that begin and end at the same spot—i.e., Loop or Out & Back— the vertical gain exactly matches the vertical descent. With a Point-to-Point route, the vertical gain and loss will most likely differ, since the start and end points most likely will be different elevations.

Note that for *simple* Out & Back trails the elevation gain and loss are for one direction only, that is, hiking in. Hiking back out, the two numbers are reversed. Adding the four numbers together will give you the total up and down you will hike. An example of this is Trail 1, Barney Lake and Peeler Lake, with the following numbers: +2730'/-310'/±6080'. Hiking up to Peeler Lake, you will climb 2730 feet and descend 310 feet. Returning to the trailhead you will descend 2730 feet and climb 310 feet. Add these four numbers and you get 6080 feet.

For *branching* Out & Back trails, the elevation gain and loss are to the farthest destination, but include the side trips that are included in the mileages. An example of this is Trail 7, Lembert Dome, Dog Dome, and Dog Lake, with the following numbers: +980'/-120'/±1810'. If you visit all of these features you will first climb up a saddle, branch over Dog Dome, then do Lembert Dome, then return to the main trail, and finally drop and climb to Dog Lake. The elevation changes for all of this are +980 feet and -120 feet, for a total of 1100 feet. But when you return, you do so directly, skipping the two domes, and the elevation changes are less, being +120 feet and

-590 feet, for a total of 710 feet. Add the going and returning totals together and you get the grand total, 1810 feet.

For Loop trails, both the gains and losses continue to accumulate until you arrive back, and together they give you the total gain and loss. An example of this is Trail 4, the Twenty Lakes Basin, with the following numbers: +900'/-900'/±1800'.

Likewise, for Point-to-Point trails, both the gains and losses continue to accumulate until you reach your end point, but because it is likely to be a different elevation than your starting point, the vertical gain and loss most likely will differ. An example of this is Trail 3, Virginia Lakes Basin to Green Creek, with the following numbers: +1720'/-3550'/±5270'. What these numbers tell you is that on this hike you ascend only about half as much as you descend.

Finally, some of the Trail Entries in the Top Trails series have an **Elevation Profile**, an easy means for visualizing the topography of the route. These profiles graphically depict the elevation throughout the length of the trail. However, since the profiles are constructed with a computer by using digital topographic maps, they tend to be short on actual mileage since these maps don't show every twist and turn of the trails, as mapped in detail by the author. Trails that are less than 3 miles in total length *and* that have less than 1000 feet of total elevation gain do not have profiles.

Top Trails Difficulty Ratings

1 A route usually less than 2 miles, generally level, that can be completed in one hour or less. Bring grandparents or grandkids.

2 A route of about 2 to 8 miles, usually with 1000 to 3000 feet of total elevation gain and loss, that can be completed in one to four hours.

3 A route of about 6 to 12 miles, usually with 2000 to 5000 feet of total elevation gain and loss, that can be completed in four to eight hours.

4 A route of about 12 to 20 miles, often with more than 5000 feet of total elevation gain and loss, that most will want to backpack with one overnight stay.

5 A route longer than 20 miles, with more than 9000 feet of total elevation gain and loss, that most will want to backpack with two or three nights' stays.

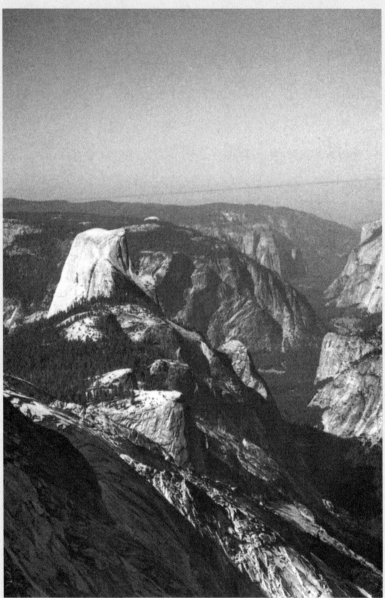

Greg Schaffer

Half Dome *from Clouds Rest*

Introduction to Yosemite National Park

Although Yellowstone was the first federal land to be set aside as a national park, in 1872, Yosemite was the first federal land to be set aside as *any* kind of park, in 1864. In that year, President Abraham Lincoln signed a bill that deeded Yosemite Valley and the Mariposa Grove of Big Trees to the State of California, and for good reason. Although the valley had been discovered only 13 years earlier, its sheer walls and magnificent waterfalls were rapidly attracting national fame, thanks to articles, paintings, photographs, and personal testimonials.

Today, visitors from around the world still come to Yosemite National Park to experience Yosemite Valley firsthand. Who can forget his or her first visit to the valley, with its enormous granite cliffs, its leaping, dashing waterfalls, and its domes? The valley's prominent features, if not etched on the mind, are recorded by camera: the monolith of El Capitan, Bridalveil Fall backdropped by the Cathedral Rocks, the Three Brothers opposite the valley from the Cathedral Spires, the giant tombstone of Sentinel Rock capped by Sentinel Dome, the Lower and Upper Yosemite Falls and adjacent Lost Arrow Spire, the lithic rainbow of Royal Arches and adjacent, vertical Washington Column, both surmounted by North Dome, and the deep, gaping Tenaya Canyon bounded on the north by Basket Dome and Mt. Watkins and on the south and east by Half Dome and Clouds Rest. Finally, there is the curved Glacier Point Apron sweeping up to a vertical cliff topped by Glacier Point. Its views of Yosemite Valley and of the wilderness lands of the high country beyond it must rank as one of the greatest natural wonders of North America, if not the world.

Geography and Topography

Yosemite National Park covers an area of 1189 square miles, all of it within two river drainages, the Tuolumne and Merced. Despite this large area, comparable to that of the San Francisco Bay Area or the greater Los Angeles metropolitan area, only a small percentage of the park's visitors backpack into the wilderness lands of the high country, which comprise the bulk of the park's area. Rather, most visitors converge on the few square miles of Yosemite Valley's floor and the square mile of the Mariposa Grove.

The Sierra Nevada has been called the "gentle wilderness," but if you've backpacked the high country of Sequoia and Kings Canyon National Park, you know that thousands of feet of ascent to a lake basin is anything but gentle. In contrast, Yosemite National Park's high country really is a gentle wilderness, its lakes reached with about half the effort. (If you consider a lake to be at least an acre in area and a pond smaller, then Yosemite has over 500 lakes and over 1000 ponds.) Part of the reason for this relative ease of backpacking is that the main river canyons, the Merced and the Tuolumne, are only about half as deep as Kings Canyon and none have a major east-side ascent comparable to those out of the Owens Valley up to the Sierran crest. More significantly, thanks to the Tioga and Glacier Point roads, most of Yosemite's trailheads are high, ranging from about 7000 feet to over 9000 feet in elevation, and since most of the lakes that are visited lie below 10,000 feet in elevation, the effort required to reach them is not that great.

In this Top Trails guide, most of the lakes described can be reached with about 1000 to 2000 feet of elevation gain. There are only three that require about 3000 feet of elevation gain: Peeler Lake (Trail 1), Lake Vernon (Trail 24), and Merced Lake (Trail 35). This is not to say there are no lakes where a major elevation change is involved—there are. Most of these lie in the northern third of the park, that is, north of the Tuolumne River's Hetch Hetchy Reservoir and the Grand Canyon of the Tuolumne River. The remainder lie in the Merced River drainage above Merced Lake. For these relatively remote lakes, you'd want to spent four or more days in the wilderness, and lengthy hikes are beyond the scope of the book. For lengthy hiking trips and for a description of virtually all of the park's approximately 800 miles of trails, consult my *Yosemite National Park: A Complete Hiker's Guide* (Berkeley, CA: Wilderness Press, 2006).

The Top Trails guide you are holding does include several stiff climbs of 3000-plus feet of elevation gain to popular, prominent summits or viewpoints: Mt. Dana (Trail 5), Upper Yosemite Fall (Trail 30), and of course Half Dome (Trail 34). Additionally, some trails, especially the longer ones, ramble up and down, and the elevation gain and loss can accumulate to impressive numbers. For example, on a map the trail from the Hetch Hetchy Dam east along the north slopes of the reservoir looks like a walk in the park (technically, I suppose, it is). Where it ends at Rancheria Falls Camp, the elevation is only about 800 feet higher than at the trailhead, but you will climb about 1500 feet and drop about 800 feet to reach the camp. The reason for this is that the north wall above the reservoir is steep and the trail's route must climb or descend from one bench to another, resulting in a rollercoaster route. Why some canyon walls of the park are very steep and why there are benches along some of these walls is the topic of geology.

Whirlwind Tour

Although this is primarily a hiking guide, if you plan to visit the park for only one day, you'll hardly have time to get out of your vehicle. Given only one day, you can best sample Yosemite's greatness by driving across it.

• Starting in Oakhurst or Fish Camp with a full tank of fuel, first drive north up Highway 41 to the entrance station, head up to the **Mariposa Grove** (consider taking a free shuttle from Wawona), and then take a tram tour past the giant sequoias.

• Next, continue north from Wawona to the Glacier Point Road, which you take east up to **Washburn and Glacier points**. Backtrack to the main road and descend to **Yosemite Valley.** Park at the **Bridalveil Fall** lot and walk up the short path toward that fall.

• Then drive through the valley and park on either side of Northside Drive west of Yosemite Village but east of shuttle stop 6. From it, take a paved path that parallels Northside Drive 0.2 mile west, to where you will see a nearby building with restrooms. From the building a path heads 0.3 mile north up to a bridge just below **Lower Yosemite Fall.**

• Leave the valley, drive up to Crane Flat, then start up the **Tioga Road.** If the Mariposa Grove was too crowded and you passed it up, head just up the road and branch left into a parking area. Make a 1-mile descent into the **Tuolumne Grove of Big Trees**, then return.

• Drive up into a red-fir forest, traverse the Yosemite Creek drainage, and then stop at **Olmsted Point**, recognizable by the presence of tourists and tour buses. It is worth it.

• Next, descend to nearby **Tenaya Lake,** seen from the point, and perhaps stop along it to savor its setting as well as to watch climbers ascend various routes on an adjacent domelike ridge. A few minutes beyond the lake, you enter **Tuolumne Meadows.** If you have a couple hours and considerable energy, make the unforgettable ascent to at least Dog Dome, if not to slightly higher Lembert Dome.

• Conclude your day by exiting via **Tioga Pass,** which in late afternoon or evening can have a backdrop of dramatic clouds.

Geology

The oldest rocks in the park's vicinity are about 540 million years old and originated as sandy sediments deposited on the ocean's floor off North America's west coast. These sandstones later metamorphosed to **quartzites**, which today straddle the park's lightly visited northern-boundary lands. Other significant remnants of metamorphic rocks stretch from the Saddlebag Lake environs south to Tioga Pass and into the northern Ritter Range. These rocks have weathered to earth tones, which add color to our area's crest lands. Additionally, the mineral-rich soil they produce results in more plant species and greater numbers of plants than grow in adjacent granitic soil.

But like most of the Sierra Nevada, most of Yosemite's lands are **granitic**—grayish rocks that once solidified from a melt (magma) several miles beneath the surface, but today are exposed, creating what John Muir called the "Range of Light." The high country of Yosemite and the rest of the High Sierra would not be very luminous if the overlying rocks intruded by molten "granite" had not been removed. Foremost, Yosemite National Park was set aside because of its renowned Yosemite Valley, arguably the world's most spectacular, which owes its origin to a unique pattern of major, nearly vertical **fracture planes** in its granitic rock that have given rise to impressive cliffs such as the faces of Half Dome and Sentinel Rock. For this joint-controlled landscape to evolve, Yosemite's lands needed first an uplift, then a collapse, some major canyon cutting, and then glaciation.

Mountain-building episodes (orogenies) occur when continental crust on one plate is compressed against continental crust on another plate, much as India once collided with today's Asia, creating the Himalayan Range. In the area covered by this book there were three orogenies, the Nevadan, named after the Sierra Nevada, being the last. Like earlier orogenies, this one metamorphosed the area's previously existing rocks. Compression and uplift may have begun about 180 million years ago, peaked from 160 to 155 million years ago, and then waned for millions of years.

Major changes were needed to create today's largely granitic range, and these were accomplished in part when the compression that brought about the Nevadan orogeny gave way to extension. Faults rifted the upper crust apart, providing space for ascending magma. Extension and plutonism went hand in hand, and from about 115 to 85 million years ago, Sierran plutonism occurred on an unprecedented scale.

Magmatism (the solidifying of molten rock beneath the earth's surface) waned in the Sierra Nevada until about 80 million years ago, when the locus of magma generation shifted far east of the range to cause the Rocky Mountains' Laramide orogeny. The Sierra Nevada now had a core composed of dozens of generally light-gray plutons. These, however, typically lay several

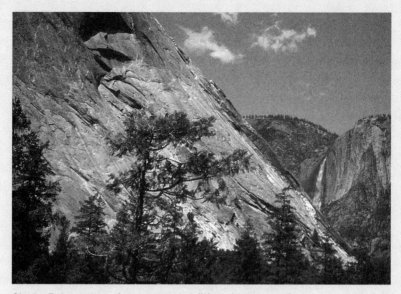

Glacier Point apron *and Upper Yosemite Fall from above Happy Isles*

miles beneath a largely volcanic landscape—definitely not the Range of Light. About 80 million years ago, major extension occurred in the range, and in perhaps only a few million years, its upper crust detached westward, exposing mainly the upper parts of plutons (granitic intrusions) but also some lower remnants of metamorphic rocks. With the removal of the upper crust, the lower crust of the Sierran block would have risen—an isostatic (stabilizing) rebound upward—although not to its original height. In this rebound, the range's bedrock was fractured, and the unique patterns of the local fractures gave rise to the modern range's drainages and topography.

Since the isostatic rebound tens of millions of years ago, the Sierra's crest has changed very little in altitude. What have changed dramatically are the range's **major canyons**. By the start of the modern Cenozoic era, 65 million years ago, the main difference from today was that the river canyons were shallower, perhaps half their present depths. In contrast, the features above the canyon rims resembled their modern equivalents. Back then Yosemite Valley was developing a generally broad U-shaped cross profile of steep slopes and a flat floor—the characteristic shape of today's tropical granitic ranges. **Ribbon, Upper Yosemite**, and **Nevada falls** may have achieved about two-thirds of their present heights. Since that time, **weathering and erosion** have removed only about 100 feet of bedrock from the most resistant summits.

Canyon cutting occurred under hot, wet climates until about 33 million years ago, when global climates began evolving toward a drier, cooler regime. About this time, surprisingly, major canyon cutting stopped. We know this because remnants of volcanic rocks that erupted as long ago as 30 million years still adhere to the floors of glaciated Sierran canyons. Obviously, no deepening has occurred, or else these ancient volcanic rocks would have disappeared. From this you can deduce two points. The first is that there has been no significant uplift in the last 30 million years, for if uplift had occurred, the rivers would have deepened their canyons. Second, because glaciers have not removed all of the volcanic rocks from the canyon floors, they performed very little erosion. Yosemite Valley actually was deeper some 30 million years ago. Since that time, rocks have fallen from its walls, and so the valley has widened over time. Since the advent of major glaciation, by at least 2 million years ago, the valley has filled in with several hundred feet of sediments.

Glacial landscapes developed best near the Sierran crest, not down in Yosemite Valley, but this was due more to mass wasting, particularly earthquake-induced rockfall, than to glacial erosion. The principal role of an alpine, or mountain, glacier in any of the world's glaciated ranges is to transport the products of mass wasting, not to erode, a process that is minimal where the bedrock is resistant. In each glacial episode, cold climates would create myriad freeze-and-thaw cycles of ice, which pried rock from steep walls to collect below as talus. As the walls gradually retreated through rockfall, the heads of canyons became broader. The canyon heads are called **cirques**; the small glaciers that occupied them are called cirque glaciers, such as below Mt. Lyell. As glaciers advanced down-canyon they excavated decomposed bedrock, leaving basins that would become lakes, which over time would accumulate sediments (on average about a foot per 1000 years). The upper lands may have been glaciated dozens of times, and each time they would have removed lake sediments.

Glaciations that occurred before 200,000 years ago collectively are called pre-Tahoe, since they preceded the well-known Tahoe glaciation. On the east side of the range, the Sherwin glaciation, which lasted from about 900,000 to 800,000 years ago, produced the oldest known glaciers. In the Yosemite area, Sherwin sediments are preserved due in large part to burial in the mammoth Long Valley eruption of about 760,000 years ago. In contrast, on the west side there is no viable evidence of Sherwin glaciers, since the slightly larger Tahoe glaciers overrode their evidence. The Tahoe and slightly smaller Tioga glaciers, which existed, respectively, about 200-130,000 and 30–15,000 years ago, were larger in the Merced River drainage than previously supposed, advancing to the lower part of Merced Gorge, about 6 miles beyond Bridalveil Meadow. Also, both glaciers were thicker than previously supposed, especially in **Little Yosemite Valley**, where they were about 2000 feet thick, not 1000. After the **Tioga glacier** left Yosemite Valley about 15,000 years ago, there was at best a swampy floor, not a lake. In the Tuolumne River drainage, the glaciers were about twice as large, about 55 miles long and up to 4000 feet thick.

Flora and Fauna

Yosemite is predominantly a landscape of forest green, and driving up through the park you'll see changes with elevation. The most obvious changes are the tree species, but shrubs, wildflowers, grasses, and animals also change with elevation. The distribution of species is controlled by a number of influences, of which climate is probably the foremost. Others include topography, soil, fire, and other species.

Of climatic influences, **temperature** and **precipitation** are the most important. Temperature decreases with increasing elevation, and precipitation increases up to mid-elevations, beyond which it decreases slowly on the approach to the crest, then rapidly beyond it. Because much of a winter's snow remains through late spring—and some remains throughout summer—most of Yosemite's vegetation has an adequate water supply. In fact, the presence of the **subalpine meadows** is due to too much water, for conifers aren't able to survive in these seasonally water-saturated soils. In contrast, on **alpine rocky slopes**, the snow often melts before the start of the growing season. On these dry slopes, then, the **wildflowers** are often dependent on summer thunderstorms for moisture. Finally, there were a lot of thick soils before glaciers removed them, and this altered the distribution of at least one notable species, the giant sequoia, which before glaciation was associated with red firs.

The presence or absence of ground fires can really alter the ecosystem, for it significantly alters the populations of ground-dwelling plants and animals and everything associated with them. Until 1971, fire suppression was a general Yosemite policy, but it led to the accumulation of thick litter, dense brush, and over-mature trees—all prime fuel for a holocaust when a fire inevitably sparked to life. Foresters now know that natural fires should not be prevented, but only regulated.

Yosemite National Park has a diverse range of species. Plants are the most conspicuous, and there are about 1200 species of **native plants**, about 160 of them rare. Of the park's vertebrate animals (ignoring insects, spiders, etc.), **birds** are the most common, about 250 species, although about 100 species are uncommon. **Mammals** are next, and depending on how you want to split **rodents** into species, there may be seven dozen species. Reptiles are represented by about two dozen species of **lizards** and **snakes**,

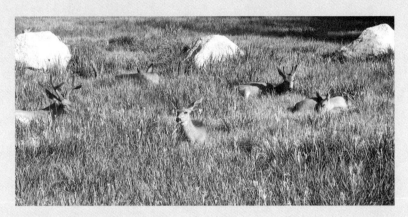

Deer *west of Twin Lakes (Trail 1)*

two of the latter notable: first, rattlesnakes because they are poisonous, and second, racers, which climb not only bushes but also steep cracks. Amphibians are not faring well here and around the world, and are down to several species. The only trout native to the area is the **rainbow trout**, but other species have been introduced and some hybridization has occurred.

In this book, plants and animals are classified according to the dominant *plant* or *plant type* simply because plants are the most readily observed life forms. Such a group of life forms is called a **plant community**, even though it includes animals. As you drive east up toward the Sierran crest, you pass through following plant communities: foothill woodland, ponderosa-pine forest, jeffrey-pine forest, red-fir/lodgepole-pine forest, mountain meadow, subalpine forest, and alpine fell-fields. If you are interested in natural history, consult the list of books at the end of this book.

When to Go: Weather and Seasons

If you are a typical hiker using this guidebook, you'll probably visit the park during the **summer** and likely will be taking trails above Yosemite Valley. Unlike most of America's mountain ranges, the Sierra Nevada is summer-dry, receiving only about 1.5 inches of precipitation. **Summer** starts about June 22, and lasts until the start of fall. For Yosemite Valley, the last cold night and/or significant storm usually has just ended by the start of summer, and the days will be in the 80s and the nights down to the 50s by the crack of dawn. Temperatures drop with elevation gain, and up at Tuolumne Meadows, which is about 4000 feet higher than the valley, the summer temperatures are about 15°F cooler.

At Tuolumne Meadows and other high-elevation areas, early summer temperatures are cool but acceptable. What limits hiker use is lingering snow. Unless the year has had above-average snowfall, by the start of summer all the park's major roads usually are open, with roads to Tamarack Flat Campground, Yosemite Creek Campground, and the May Lake trailhead opening by early or mid-July. High trails, however, may be partly to mostly snowbound, so its best to confine your hiking to below about 7500 feet elevation, such as along both rims of Yosemite Valley, up Little Yosemite Valley to Merced Lake, or up from Hetch Hetchy to Laurel Lake and Lake Vernon.

By mid-to-late July most of the area's trails will be snow-free or nearly so, and the afternoon temperatures usually warm and the nights pleasant. However, July like June is a month of copious mosquitoes, so if you backpack then, be sure to bring a tent. Furthermore, July gets its share of thunderstorms, and the closer you approach the Sierran crest, the more likely you are to experience one. These mostly occur from about midafternoon until sunset, and usually they are short-lived, drenching a local area for a few minutes before moving on. If ominous clouds are threatening you, be sure to take cover within a forest rather than staying in the open or under an isolated tree. Also by mid-to-late July, because snowmelt then is minimal, the volume of Yosemite Falls and other waterfalls is greatly diminished and they are not very photogenic.

For hikers, the first half of August is best, since chances of a major frontal storm (possibly bringing snow at high elevations) or of an isolated thunderstorm are minimal, and mosquito populations have dwindled to an acceptable level. Also, lakes, which typically reach their maximum temperatures by late July (low-to-mid 70s for the lower lakes, mid-to-high 60s for the higher lakes), are still nearly as warm and are fine for swimming. By the end of August or early September, the lakes definitely are cooling, and the Sierra may have had one or two weak frontal storms. After the Labor Day weekend the park has fewer visitors, and mosquitoes are virtually nonexistent. Should you backpack then, be sure to check the weather forecast for a possible storm, and certainly bring a tent if you will be out for more than one or two nights.

Autumn/fall starts in late September, and now the days are considerably cooler. Yosemite Valley during the first half of autumn (through early November) is a favorite time for some. Whereas the nights may be crisp, the days are ideal, and the colors of turning foliage compensate for the valley's lack of waterfalls (except for a wispy Bridalveil Fall).

Backpackers at higher elevations need to be prepared for the season's first major storm, which may strike in early October or not until early November. Although most days are fair weather, I have a rule of thumb that after October 15 I don't backpack more than a few miles from the trailhead, since if a storm does hit and drop a foot or two of snow, I can still plod back in a day's time and, hopefully, will be able to drive back home (carry chains). The Tioga Road may close briefly in a minor snowstorm, but anytime from about mid-October into November a major one usually hits, and then this road (along with Forest Service roads bordering the park) closes for the season.

November through mid-December is a time of solitude. The backcountry is virtually devoid of hikers, save for a few mountaineers. Likewise, the valley is empty, for the days are cool, the nights are nippy, and the ski season has not begun.

Winter starts in late December, and it is the season with the least amount of daylight and the lowest noontime sun. Consequently, the valley's floor stays in the shadows, although much of the north wall may be sunlit. With no sunlight on the floor, its temperatures are downright cold. Both November and December receive a lot of precipitation, and at first this is rain, but by around Thanksgiving most of it will be snow. Snow often covers the valley's floor from about mid-December to mid-February, after which the cover may be patchy. Winter is ski season, and most folks driving up to the park head to Badger Pass for downhill skiing or cross-country skiing. Buses still bring in hordes of tourists to the valley, for indeed in the deep of winter, especially after a storm, the valley is a winter wonderland. Although the four months from November through March produce the most precipitation, about 75 percent of it, most days are storm-free, and when a storm does hit, it usually clears out in a day or two.

By early March the snow is mostly gone, although you can still get a snowstorm in March and even in April. February, March, and April temperatures often get above freezing during part of the day but then drop below freezing during the night.

Spring begins in late March, and March and April can have quite variable weather, pleasant in some years, wintry in others. You may experience balmy afternoons in the 70s or cold, blustery ones in the 40s or 50s. For plants on the floor of Yosemite Valley, it is still winter. By early May, daylight is about 13.5 hours long, and with longer daylight the sun is higher in the sky, providing increasing radiation to bring spring to the valley floor. The deciduous trees produce leaves and the meadows change from matted, brown, dead vegetation to a sea of green. The added radiation also increases snowmelt, sometimes augmented by the passage of a relatively warm rainstorm, and the valley's waterfalls reach their zenith from about early May through late June. The best time to visit these falls is around mid-May, by when most of the season's storms have abated and just before the storm of tourists invade the valley, beginning around the Memorial Day weekend.

Although all of the high country still lies under snow in May, some intermediate elevations are open to hikers. In late spring, that is, through most of June, the rims of Yosemite Valley are largely snow-free, and so you can hike up the Yosemite Falls Trail to the brink of Upper Yosemite Fall. Or, you can start from Glacier Point and the Glacier Point–Panorama Trail to the floor. Finally, usually in June the Park Service opens the cable route to the summit of Half Dome.

Trail Selection

Three criteria were used during the selection of trails for this guide. Only what I consider to be premier dayhikes and overnight backpacking trips are included, based on **beautiful scenery, ease of access**, and **diversity of experience**. Because this area is Yosemite, most of the selected trails are very popular, and you can expect to see dozens to hundreds of other hikers along your route. Additionally, on trails 27 and 43 you may meet only a dozen or so hikers. For solitude in the park, you have to strike cross-country.

The great majority of the trails included in this guide are out-and-back trips, requiring you to retrace your steps back to the trailhead. About a half dozen are loop or partial loop trips (some with options for straight out-and-back), and only four are point-to-point trails that are worthy of the required shuttle. However, for three of these, public transportation is available, so you don't need two vehicles.

Features and Facilities

Top Trails books contain information about "features" for each trail, such as lakes, great views, summits, waterfalls, or wildflowers. These are listed in the margin of each trail. Just beneath each list is a list of facilities, such as restrooms, nearby phone, or tap water.

Trail Safety

One danger is getting lost, although most of the trails in this book are very obvious routes. You can lose a trail where it crosses a lengthy stretch of bedrock that is not adequately marked by a line of rocks or by small piles of stones, called ducks. Also, in early season, patches of snow can obscure enough of your route that you lose it. In both situations it can be helpful to look back and note key features you've passed, so that if you think you are getting lost, you then can recognize your way back toward the trailhead.

Most of the park's trails are safe, but some spots are potentially dangerous, and these are identified in the text.

At high elevations, especially above treeline, thunderstorms can be dangerous, since they generate lightning. If the weather looks threatening, don't venture above the forest cover, even if the lightning is several miles away. Should you find yourself above trees (don't try to hide beneath isolated ones!), get rid of all your metal gear and stoop low, and cover your head and keep your hands off the ground. These storms usually pass overhead in about 15 minutes.

Both thunderstorms and frontal storms can chill you sufficiently that you can start slipping into hypothermia, and then you begin to lose physical coordination and mental judgment. Therefore, be sure you bring sufficient clothing to protect you from rain, snow, and cold winds. Even if you are on just a dayhike, consider what you would need to survive a night, should you, say, break a leg and not get rescued until the next day.

Above 8000 feet, you may get altitude sickness if you overexert, especially after a large meal. You can minimize this through partial acclimatization by camping one night above 7000 feet elevation and then hiking the next day.

Sunburns can be particularly bad at high elevations, where the ultraviolet radiation is greater, and you can even get burned on cloudy days since the radiation penetrates clouds. Therefore, apply sunscreen to all exposed skin, even if you are just hiking for an afternoon down in Yosemite Valley.

Besides staying on route and addressing the weather (which more often than not is fine), you have to be aware of certain animals. Mosquitoes top my list as the most annoying, but so long as you have repellent, they are manageable. They are most plentiful before late July, especially around moist places such as meadows, grassy lake shores, and lodgepole-pine forests; before August you'll likely want to backpack with a tent so that you can sleep in peace.

The largest animals are black bears, which almost always leave you alone, but do want your food. Day hikers don't have to worry about bears, since it is extremely unlikely that one will rip the pack off your back. However, since backpackers stand a very good chance of being visited by a bear during the night, they are required to keep their food in a bear canister. You don't need canisters for campsites at Little Yosemite Valley and at the High Sierra Camps, which have bear-proof metal food-storage boxes. With cash or a credit card, for your backpack trip you can rent a park canister for a few dollars (plus a refundable deposit equal to the cost of the canister). Canisters are available at the Yosemite Valley and Tuolumne Meadows wilderness centers, the Big Oak Flat Information Station, the Wawona Information Station, the Hetch Hetchy Entrance Station, and the

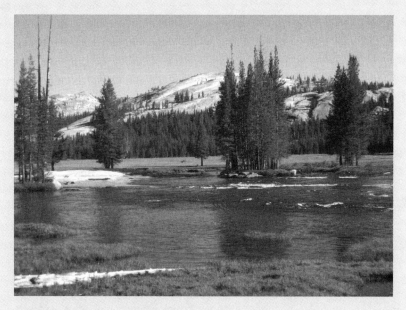

Tuolumne River *north of Pothole Dome (Trail 8)*

Crane Flat and Wawona stores. They can be returned to any of these locations, and drop bins are available for after-hour returns. Drop bins are also available in the Yosemite Valley's trailhead parking area, near Happy Isles. If you've charged your deposit on a credit card, the charge slip will be torn up. If you've used cash, which few do, then to get your money back you will have to return the canister during business hours to the site you got it from.

Whereas bears see you as bearers of food, mountain lions see you as food. Therefore, it is best not to hike alone, and if you bring children, keep them close by. Although no one has been attacked by a lion, they are getting bolder. Should you be threatened, you may have to fight back. Running away is to invite attack, since that is what prey does. About the only reason I can see to use trekking poles (and I don't) is that you can wave them threateningly at a mountain lion. Also, with them you can move a rattlesnake from your route, but I prefer to just walk around it. Your chance of meeting one on a trail is remote; of being bitten, more remote; and of dying from a bite even more so (the toxicity of their venom is overrated).

If you are going to be injured by an animal, it could be by a deer, whose front hooves are lethal weapons, so photograph them at a safe distance, not within striking distance. And avoid bites by not feeding cute rodents or any other animals. Let them get their own food, which for them is healthier than human food.

Fees, Camping, and Permits

Most hikers prefer to stay in campgrounds, and for each trail mentioned in this book, the relevant campgrounds are mentioned in the trail's introductory section, "Finding the Trail." An appendix at the end of this book lists of all of the area's campgrounds, public and private, as well as many resorts and lodges.

Not surprisingly, most trails start within Yosemite National Park, and to enter it you'll have to pay an entrance fee. Its cost depends on which type of pass you purchase. The Standard Pass is $20 per vehicle ($10 on foot, motorcycle, bicycle, or bus), and it is good for seven days. The Annual Pass is $40 per vehicle and is good for one full year from the date of purchase. Obviously, if you plan to visit the park more than twice within a 12-month period, the Annual Pass is the better deal. Should you plan to visit three or more national parks, purchase the $50 National Parks Pass. But if you plan also to visit national monuments, recreation areas, historic sites, and/or wildlife refuges, then go for the $65 Golden Eagle Pass. Finally, citizens or residents 62 and over, such as I, can get the $10 Golden Age Passport, which is good for a lifetime. (U.S. citizens or residents who are blind or permanently disabled get into all national entities for free and for life with the Golden Age Access.)

Many visitors who stay overnight in the Yosemite area would like to do so in campgrounds, which, unfortunately, are often full during the summer hiking season. Every hiking chapter includes information about nearby campgrounds and other accommodations such as resorts, motels, and lodges.

Within the park, reservations are required for sites in Yosemite Valley's North, Upper, and Lower Pines campgrounds. The Valley also offers Sunnyside Walk-in Campground, on a first-come, first-served basis, but don't count on getting a site, since climbers have a virtual monopoly on it. Other park campgrounds requiring reservations are Crane Flat, Wawona (reservations May-September), Hodgdon Meadow (reservations May-September), and half the sites of Tuolumne Meadows. The park's five other campgrounds, which are smaller and open only in the summer season, are on a first-come, first-served basis, and they fill up fast. These are Bridalveil Creek, along the Glacier Point Road, and, from west to east on or near the Tioga Road, Tamarack Flat, White Wolf, Yosemite Creek, and Porcupine Flat campgrounds.

To make reservations, phone the National Park Reservation System at (800) 436-7275 as early as possible within the given time frame. Alternatively, make reservations on the Internet at http://reservations.nps.gov. Each time frame begins on the 15th of every month, and you can reserve from as little as one day in advance to as much as five months in advance. For example, if you wanted to camp between June 15 and July 14, you could reserve as soon as February 15.

The Delaware North Companies Parks & Resorts at Yosemite, Inc. manages the park's hotels and lodges as well as the backcountry High Sierra Camps. The latter are so popular that a lottery is held each December to determine the lucky relative few reservations for the following summer. To obtain a lottery application, contact the concessionaire from early September through late November (see the appendix for contact information). In a normal year these facilities open around mid-July and close around mid-September. In years of heavy snowfall the camps may not open at all! Through Delaware North, you can reserve *up to one year and one day in advance*.

Finally, if you are going to spend one or more nights in the wilderness, be it in Yosemite National Park or in the wildernesses of adjoining Forest Service lands, you will need a wilderness permit. Every hiking chapter includes information about where to get these permits. Since the bulk of the backcountry hikes are within the park, the basic information on permits you will need for them is given below.

Yosemite National Park's backcountry has quotas from May through October, and 60 percent of each day's trailhead quota is available by reservation; the rest of the permits are given on a first-come, first-served basis. The rest of the year, virtually all of the high country will be under snow, and very few people will be backpacking, so you won't have to worry about any trailhead having its quota full.

To register in person, see "Permits" near the start of each hiking chapter. Popular destinations, such as Lyell Canyon, the Cathedral Lakes, the Vogelsang Lake area, and Little Yosemite Valley, can easily reach their quotas, especially for overnight trips beginning on a summer weekend. Therefore, you might want to get a permit well in advance if you are backpacking on a weekend from late June through late September. You can get a permit from 24 weeks to two days in advance of your trip date. If your reservation request is made less than two days or more than 24 weeks in advance, it will be rejected *without notice*.

You can also get a permit by calling the valley's Wilderness Center at (209) 372-0740, but the reservation phone lines are often busy, and you may not get through. For general information about wilderness permits and the backcountry, phone the center at (209) 372-0745. You can also make your request in writing or on the Internet at www.nps.gov/yose/wilderness. Written requests are processed simultaneously with phone requests. Write to: Wilderness Permits, PO Box 545, Yosemite, CA 95389. Include the following in your request: name, address, daytime phone, number of people in party, method of travel (i.e., ski, snowshoe, foot, horse), number of stock (if applicable), start and end dates, entry and exit trailheads, and principal destination. Include alternate dates and/or trailheads. A $5 *per person* nonrefundable processing fee is charged for all reservation requests. Payment by check or money order should be made to the Yosemite Association. Credit card payments are accepted with valid card number and expiration date.

Topographic Maps

Topographic maps of various scales exist for all areas covered in this guidebook. Several cover the entire park, including one I created by mapping the trails on foot and placing my data on a USGS topographic map (Yosemite National Park and Vicinity, 1:125,000 scale, Wilderness Press, 2004). This is particularly useful for identifying distant peaks, canyons, lakes, etc. from summits.

For more detailed maps, there are several choices, and I recommend (and have done all) three. First, you can purchase USGS 7.5-minute (1:24,000 scale) topographic quadrangles from the USGS or from other vendors, doing so either online or in person. Second, you can purchase a CD or DVD from companies such as National Geographic (TOPO!) or DeLORME, which is a sizable initial investment, but then you can print your own customized maps that cover only the area you need. Third, if you have access to a college or university, their library may have a USGS topographic map collection, and since the maps are not copyrighted, you can photocopy the section of the appropriate topographic map that you need.

In the introductory material for each chapter under "Maps" there is a list of the USGS 7.5-minute (1:24,000 scale) topographic quadrangles needed for each hike.

On the Trail

Every outing should begin with proper preparation, which usually takes only a few minutes. Even the easiest trail can turn up unexpected surprises. People seldom think about getting lost or injured, but unexpected things can and do happen. Simple precautions can make the difference between a good story and a miserable outcome.

Use the Top Trails ratings and descriptions to determine if a particular trail is a good match with your fitness and energy level, given current conditions and time of year.

Have a Plan

Choose Wisely The first step to enjoying any trail, no matter the intended activity or the degree of difficulty, is to match the trail to your abilities. It's no use overestimating your fitness or experience—know your abilities and limitations, and use the Top Trails Difficulty Rating that accompanies each trail.

Leave Word About Your Plans The most basic of precautions is leaving word of your intentions with friends or family. Leave specific information such as your trailhead location and your daily itinerary. (I also mark all of this up on map.) Many people will hike the backcountry their entire lives without ever relying on this safety net, but every year you are likely to hear news reports about missing persons in the mountains. If you get caught in an unexpected storm, you can't be rescued if first, no one knows that you are missing, and second, no one knows where you went hiking.

Prepare and Plan

- **Know your abilities and limitations**
- **Leave word about your plans**
- **Know your route and the area**

Review the Route Before embarking on any hike, read the entire description and study the map. It isn't necessary to memorize every detail, but it is worthwhile to have a clear mental picture of the trail and general area. Because virtually all of the described trails are well used and easy to follow, you really don't need a topographic map.

Carry the Essentials

Proper preparation for any type of trail use includes gathering the essential items to carry. Your own checklist will vary tremendously by trail, conditions, and your personal preferences.

Clothing, etc. In good summer weather, I prefer dayhiking and backpacking in a short-sleeved shirt or T-shirt, in shorts, and in inexpensive jogging shoes. The less you wear, the less you sweat and the less likely you'll get crotch burn. That said, I am prepared for the worst, having lightweight waterproof gear to cover my body from head to foot as well as extra clothing should I be stuck overnight on a dayhike gone astray.

Blisters can make your trip miserable, and you can avoid them two ways. First, wear broken-in, lightweight shoes, not heavy boots; second, wear two or three pairs of socks, and have at least one spare pair should your get wet feet.

Backpackers definitely will want long pants and warm clothing, since in the high country, nights and mornings can be nippy even in the height of summer. Bundle up in the morning, then shed layers of clothing as you warm up. In the high country you'll also want a lightweight sleeping bag that keeps you warm down to about 20°F. Traveling light, I'll bring a tarp that is big enough to serve as an emergency shelter to keep me and my sleeping bag dry should a storm occur. If I'm out for more than two nights or am hiking in mosquito season, I'll bring a lightweight tent.

Whether you dayhike or backpack, bring sunscreen and, to be safe, mosquito repellent. Many wear caps or hats, which are great if you are not a profuse sweater. Also, most bring dark glasses, but squinting at high elevations (even above treeline) works just as well.

Water and Its Treatment If you expect to be out for an hour or less, you can skip water. However, on longer dayhikes, you'll likely want to bring along one or more water bottles. My rule of thumb is that on a hot day I'll consume one quart for every 5 miles I walk; more, if the hike is strenuous. If you backpack, you'll need to refill from creeks and/or lakes, which *usually*

Trail Essentials

- **Dress to keep cool, but be ready for cold**
- **Carry plenty of water**
- **Have adequate food (plus a little extra)**

are safe for drinking, but on occasion may be contaminated with unseen Giardia. Should you choose not to risk giardiasis, then use a water filter.

Food Books give advice on the best food, but I say that within reason, take what you like. I know someone who backpacked about 2500 miles on hardly anything else other than candy, salami, and vitamin supplements. To each his own. If you are going to be out longer than an overnight, bring extra food just in case you get lost or stuck in the wilderness. Especially in an unexpected snowstorm, you'll want to down a lot of calories. If you want to backpack light, leave the stove and pots at home, eating only cold food, although this is not acceptable to most folks.

Gear Depending on the remoteness and rigor of the trail, there are many additional useful items to consider. Even in my day pack I carry a flashlight, pocket knife, fire source (waterproof matches and/or lighter), and first-aid supplies. On backpacks, I may throw in duct tape and straps; you never know if you have to fix something, say, a broken pack or a broken bone. Every member of your party should carry basic survival items, since groups sometimes get separated along the trail.

For most folks, a topographic map and a compass are not necessary, but with them you can identify a lot of features not shown on this book's maps. Also, should you decide to leave your trail and go cross-country, say to a nearby lake, a topographic map is extremely valuable. Wilderness Press sells the topographic map "Yosemite National Park and Vicinity," which includes all the trails covered in this book, plus many more. Handheld GPS (Global Positioning System) receivers can be useful, but in deep canyons there is no reception. The same goes for cell phones: on the trail, the ability to communicate through them is essentially zero.

Solo hikers should be even more disciplined about preparation, should be more knowledgeable about potential hazards and their avoidance, and should carry more gear. Traveling solo is inherently more risky. With a group of three or more, should one be injured, another could stay behind with that person while another goes for help.

Travel Light If you pack intelligently, then most of this book's overnight hikes can be done with a loaded pack of 20 to 25 pounds (or less). On the longest hike, Trail 15, your loaded pack still should be under 30 pounds, which for most adult males will be less than 20 percent of their body weight. And this is what you should strive for, since it can be hard to enjoy your outing if your pack weighs you down and/or its straps dig into your shoulders.

By keeping your pack light, you can hike even in inexpensive jogging shoes or walking shoes. Unless you have weak ankles, heavy boots serve no other purpose than expending more energy to help you lose weight. With a light backpack, you can skip those expensive trekking poles, which are valuable for Himalayan expeditions or if you have bad knees. On Yosemite's trails, you don't need them, and 90-plus percent of those I see with them are either carrying them or tapping the ground, neither activity doing any good for their knees. Perhaps the most compelling reason against using them is that you spend much time looking at the ground instead of at the scenery, depriving yourself of a superior outdoor experience.

Trail Etiquette

The overriding rule on the trail is **Leave No Trace**. This is especially applicable to the more popular hiking destinations in and about Yosemite National Park, where over any summer dozens of lakes will be visited by hundreds of hikers.

Never Litter If you carried it in, it's even easier to carry it out, since it weighs less. Try picking up any litter you encounter and packing it out—it's a rewarding feeling. Nature also litters, and I make it a habit to move at least a bit of debris from the trail, be it boulders, branches, or small trees. It is amazing just how large a tree a few sturdy hikers can move.

Don't Build Campsites Constructing fire rings or clearing the ground to place a tent or tarp transforms a pristine site into a human one—hardly a wilderness experience. Also, if you are going cross-country, don't mark your route. Let others do their own rewarding pathfinding just as you did.

Stay on the Trail Repeated shortcutting of switchbacks can lead to rapid erosion and time-consuming trail repair. Also, because shortcuts are steeper and have an uneven, sometimes bouldery tread, they can be dangerous, particularly for an exhausted backpacker in a hurry to get down. Don't risk broken bones or sprained ankles.

Share the Trail This book's trails attract many visitors, and you should be prepared to share the trail with others. Commonly accepted trail etiquette dictates that hikers yield to equestrians and their stock, and that ascending and descending hikers keep to their respective right side as they pass each other. Short tourist trails are severely impacted, hosting hundreds to thousands of visitors a day. You may meet an obnoxious person or two; don't become one and spoil someone else's day.

Leave It There Removal or destruction of plants, animals, and historical artifacts is both unethical and illegal.

 Trail Etiquette

- Leave no trace—Never litter
- Stay on the trail—Never cut switchbacks
- Share the trail—Use courtesy and common sense
- Leave it there—Don't disturb plants or wildlife

CHAPTER 1

Northeast Yosemite

Northeast Yosemite

A s defined in this guidebook, the Northeast Yosemite country is almost exclusively the lands extending down from the park's northeast boundary, which is a small part of the Sierra Nevada crest. Except for Trail 1 up to Barney and Peeler lakes, which traverses through an entirely granitic landscape—John Muir's "Range of Light"—all the trails traverse through landscapes that are partly to entirely metamorphic. Rather than being lands of light gray, these are vari-hued earth-tones of brown, brownish red, rust, and shades of ochre. In addition to being more colorful, metamorphic rocks weather to produce more nutrients, and so these lands support an abundance of subalpine and alpine wildflowers.

Highway 395 gives rise to roads climbing west to trailheads north and east of Yosemite's Sierran crest, and from these you can advance up canyons to the crest and then beyond into lands of the northern third of the park. This area's landscape is characterized by many parallel or nearly parallel canyons, which, generally, speaking, get progressively deeper toward the east. Many of the canyons lack trails, and the park's management is to be applauded for keeping them that way. In my opinion, this Yosemite backcountry and the adjacent Emigrant Wilderness to the west together contain the finest assemblage of cross-country routes to be found in the Sierra Nevada—a last stronghold for the true wilderness experience. However, most of these routes are not described in this book, since they tend to be long, usually 40 to 55 miles, which limits their appeal to those willing to carry relatively heavy packs for four to seven days.

Rather, shorter, popular routes are described, these being dayhikes or overnighters. Trails 1 through 4 start from eastern lands and visit lakes of the Hoover Wilderness that are east of and below the Sierran crest. Trails 5 and 6 start from Tioga Pass, which at about 9940 feet is the Sierra's highest pass that is traversed by a highway (Highway 120, also know as Tioga Road). Trail 5 ascends to the summit of Mt. Dana, within the park. Perhaps nowhere in the park or its vicinity can you obtain such expansive views of

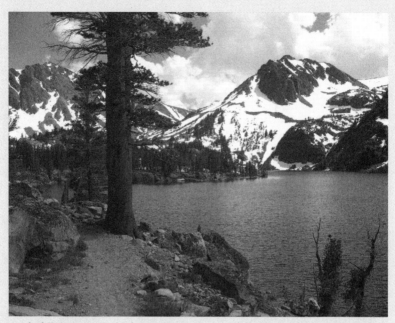

Overleaf: **Twin Lakes** *and Robinson Canyon (Trail 1). Above:* **East Lake** *(Trail 2 and 3).*

the Mono Basin and Owens Valley than from this summit. And nowhere in the Sierra Nevada can you find a more easily attained summit over 13,000 feet than Mt. Dana. Finally, Trail 6 visits popular, easily visited lakes west of and below the Sierran crest, the subalpine Gaylor Lakes.

Permits

If you want to reserve a permit, rather than get one in person, see the "Fees, Camping, and Permits" section on page 14.

In person, for Trails 1–3, get your permit at the Bridgeport Ranger Station (760-932-7070). It is on Highway 395 at the east end of Bridgeport, 1 mile east of the town's Twin Lakes Road junction. Should you wish to enter Yosemite National Park via Trail 4 through the Twenty Lakes Basin (no camping within the basin!), stop at the Lee Vining Ranger Station (760-647-3044), located 1 mile west up Highway 120 from its junction with Highway 395, at the south end of Lee Vining. Trails 4–7 are dayhikes, so wilderness permits are not needed.

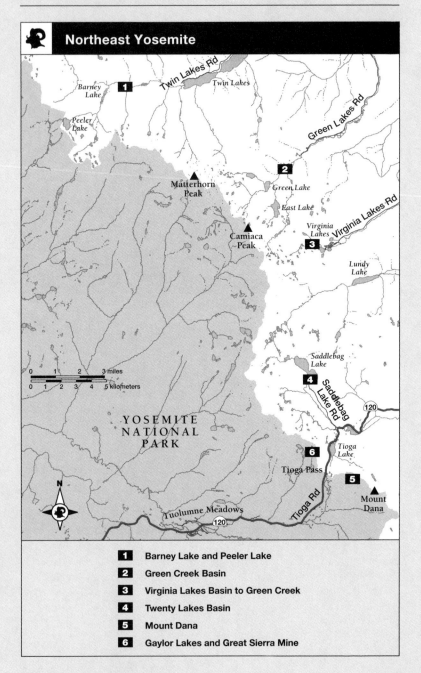

Northeast Yosemite

1 Barney Lake and Peeler Lake

2 Green Creek Basin

3 Virginia Lakes Basin to Green Creek

4 Twenty Lakes Basin

5 Mount Dana

6 Gaylor Lakes and Great Sierra Mine

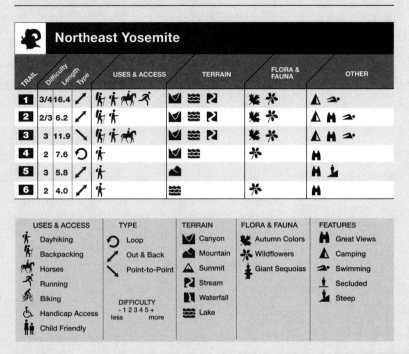

TRAIL	Difficulty	Length	Type	USES & ACCESS	TERRAIN	FLORA & FAUNA	OTHER
1	3/4	16.4	↗	🚶🎒🐎🏃	⛰ ≋ ⊠	✿ ❋	▲ ⌿
2	2/3	6.2	↗	🚶🎒🏃	⛰ ≋ ⊠	✿ ❋	▲ 🔭 ⌿
3	3	11.9	↘	🚶🎒🐎🏃	⛰ ≋ ⊠	✿ ❋	▲ 🔭 ⌿
4	2	7.6	↻	🚶	⛰ ≋	❋	🔭
5	3	5.8	↗	🚶	⛰		🔭 ⌖
6	2	4.0	↗	🚶	≋	❋	🔭

USES & ACCESS	TYPE	TERRAIN	FLORA & FAUNA	FEATURES
Dayhiking	Loop	Canyon	Autumn Colors	Great Views
Backpacking	Out & Back	Mountain	Wildflowers	Camping
Horses	Point-to-Point	Summit	Giant Sequoias	Swimming
Running		Stream		Secluded
Biking	DIFFICULTY	Waterfall		Steep
Handicap Access	- 1 2 3 4 5 +	Lake		
Child Friendly	less more			

Maps

For the Northeast Yosemite country, here are the USGS 7.5-minute (1:24,000 scale) topographic quadrangles that you will need, listed in the order that you will need them as you hike along your route.

Trail 1: Buckeye Ridge, Matterhorn Peak
Trails 2 and 3: Dunderberg Peak
Trail 4: Tioga Pass, Dunderberg Peak
Trail 5: Tioga Pass, Mount Dana
Trail 6: Tioga Pass

Northeast Yosemite

The Robinson Creek Trail is the most popular route through the Hoover Wilderness and into the Yosemite north country, and justifiably so. This relatively short, scenic trail leads quickly into breathtaking subalpine terrain, and to glittering Peeler Lake. Most folks, however, climb only as far as Barney Lake, a route that is a popular dayhike.

Large, attractive Green Lake is one of the most easily reached backpacker lakes in the North Yosemite area, and the hike up to it is memorable because of the diverse vegetation and the impressive views down-canyon from the multi-step climb. For those staying in the Bridgeport area the relatively short trail up to Green Lake (and even to East Lake) is a great dayhike.

The road up to the Virginia Lakes basin has much to offer. You can spend a relatively short time exploring the Virginia Lakes, or you can climb above them to the views at Burro Pass. Also, you can make either a long dayhike or a moderate backpack beyond the pass down to the Green Creek trailhead. And you can either dayhike to Summit Lake or backpack beyond it into upper Virginia Canyon, a classic glacier-smoothed subalpine gorge.

Twenty Lakes Basin 53

TRAIL 4

This splendid semi-loop trip from Saddlebag Lake to Helen Lake and back passes more than one lake per mile, and in doing so offers you some of the Sierra's finest subalpine scenery along an easy grade. With the high and low elevations only about 400 feet apart, there are no significant ascents and descents. Still, at over 10,000 feet, you will notice the rarefied air if you try to hurry along.

Dayhike
7.6 miles, Loop
Difficulty: 1 **2** 3 4 5

Mount Dana 59

TRAIL 5

Dark glasses and good health are both necessary for this climb to the second highest summit in Yosemite. Only Mt. Lyell exceeds it—by about 60 feet—but the Lyell summit is distant and it requires mountaineering skills. Because Dana vies with Mt. Hoffmann as Yosemite's most accessible peak, it is very popular, and on weekends you may find dozens of persons ascending it. Its summit views are among the Sierra's best.

Dayhike
5.8 miles, Out & Back
Difficulty: 1 2 **3** 4 5

Gaylor Lakes and Great Sierra Mine . .65

TRAIL 6

Five subalpine lakes and sweeping panoramas await those who take this hike and its optional side trip. You also have the option of visiting the Granite Lakes by making a short cross-country hike. Camping is not allowed in the Gaylor Lakes area, which includes the Granite Lakes.

Dayhike
4.0 miles, Out & Back
Difficulty: 1 **2** 3 4 5

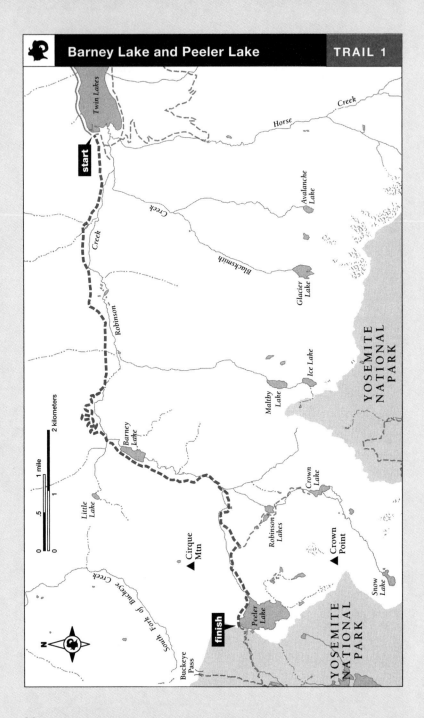

start

Twin Lakes

Horse Creek

Avalanche Lake

Creek

Creek

Robinson

Blacksmith Creek

Glacier Lake

Ice Lake

Maltby Lake

YOSEMITE NATIONAL PARK

Barney Lake

Crown Lake

2 kilometers

1 mile

Little Lake

Robinson Lakes

Crown Point

Snow Lake

Cirque Mtn

South Fork of Buckeye Creek

finish

Peeler Lake

Buckeye Pass

YOSEMITE NATIONAL PARK

N

Barney Lake and Peeler Lake

The Robinson Creek Trail is the most popular route through the Hoover Wilderness and into the Yosemite north country, and justifiably so. This relatively short, scenic trail leads quickly into breathtaking subalpine terrain. Glittering Peeler Lake, surrounded by frost-shattered and glaciated granite and windswept conifers, mirrors the region's grandeur. Intimate campsites beside its shore more than compensate for the day's tough climb. Most folks, however, climb only as far as Barney Lake, which is a popular dayhike. Finally, the Twin Lakes area is a great one for joggers, who can make a roughly 4-mile-long loop around each of the two lakes, or a 3-mile gentle ascent of the scenic Robinson Creek Trail to the start of its switchbacks.

Best Time

The trail up Robinson Creek canyon usually is snow-free by late May. Barney Lake is a desirable goal by late June, while Peeler Lake is best left for mid-July through mid-August. September, when the deciduous vegetation puts on a display of color, is a good month for Robinson Creek canyon and Barney Lake.

Finding the Trail

From Highway 395 near the west side of Bridgeport, take paved Twin Lakes Road south 13.6 miles to the entrance to Mono Village at the west end of upper Twin Lake. The Forest Service campgrounds you pass as you ascend this road are Honeymoon Flat,

TRAIL USE
Dayhike, Backpack,
Run, Horse

LENGTH
16.4 miles, 5–10 hours

VERTICAL FEET
+2730'/-310'/±6080

DIFFICULTY
- 1 2 **3 4** 5 +

TRAIL TYPE
Out & Back

FEATURES
Backcountry Permit
Lakes
Streams
Wildflowers
Camping
Swimming
Autumn Colors

FACILITIES
Resort
Campgrounds
Picnic Tables
Phone
Water
Horse Staging

Robinson Creek, Paha, Crags, and Lower Twin Lakes.

The trailhead is at road's end in Mono Village. Day hikers will see a large parking area immediately to their left, alongside the lake. Backpackers need to drive about 0.1 mile farther, to Mono Village's obvious campground entrance booth. Pay for backpacking here, which is a few dollars for your trip, regardless if it is one night's parking or many. Mileage is measured from the campground entrance booth, which is about the same distance from the trail's turnaround point as the backpackers' overnight parking lot.

Trail Description

You begin in Mono Village, ►1 a private resort with cabins and a campground at the head of upper Twin Lake. From the campground's entrance booth are two main roads, and you can take either, since they reunite in about 0.2 mile (it's a loop road). From the high end of the loop, by a meadow's edge, your route, a closed road, starts up-canyon. This goes 0.25 mile past the meadow, then 100 yards more to the start of the Robinson Creek Trail. You've done 0.5 mile to here. Just ahead, the road quickly bridges Robinson Creek. After walking west a couple of minutes, you pass low granitic outcrops, and just beyond them is a bulletin board with information on the area. The first part of your hike is open forest, dominated by Jeffrey pines on the dry slopes and aspens on wetter soils, particularly near unseen Robinson Creek. Less common trees include Fremont cottonwood and western juniper, both in more abundance up-canyon.

About 0.66 mile along the Robinson Creek Trail you reach a persistent stream, chortling down through wild-rose shrubbery from the basin

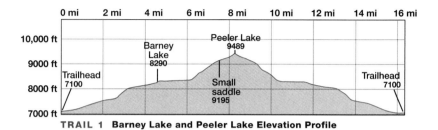

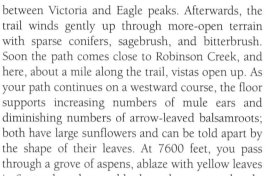

TRAIL 1 Barney Lake and Peeler Lake Elevation Profile

between Victoria and Eagle peaks. Afterwards, the trail winds gently up through more-open terrain with sparse conifers, sagebrush, and bitterbrush. Soon the path comes close to Robinson Creek, and here, about a mile along the trail, vistas open up. As your path continues on a westward course, the floor supports increasing numbers of mule ears and diminishing numbers of arrow-leaved balsamroots; both have large sunflowers and can be told apart by the shape of their leaves. At 7600 feet, you pass through a grove of aspens, ablaze with yellow leaves in September, then amble through more sagebrush, scattered junipers, and boulders to the Hoover Wilderness boundary, about 2.75 miles from Mono Village. Minutes later you re-enter white-fir cover, and can stop for a drink beside tumbling Robinson Creek. This is a good rest spot for the climb ahead.

 Stream

When you are ready to assault the canyon head-wall, gear down to accommodate more than a dozen well-graded switchbacks that lead north through head-high jungles of aspen, bitter cherry, service-berry, snowberry, and tobacco brush, staying always within earshot of unseen Robinson Creek. Above 8000 feet you step across a rivulet merrily draining the slopes of Hunewill Peak, a welcome respite abundant with wildflowers. Still climbing, you return momentarily to the creekside, then you climb rockily, bending south, in a gully under aspen shade. Half your ascent to Peeler Lake is behind you

Wildflowers

when you level out to step across a branch of Robinson Creek that drains the 10,700-foot saddle to the west.

Just ahead you reach the north end of a large flat that extends to the north shore of Barney Lake, and in times past was littered with campsites. Today, camping on the flat is discouraged, but there are sites east of the creek (sometimes a ford) on a flat behind a granitic mass at the lake's northeast corner. About 4.5 miles from Mono Village, 14-acre Barney Lake, ▶2 at 8290 feet, is nestled in a narrow, glaciated trough, rimmed on the east by the broken north spur of Kettle Peak. The lake's north shore has a sandy beach, good after a swim, and it makes a fine spot for a lunch break.

The western shoreline, which your trail follows, is a dry talus slope mixed with glacial debris. Here, a pair of switchbacks elevate the trail to an easy grade some 100 feet above Barney Lake's inlet.

After a few minutes, you descend several short switchbacks, wind through broken rock and past avalanche-twisted aspens, over two freshets draining Cirque Mountain, then come to a ford of Robinson Creek, about 0.75 mile past the lake and about 2.5 miles before Peeler Lake. This crossing can be a wet ford in early season if industrious beavers have widened the ford by damming the creek in the meadow just downstream. Rainbow and brook trout occur here, as in Barney Lake. From the far bank, you climb easily south in a pleasant forest of lodgepole pine, red fir, western white pine, and a new addition, mountain hemlock, which reflects the higher altitude. The trail soon leads back to the west bank of Robinson Creek, which you cross (using a log, if one is handy). Next the trail crosses the cascading stream from Peeler Lake, beside which you might rest before ascending a long series of switchbacks just ahead. The first set of gentle switchbacks traverses a till-covered slope to about 8800 feet,

≋ Lake

⬤ Swimming

▶ Stream

where you level off momentarily for a breather before darting north for a steeper ascent. The vistas east, to stunted whitebark pines growing on rough, ice-fractured outcrops of Kettle Peak, offer good excuses to stop frequently on this energetic climb. Eventually you come to a small saddle at 9195 feet, which has a trail bound for Rock Island Pass and Slide Canyon. ▶3

Those bound for Peeler Lake now turn northwest, walking moderately up in mixed open forest, to a small, shaded glade beside Peeler Lake creek. Step across this stream twice before switchbacking south moderately up into a narrow gully. The wind can pick up as you ascend it, a sure sign that you're nearing the ridgetop. And sure enough, about 8 miles from Mono Village, 9489-foot Peeler Lake's often windswept waters soon come into view, behind car-size granodiorite blocks that dam its outlet. A short descent leads you below this talus to dynamited trail tread on the north shore of Peeler Lake, ▶4 where its waters foreground rounded Acker and Wells peaks, in the west. Most of the good campsites, under conifers, are found as the trail undulates rockily into forest pockets along the north shore—though the east shore has some fine ones too, if a bit out of the way. The lake margin, mostly rock, does have a few stretches of meadowy beach, where you can fly-cast for rainbows and brookies. When you are ready, backtrack to the trailhead. ▶5

≋ **Lake**

⚠ **Camping**

🏊 **Swimming**

🚶	**MILESTONES**

▶1   0.0 Start at Mono Village parking area

▶2   4.6 Barney Lake

▶3   7.5 Right at small saddle

▶4   8.2 Peeler Lake

▶5 16.4 Return to Mono Village parking area

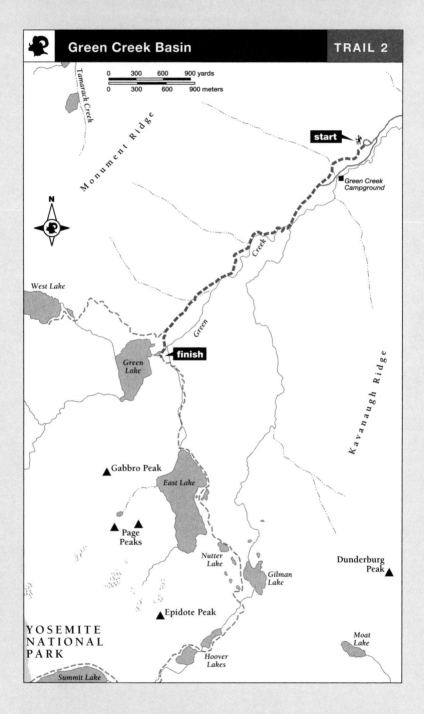

Green Creek Basin

Large, attractive Green Lake is one of the most easily reached backpacker lakes in the North Yosemite area, and the hike up to it is memorable because of the diverse vegetation and the impressive views down-canyon from the multi-step climb. You can continue on to camp at East Lake, set before a dramatic backdrop of Page and Epidote peaks. Or, from Green Lake you can make a dayhike up to alpine West Lake and even explore cross-country the isolated lakes beyond. For those staying in the Bridgeport area the relatively short trail up to Green Lake (and even to East Lake) is a great dayhike.

Best Time

The trail up Green Creek canyon usually is snow-free by late June, but snow can linger at the lakes into July, when the canyon's wildflower gardens peak. By late July, mosquitoes are abating and Green Lake is warm enough for swimming, cooling a bit by mid-August. September is a good month for Green Creek canyon, when the deciduous vegetation puts on a display of color, and most of the hikers have gone.

Finding the Trail

From Bridgeport along Highway 395, drive through the town to the Bridgeport Ranger Station, near its south edge. Continue 3.8 miles south on 395 to a junction with Green Creek Road 142. If you're traveling north, you'll meet this junction about 8.1 miles north of 395's Conway Summit with its Virginia Lakes Road junction. Take road 142 about

TRAIL USE
Dayhike, Backpack
LENGTH
6.2 miles, 2–4 hours
VERTICAL FEET
+1070'/-160'/±2460'
DIFFICULTY
- 1 **2 3** 4 5 +
TRAIL TYPE
Out & Back

FEATURES
Backcountry Permit
Lakes
Streams
Wildflowers
Great Views
Camping
Swimming
Autumn Colors

FACILITIES
Restrooms
Campground
Water

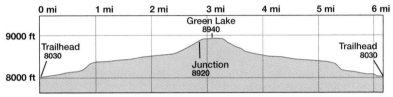

TRAIL 2 Green Creek Basin Green Lake Elevation Profile

Just past the 15-foot-high cliff is a basalt remnant that glaciers have failed to eradicate: the canyon has not deepened in more than 5 million years.

3.5 miles to a **T**. (Left, broad, well-graded Dunderberg Meadow Road 020 winds 9 miles south to a junction with Road 021. This has climbed 4.5 miles from Highway 395, and from Road 020 climbs in 1.6 miles past a pack station, resort, and campground to the Virginia Lakes trailhead. If you're making a one-way hike between the two trailheads, you'll want to take this road rather than drive all the way back down to Highway 395.) To reach the Green Creek trailhead, at the **T** you branch right, still on 142, and go for about 5 miles to an obvious trailhead parking area, with an outhouse and water spigot, on the right. Just 100 yards past this is Green Creek Campground's Group Unit, on the left, and 0.25 mile farther you enter the campground proper.

Trail Description

From the trailhead parking area, ▶1 take an obvious trail that winds and undulates up-canyon for 0.6 mile to a closed road, which has ascended about 0.25 mile from the Green Creek Campground. Start up the road, which continues for about another 0.25 mile to a creek crossing, from which a trail begins a multi-step ascent. After your first 0.1 mile you end a moderate climb at your first low step, beside a 15-foot-high cliff on your left. Whereas you started in a forest dominated by Jeffrey pines, you now ascend through a forest dominated by lodgepole pines and aspens, then take a dozen short, rocky switchbacks up to another step, which like others on your route

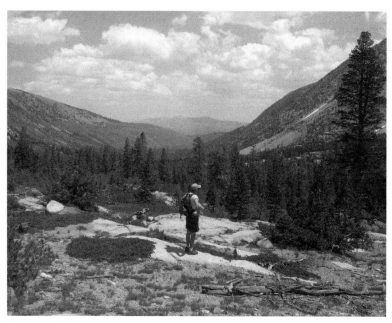

Green Creek Canyon

afford views down-canyon while you catch your breath at these subalpine elevations. [v] In this vicinity and about 1.7 miles into your hike, you enter the Hoover Wilderness, and soon early-season hikers encounter a stretch of wet trail, which may be a nuisance for some, but the trail cuts up a swath of luxuriant wildflowers that dazzle the eyes with myriad colors. By mid-season, the display can be gone, but so is the water flowing down the trail.

Great Views

As you go lower, you ascend mostly past lodgepoles and aspens, with isolated junipers adding variety, and then top out on another open step with a restful viewspot. Just ahead you'll arrive at a trail junction. ►2 To the right is a trail that provides access to the northwest shore of Green Lake and to

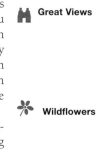 **Wildflowers**

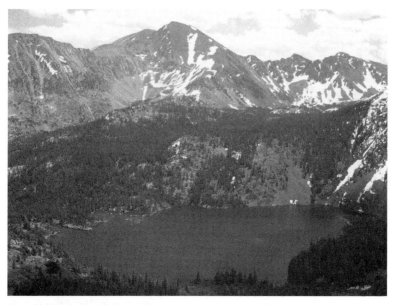

Green Lake *and Dunderberg Peak*

East Lake

OPTIONS

This is another popular and scenic lake, and from the Green Lake environs, ▶4 the 1.4-mile-long trail up to it is a moderate ascent through a relatively dense conifer forest. Part way up you'll cross the lake's outlet creek, which in early season can be swift, and a slip here will send you down its lethal, cascading course. Above, you recross it, and after about a 500-foot elevation gain you make a leisurely ascent 0.33 mile up to your last crossing of the creek, just below 9460-foot-high East Lake. This is a large subalpine lake, fully 0.75 mile long, and the trail parallels its east side for most of its length. From the outlet south to the southeast shore there are scattered, usually small campsites on granite benches shaded mostly by whitebark pines. Backpackers won't want to continue, since camping possibilities are minimal at the increasingly exposed Nutter, Gilman, and Hoover lakes.

West Lake and its western outliers. For most folks, the 1.5-mile-long trail up to this 9870-foot-high lake, with a pittance of whitebark-pine clusters and no acceptable, legal campsites, is not worth the effort.

From the trail junction virtually all users turn left and make a brief jaunt 0.2 mile to a crossing of Green Lake's outlet creek. In early season this creek can be raging, and you'll need to find a log or two to cross it. Either just before or after this creek you can head west to the nearby lake and find adequate campsites. At an elevation of 8940 feet, Green Lake ►3 can be on the nippy side for swimming, but there are slabs for drying out and sunbathing. The relatively large volume and chilly temperatures are ideal for a good-sized trout population. From here you can continue to East Lake or else backtrack to the trailhead. ►4

Caution

Lake

Swimming

🕴 MILESTONES

►1	0.0	Start at Green Creek trailhead
►2	2.9	Left at trail junction
►3	3.1	Green Lake
►4	6.2	Return to Green Creek trailhead

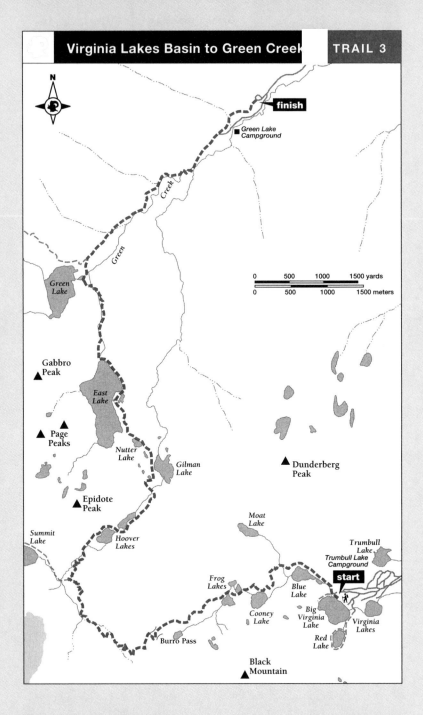

N

Green Lake
Campground

Green Creek

Green Lake

| 0 | 500 | 1000 | 1500 yards |
| 0 | 500 | 1000 | 1500 meters |

Gabbro
▲Peak

East
Lake

▲ Page
Peaks

Nutter
Lake

Gilman
Lake

▲ Dunderberg
Peak

▲Epidote
Peak

Summit
Lake

Hoover
Lakes

Moat
Lake

Trumbull
Lake
Trumbull Lake
Campground

start

Frog
Lakes

Blue
Lake

Cooney
Lake

Big
Virginia
Lake

Virginia
Lakes

Burro Pass

Red
Lake

Black
▲ Mountain

finish

Virginia Lakes Basin to Green Creek

The road up to the Virginia Lakes basin is paved, and for good reason: it attracts a lot of outdoor enthusiasts (hikers, equestrians, anglers) because there is much to offer. For the hiker there are several general possibilities. First, you can spend a relatively short time exploring one or more of the Virginia Lakes. Second, you can climb above them in rarefied air to Burro Pass to enjoy the views. Third, you can either make a long dayhike or a moderate backpack beyond the pass down to the Green Creek trailhead, passing ten lakes and several ponds along a mostly descending route. And fourth, you can either dayhike to Summit Lake or backpack beyond it down into upper Virginia Canyon, which is the easiest-to-reach classic glacier-smoothed subalpine gorge of the Yosemite north country. This is a route used by equestrians entering Yosemite.

Best Time

With a trailhead approaching 10,000 feet, this route often has snow patches well into July. You can start in early July, but late July is better, and early to mid-August is optimal. To avoid crowds, hike in September, when fall colors abound.

Finding the Trail

From Bridgeport along Highway 395, drive through the town to the Bridgeport Ranger Station, near its south edge. Continue about 12 miles south on 395 to 395's Conway Summit with its Virginia Lakes Road 021 junction. From Lee Vining you reach this

TRAIL USE
Dayhike, Backpack, Horse
LENGTH
11.9 miles, 4–8 hours
VERTICAL FEET
+1720'/-3550'/±5270'
DIFFICULTY
- 1 2 **3** 4 5 +
TRAIL TYPE
Point-to-Point

FEATURES
Backcountry Permit
Lakes
Streams
Wildflowers
Great Views
Camping
Swimming
Autumn Colors

FACILITIES
Resort
Restrooms
Campground
Phone
Water
Horse Staging

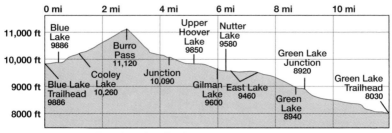

TRAIL 3 Virginia Lakes Basin to Green Lakes Elevation Profile

summit in about 12.25 miles. On this broad, paved road you climb 4.5 miles west to a junction with broad, well-graded Dunderberg Meadow Road 020, which winds 9 miles north to a junction with Green Creek Road 142, the road up to the previous trip's trailhead, and the road you take if you are doing a point-to-point hike. Road 142 goes for about 5 miles to an obvious trailhead parking area, with an outhouse and water spigot, on the right. Just 100 yards past this is Green Creek Campground's Group Unit, on the left, and .025 mile farther you enter the campground proper.

Your hike starts from the Virginia Lakes trailhead, so from road 020 you take Road 021 1.6 miles up to a moderate-size trailhead at road's end, passing along the way first the Virginia Lakes Pack Station on the right, the Virginia Lakes Resort (with cafe) on the left, and then Trumbull Lake Campground on the right.

Trail Description

From the parking area at an elevation of about 9830 feet, ▶1 the Blue Lake Trail traverses briefly west, first rounding above the shore of pretty, but sometimes crowded Big Virginia Lake, then entering a stand of aspens. In a minute or two, you turn northeast, and ascend briefly to a stand of pines, where you curve left and quickly reach a junction with a

≋ Lake

horse trail branching right, east, down to Trumbull Lake and the pack station beyond it. Under sparse subalpine shade your trail quickly passes two tarns just below you and then reaches the Hoover Wilderness boundary. Here the trail forks, the left branch dropping slightly to 9886-foot-high Blue Lake. Moments later on the higher, right-hand trail, Blue Lake comes into view, cupped in steep slopes of ruddy-brown hornfels—a metamorphic rock that lacks foliation. Beside Blue Lake, ►2 the two branches briefly merge, then you veer up from it. As you climb gently to moderately above the north shore of Blue Lake, you cross talus derived from rusty-weathered Dunderberg Peak high to your north.

≋ **Lake**

At Blue Lake's western headwall your way climbs steeply, stopping for a moment at a 9950-foot-high overlook, then rounds an immense talus fan to the verdant banks of Moat Lake's outlet stream, which descends merrily from the north together with its steeply clambering use-trail. Now your trail switchbacks southwest up a forested hillside to a switchback. Past it you arrive at the outlet of Cooney Lake, ►3 which occupies a low bench in this austere timberline upland. Good camps are found south of the inlet in wind-tortured knots of whitebark pines, reached by a footpath across the low bench. Also at a bend in the lake is a short path over to several more camps. As you leave the lake, views open to your trip's high point as barren Burro Pass (a local name) saddles the western horizon, its metamorphosed tuffs looking cream-colored against the surrounding, darker, metamorphosed lavas, such as Black Mountain, to your south.

≋ **Lake**

▲ **Camping**

About 1.25 miles into your hike, you leave often windy Cooney Lake and ascend gently west into a rocky-meadowed draw. Here you step easily across infant Virginia Creek via rocks and logs to find a second, rolling bench, which harbors a clutch of small lakelets—the Frog Lakes—named for once-numerous mountain yellow-legged frogs that formerly shared the cold, shallow waters with small eastern brook and rainbow trout. Now you swing south of the meadowy, lowest Frog Lake—a mosquito haven before mid-August—then ascend above some lush alpine turf to the highest lake, where good camps are found among scattered whitebark pines.

The next riser on your staircase ascent is steeper than those before, and has even less tree cover. Finally, the trail resolves into switchbacks, then leaves the last whitebark pines behind for a true alpine ascent along the west wall of a cirque. The relatively warm, mineral-rich, easily weathered, water-holding metavolcanic soil here supports an abundance of alpine wildflowers rarely seen elsewhere along a trail in such numbers. Views across the Virginia Lakes basin continue to improve, then after a burst of switchbacks you gain broad and relatively viewless 11,120-foot-high Burro Pass. ▶4 By walking north just a minute from the trail's high point, you can also view the Hoover Lakes, at the base of Epidote Peak, and, in the northwest, Summit Lake, at the base of Camiaca Peak.

From the barren, windswept crest, you make an initial descent south, then momentarily switchback northwest toward Summit Lake. Beside the trail you'll see tight clusters of whitebark pines, the largest cluster offering emergency shelter if you're caught in a blizzard. Your trail switchbacks northwest down through a small, stark side canyon to a sloping subalpine bench, which gives your knees a rest before you hit the third set of switchbacks. After about a 1.5-mile descent from Burro Pass, you arrive at a junction on a small bench, ▶5 with clusters of whitebark pines, just above 10,000 feet near East Fork Green Creek. Here you have a choice: head over to Summit Lake and possibly beyond, or else

 Lake

Camping

Wildflowers

Great Views

descend a popular route past a half-dozen lakes and several ponds en route to the Green Creek trailhead.

Summit Lake

From the junction ▶5 you turn southwest and drop momentarily to cross four small freshets in a seasonally verdant meadow. A steep, cobbly ascent ensues, paralleling Summit Lake's outlet stream. Soon the climb moderates, and you ascend dry sedge flats and benches past numerous good hemlock-bower campsites. Nearing the outlet of usually windswept Summit Lake, you level off. Campsites are few here, and a tent is advisable, for the scattered whitebark pines offer little wind protection. Sunset views, however, can be quite spectacular. Angling for small brookies is fair. The 0.5-mile climb to the lake is replaced with a 0.7-mile traverse curving west along the north shore to Summit Pass. On the Yosemite National Park boundary, this barely rises above the 10,195-foot-high lake. Standing at the pass, you can readily identify Virginia Peak, a pointed metamorphic summit that rises above the summits of Stanton Peak and Gray Butte.

From the junction ▶5, your Green Creek Trail starts northeast down past a tarn to an excellent overlook down-canyon to the windswept, largely desolate Hoover Lakes. Beyond, light-granitic Kavanaugh Ridge shows over the massive shoulder of Dunderberg Peak. You drop to step north across East Fork Green Creek, then traverse across talus above the west shore of upper Hoover Lake before traversing its north shore. At the northeast corner of upper Hoover Lake ▶6 you cross its wide, rocky outlet stream, and in this vicinity you could hike south briefly upslope to exposed camps on small flats above the lake's east shore. These are best viewed as emergency camps; better ones lie ahead by East Lake and the best ones are beyond at Green Lake. Lower Hoover Lake, just above which your

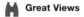 **Great Views**

≋ Lake

trail traverses via talus, has in the past contained rainbow, brook, and brown trout.

Below the lake and 1.1 miles past the trail junction, you drop easily over willowed benches, then circle above less-visited Gilman Lake to cross East Fork and Green Creek in a stand of hemlocks and whitebark pines. Soon afterward, your descent ends, and your route rises gently past easily recognized outcrops of conglomerate rocks. Soon you

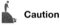 **Lake**

pass a short spur trail to Gilman Lake, ►7 followed closely by small, green Nutter Lake. ►8 Camps lie below your trail, in subalpine conifers at Nutter Lake's west end. Off-trail stealth campsites can be found just north of these two lakes. A short northwest climb from Nutter Lake on a mat-manzanita patched slope next presents East Lake, ►9 largest of the Green Creek lakes, spread 100 feet below you under the iron-stained talus skirts of crumbly Epidote Peak, Page Peaks, and Gabbro Peak. East

Lake

Lake is a large subalpine lake, fully 0.75 mile long, and the trail parallels its east side for most of its length. From the outlet south to the southeast shore there are scattered, usually small campsites on granite benches shaded mostly by whitebark pines. Finally you reach an extensive camping complex at East Lake's outlet, ►10 about 3.1 miles from the last junction. Fishing is good here for rainbow trout.

⚠ Camping

Your trail makes the first of three outlet creek crossings just below the lake, then you make an easy descent 0.33 mile to where you begin a moderate 500-foot drop in a relatively dense conifer forest to the second crossing. In early season the creek can be swift, and a slip here will send you down its lethal, cascading course. With more moderate descent, reach your third crossing, and soon

Caution

the trail levels off, and you can branch left, west, toward Green Lake ►11 and its adequate campsites. At an elevation of 8940 feet, the lake can be on the nippy side for some refreshing swimming followed

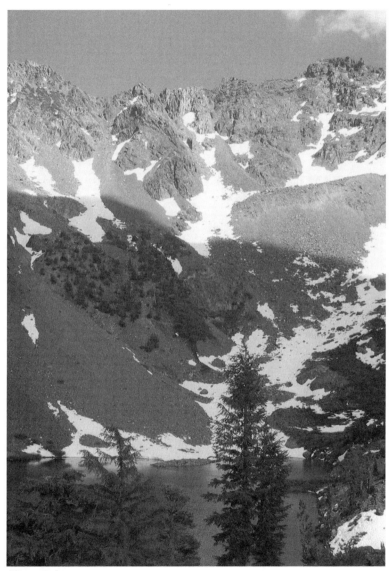

Gilman Lake

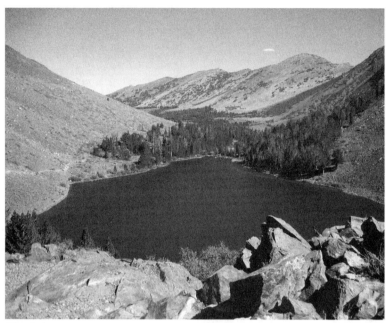

Blue Lake

 Swimming

 Caution

Wildflowers

by basking on slabs, but the lake's relatively large volume and chilly temperatures make it ideal for a good-sized trout population.

From the lake you have to cross Green Lake's outlet creek, and in early season it can be raging, so you'll need to find a log or two to cross it. Once you get back on your trail, you make a brief jaunt 0.2 mile to a junction ▶12 with a trail climbing 1.5 miles up to bleak West Lake.

From the junction, the Green Creek Trail starts a descent, and you have a great view down the Green Creek canyon, one of several to come. Next, the trail soon descends through a swath of luxuriant wildflowers that dazzle the eyes with myriad colors. By mid-season, the display can be gone, but so is the water flowing down the trail. About 1.2 miles beyond the junction you leave the Hoover Wilderness, in a forest dominated by lodgepole pines and aspens, and soon descend a dozen short, rocky switchbacks to another view. Below you, the forest is dominated by Jeffrey pines, and you complete your descent with a brief drop of 0.1 mile, down to a creek crossing. Next you make an easier descent .025 mile down a road from the Green Creek Campground, but rather, you take a trail branching left, which winds and undulates down-canyon, passing above the campground and reaching, in 0.6 mile, the parking area of the Green Creek trailhead. ►13

Great Views

☀	**MILESTONES**

►1	0.0	Start at Blue Lake trailhead
►2	0.5	Blue Lake
►3	1.2	Cooney Lake
►4	2.8	Burro Pass
►5	4.3	Right at junction
►6	5.2	Upper Hoover Lake
►7	6.0	Gilman Lake
►8	6.3	Nutter Lake
►9	6.5	East Lake
►10	7.4	East Lake's outlet
►11	8.8	Green Lake
►12	9.0	Right at junction
►13	11.9	Green Creek trailhead

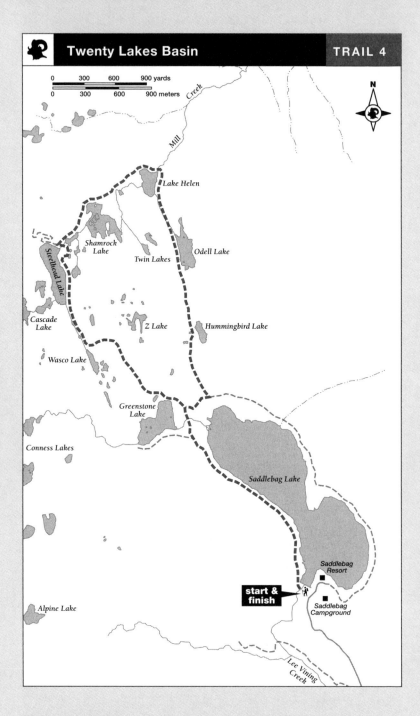

0 300 600 900 yards

0 300 600 900 meters

N

Mill Creek

Lake Helen

Shamrock Lake

Steelhead Lake

Twin Lakes

Odell Lake

Cascade Lake

Z Lake

Hummingbird Lake

Wasco Lake

Greenstone Lake

Conness Lakes

Saddlebag Lake

Alpine Lake

Saddlebag Resort

start & finish

Saddlebag Campground

Lee Vining Creek

Twenty Lakes Basin

This splendid semi-loop trip from Saddlebag Lake to Helen Lake and back passes more than one lake per mile, plus a number of ponds, and in doing so offers you some of the Sierra's finest subalpine scenery along an easy grade. With the high and low elevations only about 400 feet apart, there are no significant ascents and descents. Still, at over 10,000 feet, you will notice the rarefied air if you try to hurry along. This basin's lands are day use only; camping is not allowed other than at the campground at the trailhead.

Best Time

Because the loop trail through this basin is over 10,000 feet in elevation, snow can be long lasting. You may not want to hike before mid-July nor after mid-August, when wildflowers generally have gone to seed, and temperatures start to drop. If you dress properly, the often chilly September days can be rewarding since the summer crowds are gone.

Finding the Trail

Drive 2.1 miles north on Highway 120 (Tioga Road) down from Tioga Pass to a junction. Along this short descent you will pass Tioga Lake Campground. Or, from Highway 395 just south of Lee Vining, drive 9.8 miles west on Tioga Road up to the junction. Along this ascent you will pass the following public campgrounds: Lower Lee Vining, Cattleguard, Boulder, Moraine, Aspen Grove, Big Bend, and Ellery. From the junction beside Junction & Sawmill

TRAIL USE
Dayhike
LENGTH
7.6 miles, 3–6 hours
VERTICAL FEET
+900'/-900'/±1800'
DIFFICULTY
- 1 **2** 3 4 5 +
TRAIL TYPE
Loop

FEATURES
Lakes
Wildflowers

FACILITIES
Resort
Restrooms
Campground
Phone
Water

Lake

Wildflowers

Walk-in campgrounds, drive 2.4 miles northwest up to Saddlebag Lake, where you'll find Saddlebag Lake Campground.

Trail Description

By Saddlebag Campground is a fairly large trailhead parking area ►1 for those hiking north into the Hoover Wilderness. You can get both a wilderness permit and a fishing license at close-by Saddlebag Lake Resort. The resort's store sells fishing supplies and a few groceries, and its cafe serves breakfast and lunch, but not dinner. The resort also rents small boats, and on weekdays as well as weekends Saddlebag Lake often has quite a population of anglers in hot pursuit of the lake's brook, rainbow, and Kamloops trout. The resort also offers water-taxi service to the lake's far end. The water taxi will pick you up at your own pre-arranged time.

To get to the 10,070-foot-high lake's far end, you could hike along a closed former mining road that parallels the east shore, but a better, shorter alternative is to hike on a trail that parallels the west shore. From the trailhead parking entrance you can see a road descending to the base of the lake's dam, then climbing to the dam's west end. Head there, where the trail begins—a blocky tread cutting across open, equally blocky talus slopes. This metamorphic-rock talus may be uncomfortable to walk on, but it creates soils superior to those derived from granitic talus, and hence there is a more luxuriant growth of alpine plants.

About 0.5 mile north of the dam, your trail bends northwest, and Mt. Dana, in the southeast, disappears from view. Shepherd Crest, straight ahead across Saddlebag Lake, now captivates your attention. Among willows and a seasonally fiery field of Pierson's paintbrush, your trail ends by the former mining road at the lake's north end, ►2 and you

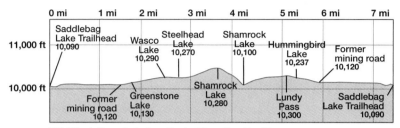

TRAIL 4 **Twenty Lakes Basin Elevation Profile**

climb west to the east shore of 10,130-foot-high Greenstone Lake. ▶3 Just before reaching the north end of Saddlebag Lake, you could have traversed west across benches to the nearby south shore of Greenstone Lake, with North Peak above it. Following the lake's shore north, you quickly meet the closed mining road that water-taxi riders will be hiking on, and above this shore your narrow road enters the Hoover Wilderness. Southwest across Greenstone Lake a granite wall sweeps up to a crest at Mt. Conness, in whose shade lies the Conness Glacier. Your tread climbs northwest, and then at the "Z" Lake outlet creek bends west over to relatively warm Wasco Lake. ▶4 Beyond the first tarn north of Wasco Lake, your trail enters the drainage of northeast-flowing Mill Creek. Then just past the second tarn you come to a junction with a former Jeep trail. ▶5

≈ **Lake**

Along the main loop you quickly arrive at the south tip of 10,270-foot-high Steelhead Lake. ▶6 From it you follow the former Jeep road north alongside deep Steelhead Lake to its outlet. ▶7 The road continues west above the lake's north shore to the Hess Mine, blocked with boulders. Higher up the road, however, is an unblocked mine that goes 50 yards into the mountainside. Just beyond it the road ends and there you have a commanding view of this "Twenty Lakes Basin," as it is sometimes

≈ **Lake**

≈ **Lake**

M Great Views

≋ Lake

≋ Lake

▲ Caution

≋ Lake

called. The large, white, horizontal dikes on North Peak stand out well, and pointed Mt. Dana pokes its summit just into view on the southeast skyline.

On the west side of Steelhead Lake's outlet—Mill Creek—you go a few yards downstream, then scramble over a low knoll as you follow a faint trail that quickly descends to the west shore of tiny Excelsior Lake. At the north end you go through a notch just west of a low metamorphic-rock knoll that is strewn with granitic glacial erratics. A long, narrow pond which, like many of the lakes, contains trout, quickly comes into view. Your trail skirts its west shore, then swings east to the north shore of adjacent, many-armed Shamrock Lake, ▶8 back-dropped by Mt. Conness.

Your ducked route—more cross-country than trail–now continues northeast over a low ridge, then goes past two Mill Creek ponds down to the west shore of Lake Helen. On a trail across talus you round this lake's north shore to Mill Creek, ▶9 where your trail dies out just below the lake's outlet—which flows through a tunnel. You go 30 yards up to the tunnel, walk across it, and begin an east-shore traverse south across blocky talus. Don't take the tantalizing trail that follows the lake's outlet creek north; it quickly becomes very dangerous.

Two creeks empty into the lake's southeast end, and you follow the eastern one up a straight, narrow gully that in early season is a snow chute rather than a wildflower garden. After 0.5 mile of southward hiking, mostly up a straight creek, you cross it at the outlet of Odell Lake. ▶10 You cross it and parallel the west shore southward while observing the lobes of slowly seasonally flowing talus just east of the lake.

Near the lake's south end an old route may still be seen climbing slightly before dying out. In contrast, your route drops to water's edge before climbing from the south shore up to Lundy Pass. ▶11 At this gap your path can become vague, but by heading south down toward a pond, you soon reach the outlet of Hummingbird Lake, ▶12 and here an obvious trail tread resumes. This tread parallels the east side of the outlet creek 0.5 mile down to the former mining road. ▶13 Here you can descend to the water-taxi dock on Saddlebag Lake and wait for the boat if you made reservations for a return trip, or, if you walk momentarily to the west, you can then retrace your steps on the west-shore trail. ▶14 Of course, for variety you can take the closed road back to the lake's south end, a route that is about 0.5 mile longer.

≋ Lake

🚶	MILESTONES	
▶1	0.0	Start at Saddlebag Lake trailhead
▶2	1.6	Former mining road
▶3	1.8	Greenstone Lake
▶4	2.5	Wasco Lake
▶5	2.7	Trail ends by former Jeep trail
▶6	2.8	Steelhead Lake
▶7	3.3	Steelhead Lake's outlet
▶8	3.7	Shamrock Lake
▶9	4.3	Mill Creek
▶10	4.8	Odell Lake
▶11	5.2	Lundy Pass
▶12	5.4	Hummingbird Lake
▶13	5.9	Reach former mining road
▶14	7.6	Return to Saddlebag Lake trailhead

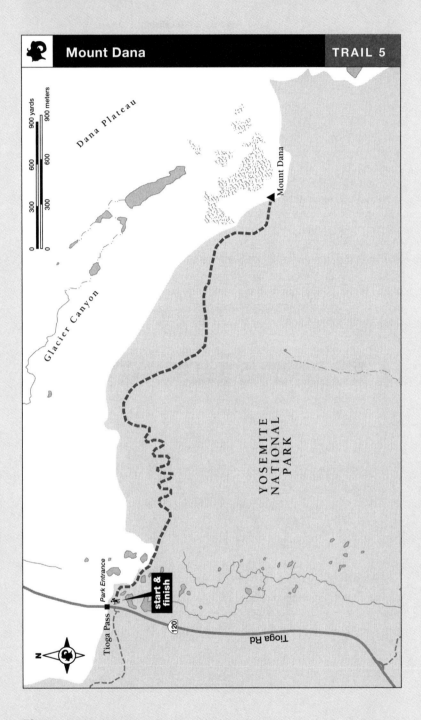

Mount Dana

TRAIL 5

900 yards
900 meters
0 300 600
0 300 600

Dana Plateau

Glacier Canyon

Mount Dana

YOSEMITE NATIONAL PARK

Park Entrance

start & finish

Tioga Pass

120

Tioga Rd

N

Mount Dana

Dark glasses and good health are both necessary for this climb to the second highest summit in Yosemite. Only Mt. Lyell exceeds it—by about 60 feet—but the Lyell summit is distant and it requires mountaineering skills. Because Dana vies with Mt. Hoffmann as Yosemite's most accessible peak, it is very popular, and on weekends you may find dozens of persons ascending it. Its summit views are among the Sierra's best, but turn back if the weather looks threatening.

Best Time

Because this route is between just under 10,000 feet and just over 13,000 feet elevation, snow can linger and obscure the trail, particularly on the lower parts. Higher up, on the windswept slopes, snow often is blown away. You won't want to hike before early July, when the start of the trail is obscured. August is perhaps best, when thunderstorms are least likely and temperatures are still warm. September is fine too, although cooler. If you dress properly, the usually chilly early and mid-October days can be rewarding since the crowds are gone.

Finding the Trail

The trail begins on Tioga Road at Tioga Pass, at the park's eastern entrance. Park buses seasonally ply the highway along the Tioga Road east up to Tioga Pass, so if you are staying in the Tuolumne Meadows Campground, check the bus schedule and perhaps take one bus up to the pass, then a later one down.

TRAIL USE
Dayhike

LENGTH
5.8 miles, 3–5 hours

VERTICAL FEET
+3260'/-40'/±6600'

DIFFICULTY
- 1 2 **3** 4 5 +

TRAIL TYPE
Out & Back

FEATURES
Summit
Great Views
Steep

FACILITIES
Resort
Restrooms
Campgrounds
Bus Stop
Entrance Station

If you ascend from Lee Vining to Tioga Pass, you will pass the following public campgrounds: Lower Lee Vining, Cattleguard, Boulder, Moraine, Aspen Grove, Big Bend, Ellery, Junction, Sawmill Walk-in, and Tioga Lake.

Logistics

The Mt. Dana and Gaylor Lakes trailheads can be accessed by parking immediately east of the Tioga Pass entrance station, thereby avoiding entrance fees.

Trail Description

From Tioga Pass, ▶1 the footpath starts due east, then meanders southeast between two ponds that are among two dozen that developed when the last major glacier retreated. About 200 yards beyond the second pond your path starts a moderate ascent, then 0.3 mile later it becomes a steep one and generally stays that way for almost 1500 feet of elevation gain. About midway up this steep stretch you can rest in an alp, which is a miniature alpine pasture. The end of the steep section is well above treeline, and the obvious path ends, just over a mile from and still 1400 feet below the summit. Up here, it's best to wear a hat and/or dark glasses and cover your skin with sunscreen.

 Steep

Several use-paths, one more prominent than the others, head up the rubbly, ancient slopes to the windblown summit. Most people climb east to a shallow saddle, at about 12,150 feet in elevation and immediately east of a crest high point, then hike southeast up the ridge to the top. Early in the hike the views west are great, but the panorama continually expands with elevation, saturating the optic nerves with overpowering vistas. When you hike southeast up the ridge, your views take on another dimension, adding to your elation. However, take

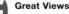 **Great Views**

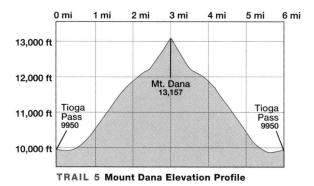

TRAIL 5 Mount Dana Elevation Profile

this ridge ascent slowly, for the atmosphere is thin and in your euphoria you can easily overexert yourself. Being above the 12,000-foot elevation, July hikers may see the sky pilot blooming, with its dense head of blue flowers.

At Mt. Dana's summit, ▶2 at about 13,157 feet, your exhausting efforts are rewarded by a stupendous 360-degree panorama. The Sierra's east escarpment can be viewed as far as the Wheeler Crest, about 40 miles to the southeast. East of it extends a long north-south mountain chain, the White Mountains. At the north end of the White Mountains stand the pale, isolated twin summits of Montgomery and Boundary peaks, both over 13,000 feet high. Gambling is legal on the Boundary Peak summit, for it is 0.25 mile in from the Nevada border.

▲ Summit

Below these twin summits rises Crater Mountain, the highest of Mono Domes' (formerly "Mono Craters") many volcanic summits, and, like most of them, less than 10,000 years old. The youthfulness of Mono Domes strongly contrasts with the age of the ancient giant, orbicular Mono Lake, directly north of them, which may be over 1 million years old. During glacial times, Mono Lake was much larger than today. At its maximum size, Lake Russell—glacial Mono Lake—was about 345

 Great Views

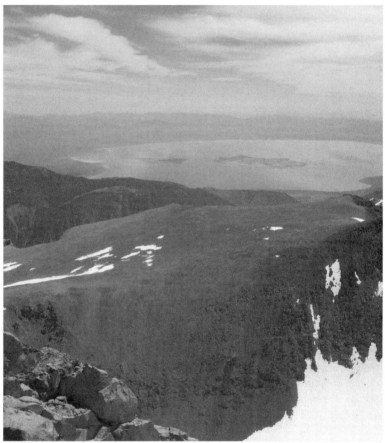

Mono Lake and Dana Plateau

square miles in area and up to 950 feet deep, versus about 86 square miles and 186 feet deep in historic time before Los Angeles started diverting water away from it.

Continuing your counterclockwise scan west, you see deep-blue Saddlebag Lake and above it, the serrated Shepherd Crest. Next comes pointed North Peak, then a true "Matterhorn," Mt. Conness.

Beyond a sea of dark-green lodgepoles lies Tuolumne Meadows and its sentinel, Lembert Dome, whose bald summit is barely visible. On the skyline above them stand Tuolumne Peak and Mt. Hoffmann, while south of these stand the craggy summits of the Cathedral Range. Examining the range counterclockwise, you can identify blocky Cathedral Peak, north-pointing Unicorn Peak, clustered Echo Peaks, and the adjacent Cockscomb plus the fin-like Matthes Crest extending south from it. A bit farther are sedate Johnson Peak, more profound Rafferty Peak, and broad Tuolumne Pass, through which former Tuolumne glaciers overflowed into the Merced drainage.

To the south-southwest stands the park's highest peak, Mt. Lyell (13,114 feet high), flanked by Mt. Maclure to the west and pointed Rodgers Peak to the southeast. Mt. Ritter and Banner Peak barely poke their summits above Kuna and Koip peaks, while Parker Peak and Mt. Wood stand above closer Mt. Gibbs, and Mt. Lewis, of intermediate distance, projects just east of them.

On your descent to your trailhead, try to retrace the way you ascended. ▶3 On any given summer's day, dozens of hikers, many naive about the danger, are tempted to zip straight down one or more snowfields, which can be iced over and treacherous, or to take an alternate route to the right or left of the general ascent route. This can lead to negotiating dangerous, steep slopes.

Caution

🚶 MILESTONES

▶1   0.0   Start at Tioga Pass
▶2   3.0 (approx.)   Mt. Dana's summit
▶3   6.0 (approx.)   Return to trailhead

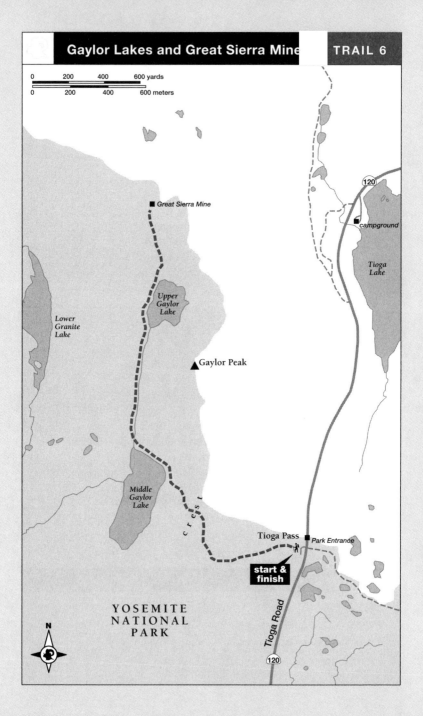

Gaylor Lakes and Great Sierra Mine

Five subalpine lakes and sweeping panoramas await those who take this hike and its optional side trip, although most visitors probably visit only Middle and Upper Gaylor Lake and perhaps the mining cabins above them. To reach the Granite Lakes, you have a cross-country hike. Camping is not allowed in the Gaylor Lakes area, which includes the Granite Lakes.

Best Time

Because this route is between about 9940 and 10,800 feet in elevation, snow can be long lasting. You can usually hike the trail by mid-July, but even then patches of trail may be under snow and stretches may be soggy. Therefore, late July through early August may be the best time for good trail tread and a maximum display of wildflowers. By late August the ground cover can begin to turn fall colors, which last through much of September. When weather permits, days of mid-September through mid-October offer brisk hikes in relative solitude.

Finding the Trail

The trail begins on Tioga Road at Tioga Pass at the park's eastern entrance. Park buses seasonally ply the highway along the Tioga Road east up to Tioga Pass, so if you are staying in the Tuolumne Meadows Campground, check the bus schedule and perhaps take one bus up to the pass, then a later one down. If you ascend from Lee Vining to Tioga Pass, you will pass the following public campgrounds: Lower

TRAIL USE
Dayhike
LENGTH
4.0 miles, 2–4 hours
VERTICAL FEET
+840'/-440'/±2560'
DIFFICULTY
- 1 **2** 3 4 5 +
TRAIL TYPE
Out & Back

FEATURES
Lakes
Wildflowers
Great Views

FACILITIES
Resort
Restrooms
Campgrounds
Bus Stop
Entrance Station

Lee Vining, Cattleguard, Boulder, Moraine, Aspen Grove, Big Bend, Ellery, Junction, Sawmill Walk-in, and Tioga Lake.

Logistics

The Mt. Dana and Gaylor Lakes trailheads can be accessed by parking immediately east of the Tioga Pass entrance station, thereby avoiding entrance fees.

Trail Description

❀ **Wildflowers**

From the restrooms by the Tioga Pass Entrance Station, ▶1 your rocky trail ascends steeply through lodgepole forest, and in season you pass a profusion of wildflowers. You may also see whitebark pines, and while its bark resembles that of lodgepoles, the former tree has two needles per bunch while the latter has five. Your steep trail begins to level off near the top of the ridge, and once atop it you have a well-earned view that includes, clockwise from the north, Gaylor Peak, Tioga Peak, Mt. Dana, Mt. Gibbs, the canyon of the Dana Fork, Kuna Peak, Mammoth Peak, Lyell Canyon, and the peaks of the

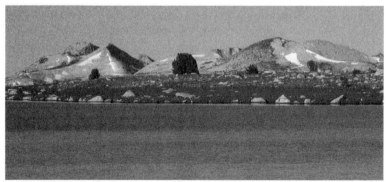

Cathedral Range peaks *peek above the rim of Middle Gaylor Lake.*

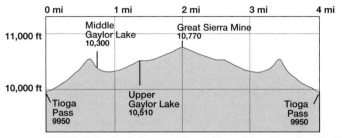

TRAIL 6 Gaylor Lakes and Great Sierra Mine Elevation Profile

Cathedral Range. From the vantage point you can see where red metamorphic rocks to the northeast are in contact with gray granites to the southwest. This division extends north to your vantage point.

Great Views

As you move west on the ridgetop, the rocks underfoot become quite purplish, a hue shared by the flowers of penstemon and lupine, which obtain their mineral requirements from these rocks. Now the trail descends steeply past clumps of whitebark pine to Middle Gaylor Lake, ▶2 and skirts the lake's north shore. On the other side, the peaks of the Cathedral Range seem to be sinking into the lake, for their summits barely poke above the water. Taking the trail up the inlet stream, you begin a short, gradual ascent to Upper Gaylor Lake. ▶3

Lake

Lake

From the upper lake you can see a rock cabin, which bespeaks the activities of a mining company that sought to tap the silver veins that run somewhere under Tioga Hill, directly north of the lake. Should you go to the cabin, you can admire the skill of the dry-rock mason who built this long-lasting house near the Sierra crest. Farther up the hill are other works—including one dangerous hole—left by the miners, in various states of return to nature. There are several other cabins in this area, and they are all that are left of the envisioned "city" of Dana, the site of the (not so) Great Sierra Mine. ▶4

Caution

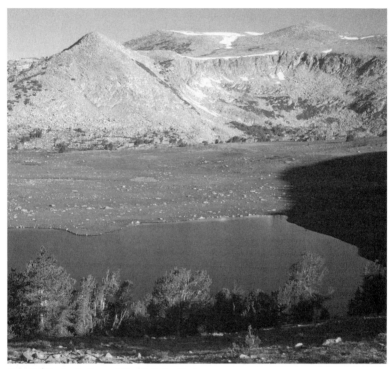

Middle Gaylor Lake *and Granite Lakes Basin*

Great Views

Atop Tioga Hill, which is just beyond the cabins, you have all the earlier views plus a view down into Lee Vining Canyon. A scant mile northeast of and below Tioga Hill is another "city," Bennettville, which in the 1880s sprang up near the mouth of a tunnel being dug to exploit the silver lodes. Its founder projected a population of 50,000! From this vicinity, most folks return to the trailhead, ▶5 but with map in hand, you could navigate over to relatively close-by and alpine Lower Granite Lake.

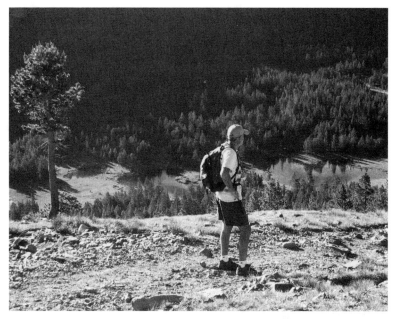

Above Tioga Pass

🚶	MILESTONES

▶1   0.0 Start at Tioga Pass
▶2   0.8 Middle Gaylor Lake
▶3   1.4 Upper Gaylor Lake
▶4   2.0 Great Sierra Mine
▶5   4.0 Return to Tioga Pass

CHAPTER 2

Tuolumne Meadows

Tuolumne Meadows

Except for Little Yosemite Valley, an outlier of Yosemite Valley, no other area in the park receives such intensive backpacker use. Consequently, you should get a wilderness permit long before you start your overnight hike. The extreme popularity of this area is due in part to its supreme scenery, which is dominated by the Cathedral Range and the Sierra crest. In part its popularity is also due to its accessibility, thanks to the Tioga Road (also known as Highway 120) which traverses east-west along the meadows. From the meadows' trailheads, you can easily hike in a few hours' time to crest passes and subalpine lakes. How can one forget the alpenglow on the metamorphic Sierra crest? The form of twin-towered Cathedral Peak? The beauty of an alpine wildflower garden? The dashing waterfalls and cascades above and below Glen Aulin? These and many other sights continue to lure backpackers and dayhikers to this area year after year.

The Top Trails I've selected for Tuolumne Meadows are mostly relatively easy and short, ranging from an hour or two to a day or two in length. The only exception is Trail 15, which is the longer part of the High Sierra Camps Loop, which lies south and east of the Tioga Road, and is usually hiked in four days.

Trails 14 and 15, when combined, comprise the entire 50.6-mile High Sierra Camps Loop. Along this loop are six High Sierra camps, each spaced a convenient day's hike from the next. Many visitors make this loop on horseback. Others hike the trail carrying little more than a day pack, since the camps provide meals and bedding. Unfortunately the camps are so popular that a lottery is held each December to determine the lucky relative few who are allowed reservations for the following summer. To obtain a lottery application, phone the camp-management company at (559) 253-5674 between October 15 and November 30.

I've omitted longer hikes, which are less popular principally because most hikers do two- to three-day weekend hikes. The most famous omission is the stretch of the tri-state Pacific Crest Trail that leaves Tuolumne

Overleaf: *Tuolumne Meadows looking east from Pothole Dome*

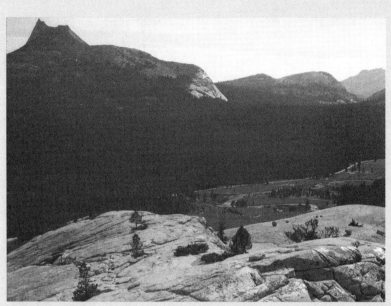

Tuolumne Meadows and Unicorn Peak *from Dog Dome*

Meadows, bound for Sonora Pass some 77 miles away. This trek requires a very long vehicle shuttle. Additionally, since most hikers are not ultralight backpackers, they will find their packs uncomfortably heavy for the six to eight days they might take. Since the park requires you to store your food in bear-proof canisters, and these hold only about three to four days of food, you would have to carry two of these containers, adding bulk and weight to your pack.

Permits

If you want to reserve a permit, rather than get one in person, see the "Fees, Camping, and Permits" section on page 14.

In person, for all of this chapter's trails, get your permit at a booth in the parking lot a short way down the Tuolumne Meadows Lodge spur road. From late June through the Labor Day weekend this booth is open on Friday nights, and it opens as early as 6 a.m. on Saturdays. After the Labor Day weekend, get your permits at the meadows' Information Center.

Tuolumne Meadows

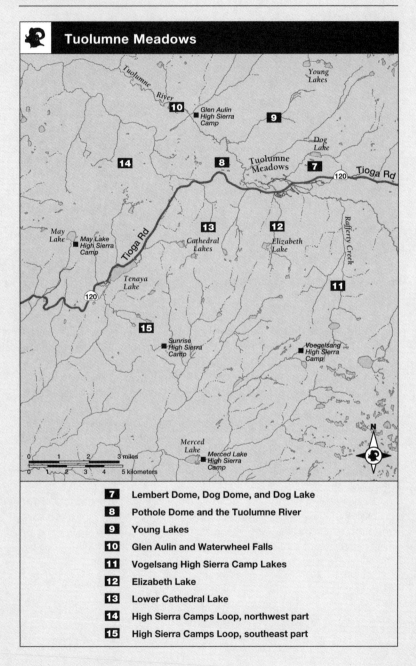

7	Lembert Dome, Dog Dome, and Dog Lake
8	Pothole Dome and the Tuolumne River
9	Young Lakes
10	Glen Aulin and Waterwheel Falls
11	Vogelsang High Sierra Camp Lakes
12	Elizabeth Lake
13	Lower Cathedral Lake
14	High Sierra Camps Loop, northwest part
15	High Sierra Camps Loop, southeast part

Tuolumne Meadows

TRAIL	Difficulty	Length	Type	USES & ACCESS	TERRAIN	FLORA & FAUNA	OTHER
7	2/3	4.6	Out & Back	Dayhiking, Horses	Summit, Lake		Great Views, Camping, Swimming
8	1	3.0	Out & Back	Dayhiking, Child Friendly	Summit, Stream		Great Views, Swimming, Child Friendly
9	4	16.4	Loop	Backpacking, Dayhiking, Horses	Lake, Stream	Wildflowers	Great Views, Camping, Swimming
10	3	12.0	Out & Back	Backpacking, Dayhiking, Horses, Running	Canyon, Stream, Waterfall		Great Views, Camping, Swimming
11	4	15.4	Out & Back	Backpacking, Dayhiking, Horses	Canyon, Lake, Stream	Wildflowers	Camping, Swimming
12	2	5.0	Out & Back	Backpacking, Dayhiking	Lake, Stream	Wildflowers	Camping
13	2	7.6	Out & Back	Backpacking, Horses	Lake, Stream		Camping, Swimming
14	4	17.6	Point-to-Point	Backpacking, Dayhiking, Horses, Running	Canyon, Lake, Stream, Waterfall		Great Views, Camping, Swimming
15	5	33.0	Point-to-Point	Backpacking, Horses	Canyon, Lake, Stream	Wildflowers	Great Views, Camping, Swimming

Legend

USES & ACCESS
- Dayhiking
- Backpacking
- Horses
- Running
- Biking
- Handicap Access
- Child Friendly

TYPE
- Loop
- Out & Back
- Point-to-Point

DIFFICULTY
- 1 2 3 4 5 +
less   more

TERRAIN
- Canyon
- Mountain
- Summit
- Stream
- Waterfall
- Lake

FLORA & FAUNA
- Autumn Colors
- Wildflowers
- Giant Sequoias

FEATURES
- Great Views
- Camping
- Swimming
- Secluded
- Steep

Maps

For Tuolumne Meadows, here are the USGS 7.5-minute (1:24,000 scale) topographic quadrangles that you will need, listed in the order that you will need them as you hike along your route. Quadrangles in parentheses are for suggested side trips that go off the quadrangles that you need for the principal hike.

 Trail 7: Tioga Pass
 Trail 8: Falls Ridge
 Trail 9: Tioga Pass, Falls Ridge
 Trail 10: Falls Ridge
 Trail 11: Tioga Pass, Vogelsang Peak, Tenaya Lake
 Trail 12: Vogelsang Peak (Tenaya Lake)
 Trail 13: Tenaya Lake
 Trail 14: Tioga Pass, Falls Ridge, Tenaya Lake
 Trail 15: Tenaya Lake, Merced Peak, Vogelsang Peak, Tioga Pass

Tuolumne Meadows

This is perhaps the finest dayhike you can take in the Tuolumne Meadows area. If you have just an hour or two, then hike only to the top of Lembert Dome or Dog Dome. However, don't overexert yourself, for at this area's elevation you can easily get altitude sickness. This entire route, being within a mile of Tioga Road, is off-limits to backcountry camping.

Because Pothole Dome is Yosemite's most accessible dome, more people climb it than almost any other in the park. Its upper slopes and summit provide outstanding views of Tuolumne Meadows and the surrounding peaks and domes. Also, a few find this use-trail a more-scenic and mile-shorter route to Glen Aulin and Waterwheel Falls.

The Young Lakes are the only reasonably accessible lakes north of Tuolumne Meadows at which camping is allowed. This isolated cluster of lakes is quite popular. Most visitors will backpack to the Young Lakes, but those in good shape can dayhike to and from them. If you visit only the lowest lake, you can shave 2.0 miles off the total distance.

Glen Aulin and Waterwheel Falls 101

This trail comprises the easiest section of the High Sierra Camps Loop Trail. This popular hike to Glen Aulin is noted for the scenic pools, rapids, cascades, and falls it passes. Because the hike is mostly downhill, it is ideal for hikers unaccustomed to high elevations.

TRAIL 10

Dayhike, Backpack,
Run, Horse
12.0 miles, Out & Back
Difficulty: 1 2 **3** 4 5

Vogelsang High Sierra Camp Lakes ...109

At about 10,130 feet in elevation, subalpine Vogelsang is easily the highest of the park's High Sierra camps. One plus is that in thin air you are treated to very starry nights. While you can stay at the camp, most folks stay overnight in its adjacent backpackers' campground. Strong hikers can dayhike to and from this camp. You should get a wilderness permit long before you start your overnight hike.

TRAIL 11

Dayhike, Backpack,
Horse
15.4 miles. Out & Back
Difficulty: 1 2 3 **4** 5

Elizabeth Lake 115

Due to its accessibility, Elizabeth Lake ranks with Dog Lake in popularity. Dog Lake is certainly better for swimming, Elizabeth Lake for scenery.

TRAIL 12

Dayhike, Backpack
5.0 miles, Out & Back
Difficulty: 1 **2** 3 4 5

Lower Cathedral Lake 119

Justifiably popular Lower Cathedral Lake receives so much backpacker use that those who can visit this scenic lake in only one day—an easy task—should do so. Another option is to visit Medlicott and Mariuolumne domes, worthy goals in themselves.

TRAIL 13

Dayhike, Backpack,
Horse
7.6 miles, Out & Back
Difficulty: 1 **2** 3 4 5

TRAIL 14

Dayhike, Backpack,
Run, Horse
17.6 miles,
Point-to-Point
Difficulty: 1 2 3 **4** 5

High Sierra Camps Loop, northwest part

The High Sierra Camps Loop hike became very popular years ago, not surprisingly, since the five backcountry camps are spaced about 6 to 10 miles apart. I've broken the loop into two parts. If you can, you might try dayhiking this part, which takes about as much energy as does the popular Half Dome hike, which hundreds do daily on fair-weather summer weekends.

TRAIL 15

Backpack, Horse
33.0 miles,
Point-to-Point
Difficulty: 1 2 3 4 **5**

High Sierra Camps Loop, southeast part

As noted above, the High Sierra Camps Loop hike became very popular years ago. This southeast part is about twice as long as the Trail 14 loop, and it has more lakes and more scenery. Most will hike it in four days, spending a night at each of the three camps and then exiting on the fourth day. Strong backpackers might do it in two or three days, while those in great shape might try dayhiking this part.

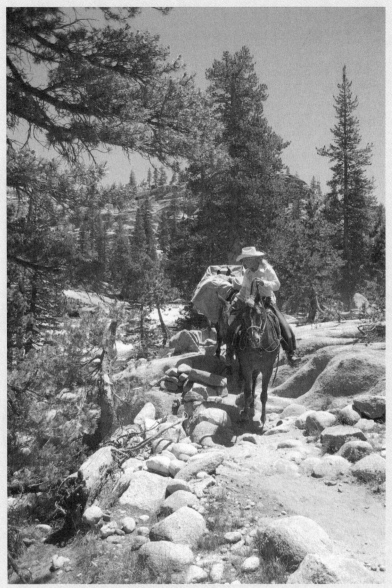

Packer *on trail to Glen Aulin High Sierra Camp*

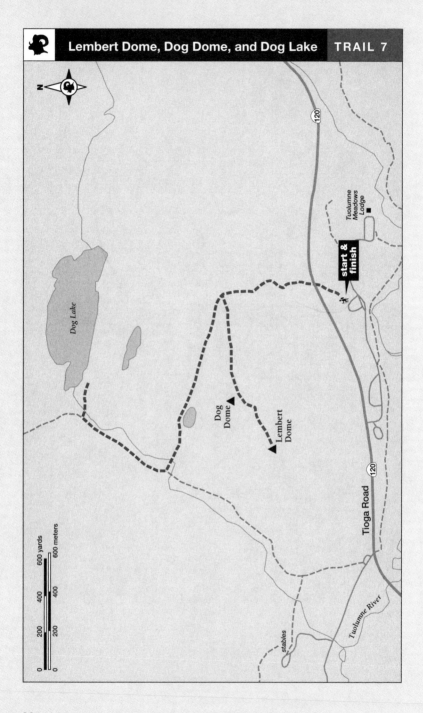

N

120

Tuolumne Meadows Lodge

start & finish

Dog Lake

Dog Dome

Lembert Dome

Tioga Road

120

600 yards

600 meters

400

400

200

200

0

0

stables

Tuolumne River

Lembert Dome, Dog Dome, and Dog Lake

This is perhaps the finest dayhike you can take in the Tuolumne Meadows area. If you have only an hour or two to spare, then hike only to the top of Lembert Dome or Dog Dome. However, don't overexert yourself, for at this area's elevation you can easily get altitude sickness. If you hike only to the top of the two domes, the round-trip distance is 2.6 miles; if only to the lake, then the round-trip distance is 3.2 miles. This entire route, being within a mile of Tioga Road, is off-limits to backcountry camping.

Best Time

Although the Tioga Road usually opens by late June, this hike is likely to have snow patches well into mid-July, and then the trail can be hard to follow, especially on the relatively flat lands between Lembert Dome and Dog Lake, where abundant snow can accumulate and, where under forest cover, can persist even longer. Around the Dog Lake environs, mosquitoes can be abundant through July, diminishing by early August. Should you want to swim at the lake, early to mid-August is optimal; beyond that, this subalpine lake begins to cool considerably. Non-swimmers can appreciate the lake mosquito-free from about late August through late September. Beyond that, air temperatures are on the cold side, though tolerable for those who dress appropriately.

TRAIL USE
Dayhike
LENGTH
4.6 miles, 2–4 hours
VERTICAL FEET
+980'/-120'/±1810'
DIFFICULTY
- 1 **2 3** 4 5 +
TRAIL TYPE
Out & Back

FEATURES
Lake
Summit
Great Views
Swimming

FACILITIES
Resort
Store
Visitor Center
Restrooms
Campground
Bus Stop
Phone
Water
Horse Staging

Finding the Trail

Start from the large parking lot for hikers and backpackers 0.33 mile west of the Tuolumne Meadows Lodge parking lot. To reach this lot from Tuolumne Meadows Campground (the only campground in the area), drive 0.6 mile northeast on the Tioga Road, turn right on the Tuolumne Lodge spur road and follow it 0.4 mile to the lot, on your left. If you are descending from Tioga Pass, drive 6.4 miles southwest to the only road that branches left before you reach Tuolumne Meadows.

Trail Description

From the north end of the parking lot, ►1 you make a brief, moderate climb up an obvious trail to a crossing of the Tioga Road. Onward, you switchback at a generally moderate grade up to a junction, about 0.66 mile into your route and just 80 yards shy of a broad, lodgepole-forested saddle. ►2 To climb Lembert Dome, branch left and ascend westward on a trail that at first stays just below the crest. In about 0.33 mile it reaches a minor gap, ►3 from which you can make a brief, safe ascent north to the adjacent summit of Dog Dome, ►4 with its precipitous north face.

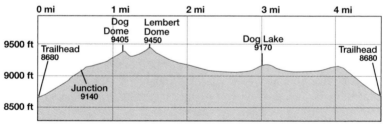

TRAIL 7 Lembert Dome, Dog Dome and Dog Lake Elevation Profile

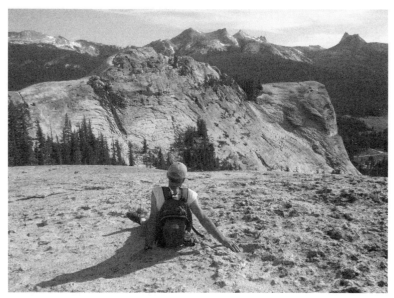

Lembert Dome *and Cathedral Range from Dog Dome*

To reach the summit of Lembert Dome, return to the minor gap, ▶5 and then head about 0.2 mile up the bedrock slopes to its summit. ▶6 While you can tackle it head-on up a steep slope, most hikers first veer to the left and then arc right up to it. Both routes are somewhat intimidating, so if you feel unsure, don't do it! Your view from 150-foot-higher Lembert Dome is nearly identical to that from Dog Dome. After exploring the glaciated Lembert Dome summit, retrace your steps first to the minor gap and then to the junction just shy of the forested saddle. ▶7

Caution

Great Views

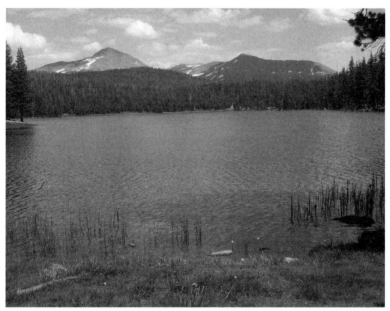

Dog Lake, *with Mt. Dana and Mt. Gibbs on the eastern horizon*

To reach Dog Lake, turn sharply left and in 80 yards reach the aforementioned forested saddle. Beyond it you drop briefly west-northwest, then traverse in the same direction, having a view of the north cliffs of Dog Dome and skirting a pond that in midsummer has wild onions growing in wet ground near its shore. Just 100 yards beyond it you cross the outlet creek of an unseen, sedge-filled pond, then in 150 yards reach a trail junction. ▶8

Alternate Return

OPTIONS

▶8 A less-desirable, longer return route to your trailhead is to descend this overly steep trail southwest to a parking lot at the foot of Lembert Dome, then cross the Tioga Road and follow a trail back to your starting point.

To reach Dog Lake, first head about 230 yards northwest up this trail, to a junction from where a trail continues about 5 miles to the first of three Young Lakes (Trail 9). Veer right ▶9 and make an easy ascent 0.25 mile to the outlet of Dog Lake, at its western end. ▶10 The official trail ends here, but you could go either right, along the lake's south shore, or left, along its north shore. Encircling the lake is difficult, due to boggy ground by its eastern end. No camping is allowed here since the lake is within 1 mile of the Tioga Road.

≋ Lake

From the lake's west shore just north of the outlet creek, you obtain views of Mt. Dana, Mt. Gibbs, and also Mt. Lewis. A long peninsula extends east into the lake from your shoreline, and on it you can walk—usually in knee-deep water—well out into the middle of this large but shallow lake. Because it is shallow, it is one of the high country's warmest lakes, suitable for swimming and for just plain relaxing. Leaving Dog Lake, retrace your steps back to your trailhead. ▶11

◢• Swimming

🚶	**MILESTONES**
▶1	0.0 Start at parking area on spur road
▶2	0.6 Left at junction just before forested saddle
▶3	1.0 Right from minor gap
▶4	1.1 Dog Dome summit
▶5	1.2 Back at minor gap
▶6	1.4 Lembert Dome summit
▶7	2.0 Back at junction just before forested saddle
▶8	2.6 Right at junction just beyond pond
▶9	2.7 Keep right at trail to Young Lakes
▶10	3.0 Dog Lake
▶11	4.6 Return to parking area on spur road

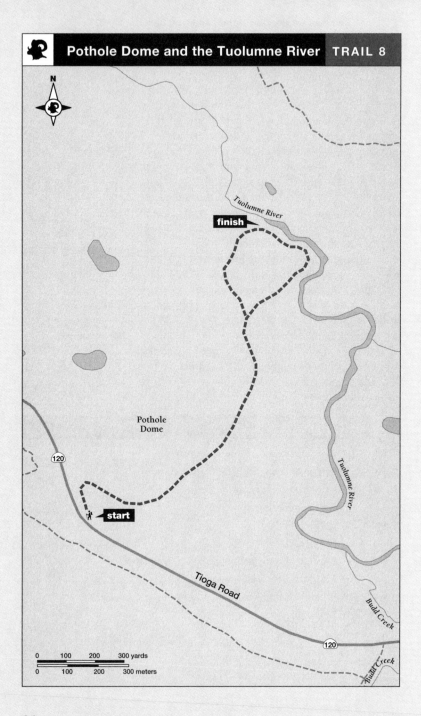

Pothole Dome and the Tuolumne River **TRAIL 8**

N

Tuolumne River

finish

Pothole Dome

120

start

Tioga Road

120

Tuolumne River

Budd Creek

Budd Creek

| 0 | 100 | 200 | 300 yards |
| 0 | 100 | 200 | 300 meters |

Pothole Dome and the Tuolumne River

Because Pothole Dome is Yosemite's most accessible dome, more people climb it than any other in the park except perhaps Lembert Dome (Trail 7), Half Dome (Trail 34), or Sentinel Dome (Trail 38). Its upper slopes and summit provide outstanding views of Tuolumne Meadows and the surrounding peaks and domes. Not all visitors climb the dome; many instead take a nearly level use-trail to granite slabs along a very scenic stretch of the Tuolumne River, and a few geologically inclined visit Little Devils Postpile, named for its larger and more famous analog, Devils Postpile, about 12 miles beyond the park's southeast boundary. Also, a few find this use-trail a more scenic and mile-shorter route to Glen Aulin and Waterwheel Falls (Trail 10). However, it is not recommended for backpackers since you encounter several brief stretches across sloping (and sometimes polished) bedrock where you could slip and possibly slide into the river should your pack throw you off balance.

Best Time

If you plan only to climb Pothole Dome, its approach is mostly snow-free by early July, and if you hurry, you can keep ahead of the swarming mosquitoes. Once away from the soggy meadow and on bedrock, your ascent is essentially mosquito-free. Mosquitoes can be prevalent through July, so if you can plan a hiking date, try one in August. This applies also to the Tuolumne River, which many years can be a life-threatening torrent through mid-July, but almost always will be safe for frolicking in

TRAIL USE
Dayhike
LENGTH
3.0 miles, 1–2 hours
VERTICAL FEET
+320'/-360'/±920'
DIFFICULTY
- **1** 2 3 4 5 +
TRAIL TYPE
Out & Back

FEATURES
Resort
Store
Visitor Center
Child Friendly
River
Cascades
Summit
Great Views
Swimming

FACILITIES
Bus Stop

its brisk water in August. If you just want a leisurely stroll, then September is fine, although the river's diminished flow is not as picturesque.

Finding the Trail

Park opposite Pothole Dome at a turnout at the westernmost edge of Tuolumne Meadows, 1.25 miles west from the Tuolumne Meadows Visitor Center. The only campground in the area is the Tuolumne Meadows Campground, just east of the visitor center.

Trail Description

From the trailhead, ▶1 take a trail that starts northwest along an often boggy meadow, then from its tip heads east along the base of the dome. From the trail you can climb initially steep slopes to the dome's summit wherever you feel it is safe. Like other glaciated Yosemite domes, Pothole Dome has gentle up-canyon slopes and steep down-canyon slopes, as do most unglaciated domes of the Sierra Nevada. Along the dome's base you'll see one or more large potholes, whence the dome's name. These formed over time as high-velocity streams beneath former glaciers turbulently churned boulders that over time drilled progressively deeper into the bedrock.

The safest routes up to the low dome's summit begin after 0.3 mile from the start, where your trail curves from southeast to northeast. ▶2 (Once the boggy meadow becomes less waterlogged, you can reach this point quicker by starting from a parking area about 200 yards off the official one and taking a trail directly north to it. Do not make your own path across this fragile meadow.)

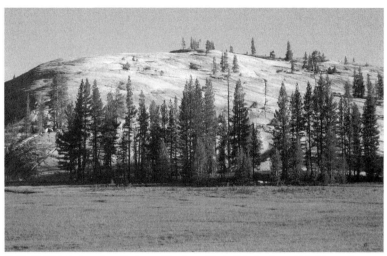

Pothole Dome *rises above Tuolumne Meadows. The trail to the dome skirts this meadow.*

From this spot or any spot north of it, an ascent of Pothole Dome is only a walk-up, with an average gradient of about 20 percent. This is the gradient you'd find on a very steep trail, and because you are over 8500 feet in elevation, the air is thin and the ascent is an effort. A beeline to the summit would be 0.25 mile long, but the ascent is easier if you switchback up the open bedrock. You need not go all the way to the summit, for after about 200 yards of ascent you are above the tops of the lodgepoles along the dome's base and have an unobstructed view across Tuolumne Meadows as well as views north, east, and south toward the high peaks beyond the meadows. ▶3 From the actual summit you have a 360-degree panorama that includes most of the park's north country. With map and compass, you should be able to identify many prominent peaks and domes.

 Great Views

To reach the Tuolumne River, return to the trail beyond its curve from southeast to northeast, ▶4 traversing along the dome's base. You are likely to see two parallel trails, one just above the base of the dome and the other along the west edge of the meadow. In 0.4 mile the slightly higher trail heads northwest, and in 0.25 mile crosses a very minor divide, and this is the route to take when the Tuolumne River is flowing swiftly, usually until mid-July, since the route straight ahead in spots traverses just above the river. Ahead your use-trail may be ill defined, so if you can't follow it, curve north over to the often-audible river. ▶5 This stretch has pools and rapids, and when the water is low, the pools may be safe for swimming, but not when the flow is swift. The water is never warm, but summer days often are, and allow you to warm up on glacier-smoothed slabs after a brisk swim. The more scenic, slightly lower trail reaches the pools and rapids by continuing north along the meadow's edge to the Tuolumne River; it then traverses for about 200 yards downstream along the lower slopes of an obvious knoll. Because these slopes are water polished in spots, and therefore slippery, don't take the upper trail in time of high water, when a slip into the raging river could be fatal. After a pleasant stay, return to the trailhead. ▶6

 Stream

 Caution

Caution

🚶	MILESTONES

▶1 0.0 Start at Pothole Dome trailhead
▶2 0.3 Trail curves from southeast to northeast
▶3 0.6 Pothole Dome summit
▶4 0.9 Back at where trail curves from southeast to northeast
▶5 1.8 Tuolumne River
▶6 3.0 Return to Pothole Dome trailhead

Tuolumne River and Little Devils Postpile

Most folks don't go beyond the initial stretch of pools and rapids, so if you continue down-river, you generally have the terrain all to yourself. In about 1.8 miles you'll reach Little Devils Postpile, and then about 0.2 mile farther, the Pacific Crest Trail. Basically you parallel the river's edge past more pools and rapids for about 0.5 mile to where you reach the edge of large meadow and the river veers from west to north. The meadow becomes increasingly boggy toward its far side, so before early or mid-August, stay near its southern edge as you traverse west for about 0.3 mile to the edge of a lodgepole forest. Within it, you stay near the base of some slopes as you traverse northwest for a similar distance to a low, narrow, obvious ridge. You then traverse about 0.25 mile northwest back to the river's edge and again briefly traverse glacier-and-water-polished slopes at the base of descending ridge. Just beyond the base you see **Little Devils Postpile**, reached in an equally short traverse. This is a remnant of a 9.4-million-year-old lava flow, similar to the more-famous Devils Postpile.

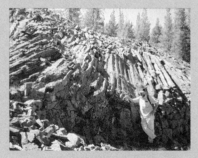

Those bound for Glen Aulin and beyond traverse across Little Devils Postpile, which is about 100 yards in diameter, and immediately confront a brief traverse along a use-path across a 30-degree slope. You don't want to slip and fall into the river below, especially if it is raging. If the traverse bothers you, either don't do it or head up the slope to safer ground and then traverse. Beyond the traverse, you walk on a flat for about 100 yards, passing a campsite on your left aboutmidway to the Pacific Crest Trail (Trail 10) where it bridges the Tuolumne River.

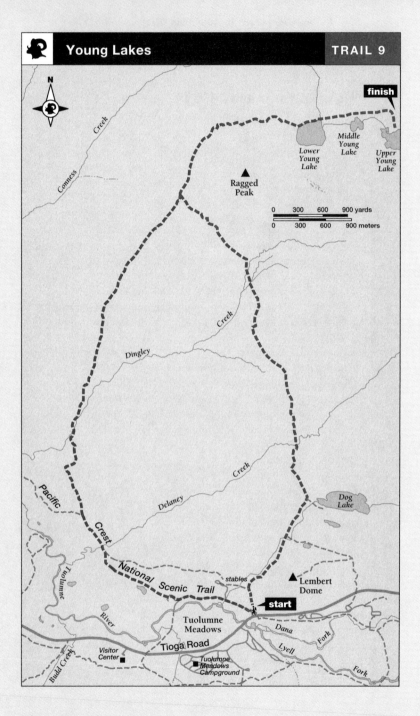

Young Lakes

The Young Lakes are the only reasonably accessible lakes north of Tuolumne Meadows at which camping is allowed. This isolated cluster of lakes, backdropped by the scenic Ragged Peak crest, is quite popular, though not overcrowded like the Cathedral Lakes and the lakes near Vogelsang High Sierra Camp. Whereas most visitors will backpack to the Young Lakes, those in good shape can dayhike to and from them. This is a relatively long dayhike, but the lakes are only about 1500 feet above the trailhead, and for most of the ascent the trail gradient is relatively easy. The advantages of dayhiking are first, that you don't need a wilderness permit (and the lakes on busy weekends can reach their backpacking quotas); and second, that you don't have to carry a heavy pack. If you visit only the lowest lake, you can shave 2.0 miles off the total distance.

Best Time

Although the Tioga Road usually opens by late June, this hike is likely to have snow patches well into mid-July. In the Young Lake environs, mosquitoes can be abundant through July, diminishing by early August. Should you want to swim at these rather cool lakes, late July through early August is optimal; beyond that, these subalpine lakes begin to cool considerably. The lakes are mosquito-free from about late August through late September. Beyond that, air temperatures are on the cold side, though tolerable for those who dress appropriately.

TRAIL USE
Dayhike, Backpack, Horse
LENGTH
16.4 miles,
8 hours–2 days
VERTICAL FEET
+3030'/-3030'/±6060'
DIFFICULTY
- 1 2 3 **4** 5 +
TRAIL TYPE
Loop

FEATURES
Backcountry Permit
Lakes
Streams
Wildflowers
Great Views
Camping
Swimming

FACILITIES
Resort
Store
Visitor Center
Restrooms
Campground
Bus Stop
Picnic Tables
Phone
Water
Horse Staging

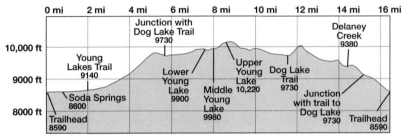

TRAIL 9 Young Lakes Elevation Profile

Finding the Trail

John Lembert sold the Soda Springs lands to the Sierra Club in 1912, and for 60 years Club members enjoyed their own private campground in Tuolumne Meadows.

Drive along the Tioga Road to a dirt road starting west from the base of Lembert Dome, which is at the east end of Tuolumne Meadows and immediately north of the Tuolumne River. Just south of the river is the Tuolumne Meadows Campground, which is the only campground in the area. Alternatively, from the trailhead parking area at this spot you can drive 0.33 mile west on the dirt road to a gate, from where the main road turns north, bound for the nearby stables, which will save you 0.33 mile each way. The mileage is measured from the trailhead parking area.

Trail Description

From the Lembert Dome parking area west of the Tioga Road ▶1 you first walk west 0.33 mile along a dirt road to its bend, and then continue west on a gated service road that contours the lodgepole-dotted flank of Tuolumne Meadows. On it you are treated to fine views south across them toward Unicorn Peak, Cathedral Peak, and some of the knobby Echo Peaks. After about 0.25 mile you meet a trail heading northeast to the horse stables, and about 200 yards past this junction you face a split. The left branch heads over to a bridge across the nearby Tuolumne River, but your road veers right, slightly uphill, and quickly encounters a trail that leads to the still-bubbling natural Soda Springs. ►2 You can take this trail west across this vicinity to your road, or take the road that arcs counterclockwise across the former site of the old Soda Springs Campground.

Westward, your trail undulates through a forest of sparse, small lodgepole pines, and in just under one mile descends to Delaney Creek, reached about 100 yards after a stock trail from the stables back in the meadows comes in on the right. In early season, look for a log to cross it; later on, boulder-hopping will do. After 0.33 mile you reach the Young Lakes Trail, ►3 on which you branch right, north.

Turning right, you ascend slightly and cross a broad expanse of boulder-strewn, grass-pocketed, glaciated sheet granite. An open spot affords a look south across broad Tuolumne Meadows to the line of peaks from Fairview Dome to the steeple-like spires of the Cathedral Range. After ascending the open, glacier-polished granite, following a line of boulders that mark the trailless route, the trail tread resumes and climbs northward up a tree-clothed slope, the first 2 miles moderately, the next mile gently, to a ridge. On the other side of the ridge a new panoply of peaks appears in the north— majestic Tower Peak, Doghead and Quarry peaks, the Finger Peaks, Matterhorn Peak, Sheep Peak, Mt. Conness, and the Shepherd Crest. From this high viewpoint a moderate descent leads 0.33 mile down, to a ford of a usually flowing tributary of Conness Creek. Just 60 yards up from this tributary is a junction with a southeast-climbing trail, the Dog Lake Trail, your return route. ►4

Great Views

Now you start a roller-coaster traverse northeast through a forest of mountain hemlocks and lodge-pole and western white pines. On a level stretch of trail you cross a diminutive branch of Conness Creek, and then switchback 0.25 mile up to a

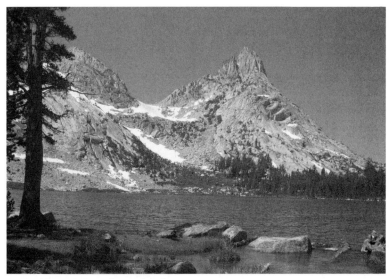

Lower Young Lake *and Ragged Peak*

≋ Lake

≋ Lake

▲ Camping

plateau from where the view is fine of the steep northwest face of Ragged Peak. After rounding the edge of a meadow, you descend to lower Young Lake, ▶5 whose north shore easily has the most campsites of the three lakes—and some hikers go no farther. At about 9900 feet in elevation, lower Young Lake lies in the subalpine realm, but still has sufficient trees for shade and to diminish the sometimes strong late afternoon winds. From the lake's northeast corner you can hop its outlet creek—a possibly wet ford in early season if logs aren't available—and take a trail east. The route parallels the creek about 0.25 mile east moderately up to relatively small Middle Young Lake. ▶6 As at the lower lake, you can camp on a rocky ridge above the middle lake's north shore. If you camp at either lake, bring a tent, since at both lakes there can be hordes of mosquitoes in the morning and evening until late July or early August. Furthermore, afternoon-to-evening thunderstorms can occur near the Sierran crest, and you are only a couple of miles from it.

You may see a use-trail following a creek to the upper lake, but avoid it. A better, if sometimes cryptic use-trail stays farther to the north, meandering eastward up to benchlands across which you make an easy, nearly level, open, scenic traverse southeast to Upper Young Lake. ▶7 At about 10,220 feet elevation, it lies in the lower alpine realm, and small clusters of whitebark pines offer little protection from the elements. You could camp above its north shore, but the small sites are marginal and the alpine turf is fragile.

Lake

After exploring the Young Lakes area, retrace your steps to the Dog Lake Trail junction. ▶8 Turn left and make a steep ascent up a boulder-dotted slope under a forest cover of lodgepoles and hemlocks. As the trail ascends, the trees diminish in density and change in species to a predominance of whitebark pines. From the southwest shoulder of Ragged Peak the trail quickly enters and then descends through a very large, gently sloping meadow. This broad, well-watered expanse is a wildflower garden in season, laced with meandering brooks. Species of wildflowers in the foreground set off the marvelous views of the entire Cathedral Range, strung out on the southern horizon.

Wildflowers

Great Views

Near the lower edge of the meadow you cross the headwaters of Dingley Creek and then descend to a seasonal creek, steeply at times, some 300 feet past exfoliating Peak 10410 through a moderately dense forest of lodgepoles and a few hemlocks. Another seasonal creek is crossed in 0.33 mile, and then you make a short but noticeable climb up to the crest of a large, bouldery ridge. Down its gravelly slopes you descend to a very large, level meadow above which the reddish peaks of Mt. Dana and Mt. Gibbs loom in the east. Here Delaney Creek

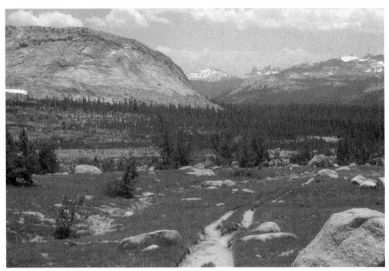

Dog Lake Trail *toward Dingley Creek Basin*

meanders lazily through the sedges and grasses, and
in early season it usually is a wet, deep crossing. ▶9
Look for shallower fords up- or downstream or, particularly downstream, a spot you can jump across.

After climbing briefly over the crest of a second
bouldery ridge, your route drops once more toward
Tuolumne Meadows. Lembert Dome can be
glimpsed through the trees along this stretch of trail.
After 0.4 mile of easy descent east, your trail levels
off in a small, linear meadow and turns south to parallel it. Should you wish to visit Dog Lake, which
definitely is worthwhile, the quickest way is to leave
the trail at this bend and continue east to reach it in
under 200 yards. By adhering to the trail, you'll parallel the linear meadow for about 250 yards, south

to a junction with the ascending, 0.25-mile lateral to
Dog Lake (Trail 7). ▶10 No camping is allowed in
this vicinity since the lake is within 1 mile of the
Tioga Road.

〰 **Lake**

About 230 yards below the junction your route
passes another junction, this with a trail that leads
east along the north side of Dog Dome, the lower
adjunct of Lembert Dome. You keep southwest, parallel a creek from Dog Lake, and begin a 450-foot
switchbacking, dusty descent on this overly steep
section. At the bottom the trail splits into two paths.
The right one leads west to the stables, the left one
south to the west side of the Lembert Dome parking
area. ▶11 Just before the parking area is a second lateral to this stables, first branching west and quickly
turning northwest.

⚐ MILESTONES

▶1	0.0	Start at Lembert Dome trailhead
▶2	0.8	Soda Springs
▶3	2.0	Right at Young Lakes Trail
▶4	5.7	Straight at Dog Lake Trail
▶5	7.6	Lower Young Lake
▶6	8.0	Middle Young Lake
▶7	8.6	Upper Young Lake
▶8	11.5	Back to Dog Lake Trail
▶9	14.3	Delaney Creek
▶10	15.1	Straight at lateral to Dog Lake
▶11	16.4	Return to Lembert Dome trailhead

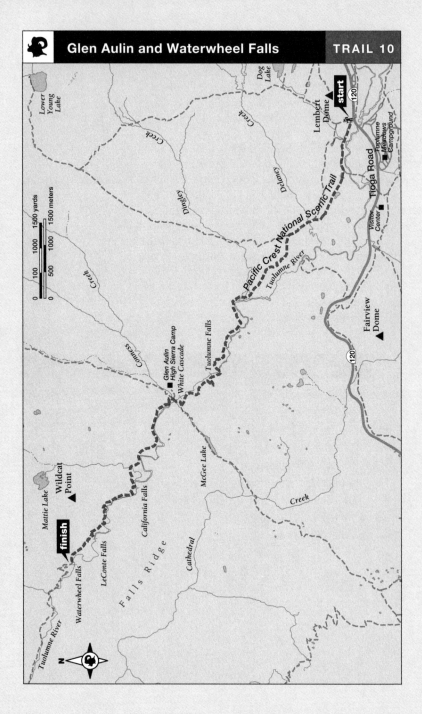

Glen Aulin and Waterwheel Falls

TRAIL 10

Lower Young Lake

Dog Lake

start

120

Lembert Dome

Tuolumne Meadows Campground

Tioga Road

Creek

Creek

Dingley

Delancy

Pacific Crest National Scenic Trail

Visitor Center

Tuolumne River

1500 yards
1500 meters

1000

1000

500

100

100

0

0

Creek

Fairview Dome

120

Tuolumne Falls

Glen Aulin High Sierra Camp
White Cascade

Cockscomb

Mattie Lake

Wildcat Point

California Falls

McGee Lake

Creek

finish

LeConte Falls

Falls Ridge

Cathedral

Waterwheel Falls

Tuolumne River

N

Glen Aulin and Waterwheel Falls

This trail comprises the easiest section of the High Sierra Camps Loop Trail (Trail 14). It is also a section of both the Pacific Crest and Tahoe–Yosemite trails. Scenically, this popular hike to Glen Aulin is noted for the scenic pools, rapids, cascades, and falls it passes. Because the hike is virtually all downhill, it is ideal for hikers unaccustomed to high elevations. Spending a night at Glen Aulin gets you partly acclimated, preparing you for the hike back up to your trailhead.

If you are hiking when the river is still swift, which usually is before mid-July, then it is worth your while to descend an additional 3.3 miles to Waterwheel Falls, which are most dramatic during maximum runoff. Strong hikers can make the trip to Waterwheel Falls in six to eight hours or less, particularly if they take Trail 8's alternate route to Glen Aulin, which results in about a 16-mile round trip instead of about an 18-mile one via the official trail. Descending from Glen Aulin to Waterwheel Falls and ascending back to it gives you an overall elevation gain and loss of about 2550 feet, which effectively doubles the elevation gain and loss along the trip to and from Glen Aulin.

Best Time

Although the Tioga Road usually opens by late June, this hike is likely to have snow patches well into mid-July. This is unfortunate, since the falls and cascades above and below Glen Aulin are at their best from about mid-June into early July, when Tuolumne Meadows' mosquitoes can swarm in

TRAIL USE
Dayhike, Backpack,
Run, Horse
LENGTH
12.0 miles, 4–6 hours
VERTICAL FEET
+310'/-1020'/±2660'
DIFFICULTY
- 1 2 **3** 4 5 +
TRAIL TYPE
Out & Back

FEATURES
Backcountry Permit
River
Waterfalls
Great Views
Camping
Swimming

FACILITIES
Resort
Store
Visitor Center
Restrooms
Campground
Bus Stop
Picnic Tables
Phone
Water
Horse Staging

Little Devils Postpile, a 9.4-million-year-old remnant of a lava flow, exists as mute testimony to the impotence of glaciers' ability to erode hard rock.

unbelievably high numbers. They diminish to acceptable numbers by early August, but so too does the volume of the Tuolumne River. Lower water makes for great, if brisk, swimming in its pools, but also for disappointing cascades and falls, which can be gliding down slopes versus roaring and dashing down them. Should you want to see Waterwheel Falls in all its glory, you'll have to visit it before mid-July. If you shun mosquitoes and don't mind a second-rate performance of cascades and falls, then mid-August through mid-September are optimal. After that, Glen Aulin's High Sierra Camp shuts down, the summer crowds leave, and you pretty much have the backpacker camp to yourself and a few other hardy souls who don't mind the early morning's freezing temperatures.

Finding the Trail

Drive along the Tioga Road to a dirt road starting west from the base of Lembert Dome, this spot located at the east end of Tuolumne Meadows and immediately north of the Tuolumne River. Just south of the river is the Tuolumne Meadows Campground, which is the only campground in the area. Alternatively, from the trailhead parking area at this spot you can drive 0.33 mile west on the dirt road to a gate, from where the main road turns north, bound for the nearby stables, which will save you 0.33 mile each way. The mileage is measured from the trailhead parking area.

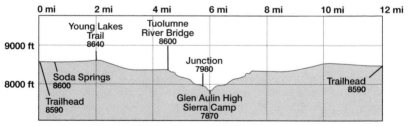

TRAIL 10 Glen Aulin Elevation Profile

Trail Description

The first 4-plus miles are nearly level, which makes it ideal for joggers. Should you jog, get acclimatized first or else take it very easy when you start.

From the Lembert Dome parking area west of the Tioga Road ►1 you first walk west 0.33 mile along a dirt road to its bend, and then continue west on a gated service road that contours the lodgepole-dotted flank of Tuolumne Meadows. On it you are treated to fine views south across them toward Unicorn Peak, Cathedral Peak, and some of the knobby Echo Peaks. You may also see an occasional marmot foraging for food, or Belding ground squirrels standing upright by their rodent holes. After about 0.25 mile you meet a trail heading northeast to the horse stables, and about 200 yards past this junction you face a split. The left branch heads over to a bridge across the nearby Tuolumne River, which proffers inspiring views. Your road veers right, slightly uphill, and quickly encounters a trail that leads to the still-bubbling natural Soda Springs. ►2 You can take this trail west across this vicinity to your road, or take the road, which arcs counter-clockwise across the former site of the old Soda Springs Campground. Once this campground, open through 1975, was the private holding of John Lembert, namesake of Lembert Dome.

From the effervescent Soda Springs, your west-bound trail undulates through a forest of sparse, small lodgepole pines, and in just under 1.0 mile descends to Delaney Creek, reached about 100 yards after a stock trail from the stables back in the meadows comes in on the right. In early season, look for a log to cross it; later on, boulder-hopping will do. After 0.33 mile you reach the Young Lakes Trail, ►3 on which those taking Trail 9 will branch right, north.

Great Views

Stream

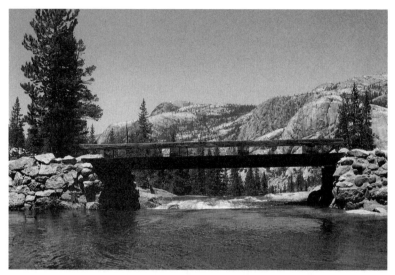

A sturdy Tuolumne River bridge *near Little Devils Postpile overlooks Glen Aulin.*

Leaving this trail, you continue westward on your rambling traverse, and after more winding through scattered lodgepoles, it descends some bare granite slabs and enters a flat-floored forest. A mile's pleasant walking since the last junction brings you to the bank of the Tuolumne River, just before three branches of Dingley Creek, near the west end of the huge meadows. From here, the nearly level trail often runs along the river, and in these stretches by the stream there are numerous glacier-smoothed granite slabs on which to take a break—or dip, if the river's current is slow.

After a mile-long winding traverse, the trail leaves the last slabs to climb briefly up a granite outcrop to get around the river's gorge. You can leave the trail and walk toward a brink, from where you'll see, on the south side of the gorge below you, Little Devils Postpile, which is a 9.4-million-year-old lava remnant. Back on the trail you wind down eventually toward a sturdy Tuolumne River bridge. ▶4

Immediately beyond the bridge you can look north up long Cold Canyon to Matterhorn Peak and Whorl Mountain, and, to their right, Mt. Conness. As the river soon approaches nearby Tuolumne Falls, it flows down a series of sparkling rapids separated by large pools and wide sheets of water spread out across slightly inclined granite slopes. **Waterfall** Beyond this beautiful stretch of river the trail descends, steeply at times, past Tuolumne Falls and White Cascade to a junction with the trail to May Lake ▶5 (Trail 14). From here it is only a few minutes' walk to Glen Aulin High Sierra Camp, reached **Waterfall** by crossing the river on a bridge below roaring White Cascade. ▶6 During high runoff, you may have to wade just to reach this bridge! From the camp is a short trail to sites in the heavily used Glen Aulin backpackers' camp, complete with bear-proof food-storage boxes, which are found at all the High Sierra Camps. Only 15 yards beyond the spur trail, across Conness Creek to Glen Aulin High Sierra Camp, is the Tuolumne Canyon Trail, going left.

If the cascades and waterfalls you've seen so far **Camping** have been impressive, then you ought to continue 3.3 miles down to Waterwheel Falls (described below) for an even more spectacular display of the dashing waters of the Tuolumne River at high volume (before late July).

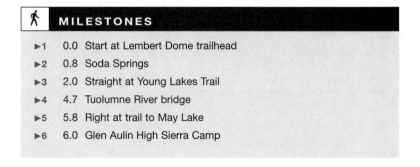

⫪ MILESTONES

▶1	0.0	Start at Lembert Dome trailhead
▶2	0.8	Soda Springs
▶3	2.0	Straight at Young Lakes Trail
▶4	4.7	Tuolumne River bridge
▶5	5.8	Right at trail to May Lake
▶6	6.0	Glen Aulin High Sierra Camp

Continuing to Waterwheel Falls

The Tuolumne Canyon Trail leaves the northbound Pacific Crest and Tahoe-Yosemite trails and climbs over a low knoll that sports rust-stained metamorphic rocks. From the knoll is an excellent view west down the flat-floored, steep-walled canyon.

Leaving the low knoll, you switchback quickly down into **Glen Aulin** proper, and paralleling the Tuolumne River through a lodge-pole-pine forest, soon reach a backpackers' camp. Between here and Waterwheel Falls are several dwarfish, generally cryptic near-trail camps, and at any along this trail you can expect a nighttime visit by a local bear. You tread the gravelly flat floor of the glen for more than a mile, and then, on bedrock, quickly arrive at the brink of cascading **California Falls**, perched at the base of a towering cliff. Be cautious around these falls and other falls downstream, for the bedrock often is polished and slippery, even when dry.

Switchbacking down beside the cascade, you leave behind the glen's thick forest of predominantly lodgepole pines with associated red firs and descend past scattered Jeffrey pines and junipers and through lots of brush. At the base of the cascade, lodgepoles, western white pines, and red firs return once more as you make a gentle descent north. Near the end of this short stretch you parallel a long pool, which is a good spot to break for lunch or perhaps take a swim. However, stay away from the pool's outlet, where the Tuolumne River plunges over a brink.

The trail parallels this second cascade as it generally descends through brush and open forest. On this descent, notice that red firs have yielded to white firs. Sugar pines also put in their first appearance as you reach the brink of broad **Le Conte Falls**, which cascades down fairly open granite slabs. On a flat-floored section of canyon, incense-cedar joins the ranks of white fir, Jeffrey pine and sugar pine, with few if any lodgepoles to be found. In this forest you reach your fifth and final cascade, extensive **Waterwheel Falls**. This cascade gets its name from the curving sprays of water tossed into the air that occur when the river is flowing with sufficient force. The cascade's classic views are from midway between its brink and its base. You'll probably spot a use-trail out to this vicinity. On the slabs the falls descend, use extreme caution even where the rock is dry.

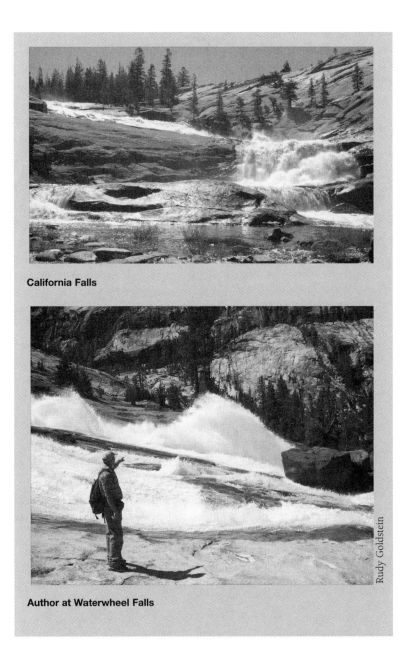

California Falls

Author at Waterwheel Falls

Rudy Goldstein

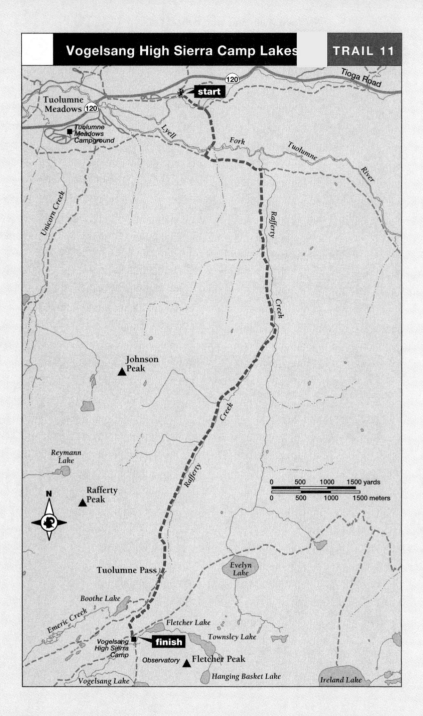

Tioga Road

120

start

Tuolumne
Meadows 120

Tuolumne
Meadows
Campground

Lyell

Fork

Tuolumne

River

Rafferty

Creek

Unicorn Creek

Johnson
Peak

Creek

Reymann
Lake

N

Rafferty
Peak

0   500   1000   1500 yards
0   500   1000   1500 meters

Tuolumne Pass

Evelyn
Lake

Boothe Lake

Emeric Creek

Fletcher Lake

Townsley Lake

Vogelsang
High Sierra
Camp

finish

Observatory

Fletcher Peak

Vogelsang Lake

Hanging Basket Lake

Ireland Lake

Vogelsang High Sierra Camp Lakes

At about 10,130 feet in elevation, subalpine Vogelsang is easily the highest of the park's High Sierra camps. At such a high elevation, nights and mornings can be brisk. A plus of high elevation is that in thin air you are treated to very starry nights, especially around the time of a new moon, when a section of our Milky Way galaxy streams across the sky. While you can stay in the camp (reservations up to about a year in advance—see "Fees, Camping, and Permits, p. 14), most folks stay overnight in its adjacent backpackers' campground. On weekends this vicinity's camping quota usually is full, so plan to visit it on weekdays, if possible. Alternatively, strong hikers can dayhike to and from this camp and its adjacent lakes.

Best Time

Although the Tioga Road usually opens by late June, this hike is likely to have snow patches well into mid-July, and then the trail can be hard to follow. Be forewarned that mosquitoes can be very abundant through July along the entire route. Additionally, July tends to be the month with the most near-crest thunderstorms, and Vogelsang is near the Sierran crest. Therefore, August is optimal, especially the latter half. Crowds are usually gone after the Labor Day weekend, and September can be a fine time to hike the trail—but be prepared for sub-freezing nights and mornings.

TRAIL USE
Dayhike, Backpack, Horse
LENGTH
15.4 miles, 5–8 hours
VERTICAL FEET
+1770'/-230'/±4000'
DIFFICULTY
- 1 2 3 **4** 5 +
TRAIL TYPE
Out & Back

FEATURES
Backcountry Permit
Lakes
Streams
Wildflowers
Camping
Swimming

FACILITIES
Resort
Store
Visitor Center
Restrooms
Campground
Bus Stop
Phone
Water
Horse Staging
Patrol Cabin

Finding the Trail

Vogelsang High Sierra Camp, at 10,130 feet, is easily the highest of the park's five backcountry High Sierra Camps.

Start from the large parking lot for hikers and back-packers 0.33 mile west of the Tuolumne Meadows Lodge parking lot. To reach this lot from Tuolumne Meadows Campground, which is the only campground in the area, drive 0.6 mile northeast on the Tioga Road, turn right on the Tuolumne Lodge spur road and follow it 0.4 mile to the lot, on your left. If you are descending from Tioga Pass, drive 6.4 miles southwest to the only road that branches left before you reach Tuolumne Meadows.

Trail Description

Start on the Pacific Crest Trail (which doubles as the John Muir Trail). ▶1 The trail runs beside the Dana Fork of the Tuolumne River just yards south of the Tuolumne Meadows Lodge road. On the trail you hike 0.33 mile east up the Dana Fork to a junction ▶2 with a spur trail that shortly goes to the west end of the lodge's parking lot. From this junction you bridge the Dana Fork and after a brief walk upstream reach a junction ▶3 with a trail to the Gaylor Lakes.

Veering right, the Pacific Crest Trail leads over a slight rise and descends to the Lyell Fork, where there are two bridges. About 70 yards past the bridges you meet a trail that heads 0.75 mile west down the river to the east end of the Tuolumne Meadows Campground. ▶4 The PCT turns left (east), and skirts around a long, lovely section of the meadow. Going through a dense forest cover of lodgepole pine, your route reaches a junction on the west bank of Rafferty Creek, from where the PCT/JMT continues its traverse east.

Your route, the Rafferty Creek Trail, ▶5 turns right and immediately begins a climb whose grade is moderate as often as it is steep. Fairly well shaded by

Stream

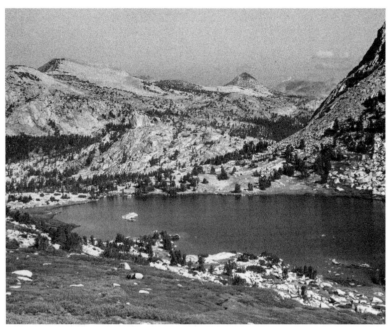

Vogelsang Lake *is a short hike south from the High Sierra Camp.*

lodgepole pines, the climb eases after well under a mile. Then, as the ascent decreases to a gentle grade, you pass through high, boulder-strewn meadows that offer good views eastward to reddish-brown Mt. Dana and Mt. Gibbs, and gray-white Mammoth Peak. Soon the trail dips close to Rafferty Creek, and after 2 miles of near-creek hiking, the gently climbing trail passes near the edge of a large meadow and continues its long, easy ascent through a sparse forest of lodgepole pines.

In the next mile you cross several seasonal creeks, and, about 3.5 miles up the Rafferty Creek Trail, reach an even larger meadow. Through this you ascend easily up-canyon, having backward views north to the Sierra crest between Tioga Pass and Mt. Conness, and views ahead to cliff-bound, dark-banded Fletcher Peak and Vogelsang Peak to the right of it. After about 1.5 miles you reach Tuolumne Pass, a major gap in the Cathedral Range. ▶6 At the pass some lodgepole pines and a few whitebark pines diminish the force of winds that often sweep through it. If you wanted to swim at any lake in the Vogelsang vicinity, you would take a trail that descends 0.5 mile to Boothe Lake. At 9850 feet elevation, it is the lowest and warmest lake, but still the temperatures are usually in the low 60s at best. Camping is forbidden at this lake.

To reach Vogelsang from the pass, keep to the main trail, which traverses across a moderately steep slope above Boothe Lake and its surrounding meadows. After about 0.75 mile your trail makes a short climb and reaches the tents of Vogelsang High Sierra Camp, spread out at the foot of Fletcher Peak's rock glacier. ▶7 At Vogelsang High Sierra Camp a few snacks may be bought, or dinner or breakfast if you have a reservation. Dispersed camping is not allowed. Rather, use a designated camping area just to the northeast at (Upper) Fletcher Lake. (There is no Lower Fletcher Lake; on the newer 7.5' topo maps, the former "Upper Fletcher Lake" has been changed, appropriately, to "Fletcher Lake.") Backpackers, like camp visitors, must use the bear-proof food-storage boxes.

≋ **Lake**

◢• **Swimming**

▲ **Camping**

≋ **Lake**

🚶	MILESTONES	
▶1	0.0	Start at parking area on spur road
▶2	0.3	Straight at trail to Tuolumne Meadows Lodge
▶3	0.4	Straight at trail to Gaylor Lakes
▶4	1.0	Left at trail to Tuolumne Meadows Campground
▶5	1.7	Right on Rafferty Creek Trail
▶6	6.9	Tuolumne Pass
▶7	7.7	Vogelsang High Sierra Camp

Emeric Lake

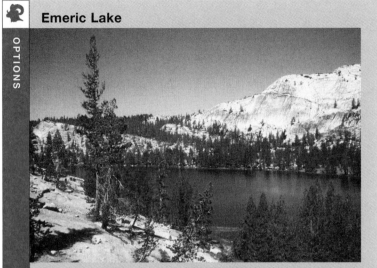

If you camp in this area you might also take the time to explore several lakes. Perhaps the most popular one is **Emeric Lake,** my favorite. From the camp you'd descend 2.3 miles southwest, most of it along Fletcher Creek, to a scissors junction. The main trail continues in that direction down along the creek and also up to Boothe Lake. You, however, cross it and walk only 0.5 mile to the east shore of Emeric Lake, vaulting a low bedrock ridge between the junction and the lake. Along the descent to this lake you'll lose about 800 feet, which you'll have to make up on the way out. At 9338 feet elevation, this somewhat isolated lake is the lowest one mentioned along this hike, and from about mid-July through early August swimming is quite pleasant. Should you camp here, look for sites above the lake's northwest shore.

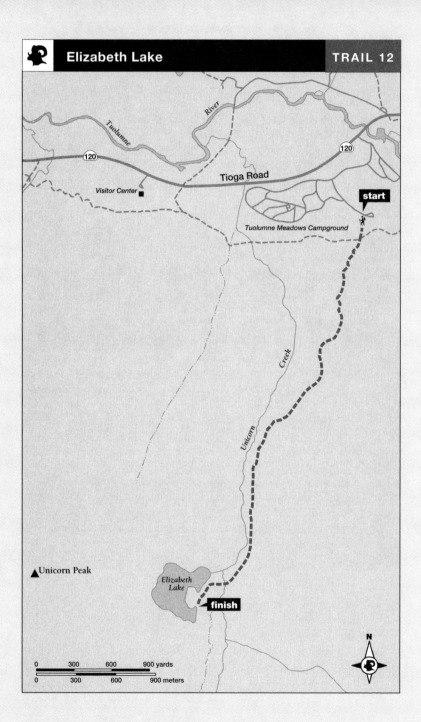

Elizabeth Lake

TRAIL 12

Tuolumne

River

120

120

Tioga Road

Visitor Center ■

start

Tuolumne Meadows Campground

Unicorn Creek

▲Unicorn Peak

Elizabeth
Lake

finish

| 0 | 300 | 600 | 900 yards |
| 0 | 300 | 600 | 900 meters |

N

Elizabeth Lake

Due to its accessibility, Elizabeth Lake ranks with Dog Lake (Trail 7) in popularity. Dog Lake is certainly better for swimming, Elizabeth Lake for scenery.

Best Time

Although the Tioga Road usually opens by late June, this hike is likely to have snow patches well into mid-July, and then the trail can be hard to follow. Be forewarned that mosquitoes can be very abundant through July along the entire route. Therefore, August is optimal, especially the latter half. Crowds are usually gone after the Labor Day weekend, and September can be a fine time to hike the trail, but be prepared for sub-freezing nights and mornings.

Finding the Trail

If you are driving up the Tioga Road, drive east through Tuolumne Meadows to its east end, where you'll find the entrance to the Tuolumne Meadows Campground, which is the only campground in the area. The entrance has a map of its layout, and after studying it, walk through the campground and find the trailhead just past campsite B49.

Trail Description

The signed Elizabeth Lake Trail in the campground ▶1 goes about 100 yards and then crosses a trail that heads east to Lyell Canyon and west to Tenaya Lake. You continue straight ahead for a steady southward

TRAIL USE
Dayhike, Backpack
LENGTH
5.0 miles; 2–3 hours
VERTICAL FEET
+820'/-40'/±1720'
DIFFICULTY
- 1 **2** 3 4 5 +
TRAIL TYPE
Out & Back

FEATURES
Backcountry Permit
Lakes
Streams
Wildflowers
Camping

FACILITIES
Resort
Store
Visitor Center
Restrooms
Campground
Bus Stop
Phone
Water

115

≋ **Lake**

ascent. Along this lodgepole-pine-shaded climb the trail crosses several runoff streams, which dry up by late summer. Before then, expect lots of mosquitoes. More than a mile out and some considerable exertion since you are now over 9000 feet, the trail veers near Unicorn Creek. After rising 800 feet from its start, the trail levels off, and lodgepoles now are both stunted and spaced farther apart. You emerge at the foot of a long meadow, and part way through it take a short spur trail southwest. ►2 Under optimal conditions, this leads momentarily to Elizabeth Lake. ►3 Unfortunately, at times there have been a number of use-paths, and folks, especially in the high water before late July, often go up and down the east bank looking for a narrow spot to jump across.

Few places in Yosemite give so much for so little effort as this lovely subalpine lake, situated at 9508 feet elevation. Backdropped by Unicorn Peak, Elizabeth Lake faces the snow-topped peaks of the Sierra crest north of Tuolumne Meadows. From the east and north sides of the lake, the views across the waters to Unicorn Peak are classic. The glacier-carved lake basin is indeed one of the most beautiful in the Tuolumne Meadows area. Should you wish to camp in this vicinity, something I discourage due to heavy use, then check out the forested bench rising above the lake's northwest corner.

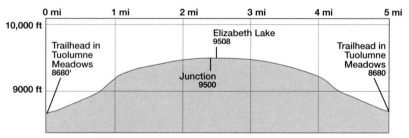

TRAIL 12 Elizabeth Lake Elevation Profile

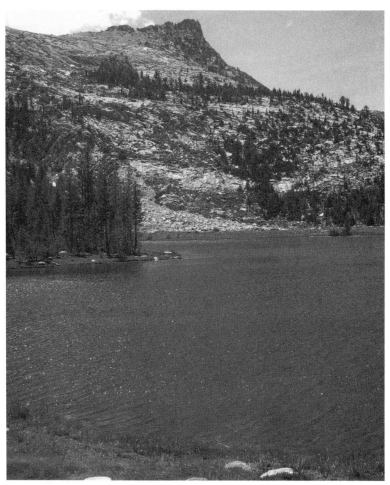

Unicorn Peak and Elizabeth Lake

🚶 **MILESTONES**

▶1   0.0 Start in Tuolumne Meadows Campground
▶2   2.4 Right on spur trail
▶3   2.5 Elizabeth Lake

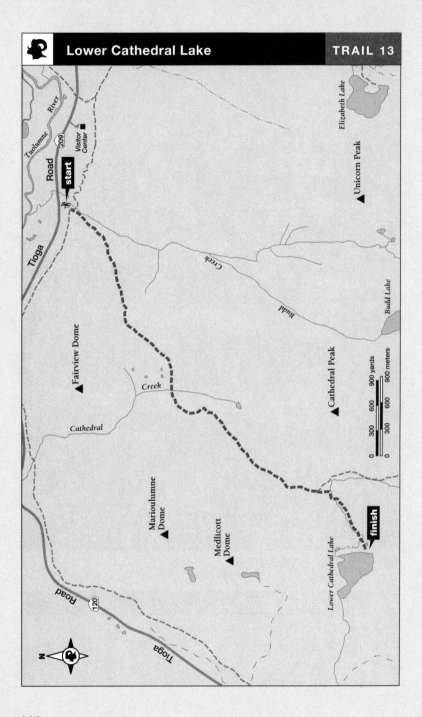

Tuolumne River

Road

209

Visitor Center

start

Tioga

Elizabeth Lake

Unicorn Peak

Budd Creek

Budd Lake

Fairview Dome

Creek

Cathedral Peak

Cathedral

900 yards

300   600   900 meters

0   300   600

Mariuolumne Dome

Medlicott Dome

finish

Lower Cathedral Lake

Road

120

Tioga

N

Lower Cathedral Lake

Justifiably popular Lower Cathedral Lake receives so much backpacker use that those who can visit this scenic lake in only one day—an easy task—should do so. Another option is to visit Medlicott and Mariuolumne domes, worthy goals in themselves. Since free shuttle buses operate between Tuolumne Meadows and Tenaya Lake, strong dayhikers have another option: after visiting Lower Cathedral Lake, follow the John Muir Trail 4.7 miles to Sunrise High Sierra Camp, then head out and down 5.8 miles to Tenaya Lake, for a grand total of about 15 miles. Then take the shuttle bus back to your trailhead.

Best Time

Although the Tioga Road usually opens by late June, this hike is likely to have snow patches well into mid-July, and then the trail can be hard to follow. Be forewarned that mosquitoes can be very abundant through July along the entire route. Therefore, August is optimal, especially the latter half. Crowds are usually gone after the Labor Day weekend, and September can be a fine time to hike the trail—but be prepared for sub-freezing nights and mornings.

Finding the Trail

In Tuolumne Meadows, drive 1.5 miles west on the Tioga Road from the entrance to the Tuolumne Meadows Campground, which is the only camp-ground in the area. Or drive about 0.75 mile east on the Tioga Road from the Pothole Dome parking area. On some summer weekends, vehicles are parked

TRAIL USE
Dayhike, Backpack,
Horse
LENGTH
7.6 miles, 3–4 hours
VERTICAL FEET
+1070'/-350'/±2840'
DIFFICULTY
- 1 **2** 3 4 5 +
TRAIL TYPE
Out & Back

FEATURES
Backcountry Permit
Lake
Streams
Camping
Swimming

FACILITIES
Visitor Center
Resort
Store
Visitor Center
Bus Stop
Water

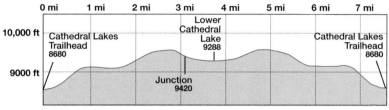

TRAIL 13 Lower Cathedral Lake Elevation Profile

along quite a lengthy stretch of the Tioga Road, which of course adds to your hiking distance.

Trail Description

From a trailhead beside Budd Creek, ▶1 walk southwest 120 yards to a junction with the Tuolumne Meadows–Tenaya Lake Trail. East, this trail goes about 1.2 miles to the southwest corner of Tuolumne Meadows Campground. West, it traverses a generally viewless 8.1 miles down to a trailhead by the southwest shore of Tenaya Lake.

Now on the John Muir Trail, which has come west to this junction, you climb moderately up a stretch that can at times be objectionably dusty due to humus mixing with the abundance of glacial deposits. Lodgepoles dominate your 0.75-mile ascent to the crest of a lateral moraine, from which the trail briefly descends west before turning southwest.

The John Muir Trail traverses southwest 0.5 mile to a creeklet, which you cross, and then ascend short, moderate-to-steep switchbacks beneath the shady cover of lodgepole pines and mountain hemlocks. After 300 feet of climbing, your trail's gradient eases and you traverse along the base of largely unseen Cathedral Peak, a mass of granodiorite towering 1400 feet above you that is the realm of the mountain climber. Your traverse leaves the Tuolumne River drainage for that of the Merced River, and soon, after a brief descent, you come to a junction with the lower Cathedral Lake Trail. ▶2

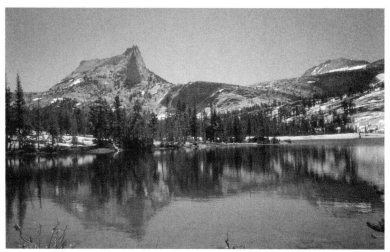

Lower Cathedral Lake *and Cathedral Peak*

This spur trail descends 0.66 mile to the bedrock east shore of lower Cathedral Lake. ►3 A rust-stained waterline on the meadow side of the bedrock marks the high-water level to which the meadow floods in early season. Bear-frequented campsites abound on both the north and south shores, the northern ones being roomier. Campfires are not allowed. Due to high angler use, fishing for brook trout is likely to be poor. Because of the relative shallowness of this fairly large lake, swimming in it is tolerable despite its 9300+ foot altitude. From the lake's outlet you can look across to Polly Dome, standing high above Pywiack Dome. Also visible are Mt. Hoffmann and a bit of Tenaya Lake, nestled between Tenaya Peak and Polly Dome.

 Lake

Swimming

🚶	**MILESTONES**

►1	0.0	Start at Cathedral Lakes trailhead
►2	3.1	Right on Lower Cathedral Lake Trail
►3	3.8	Lower Cathedral Lake

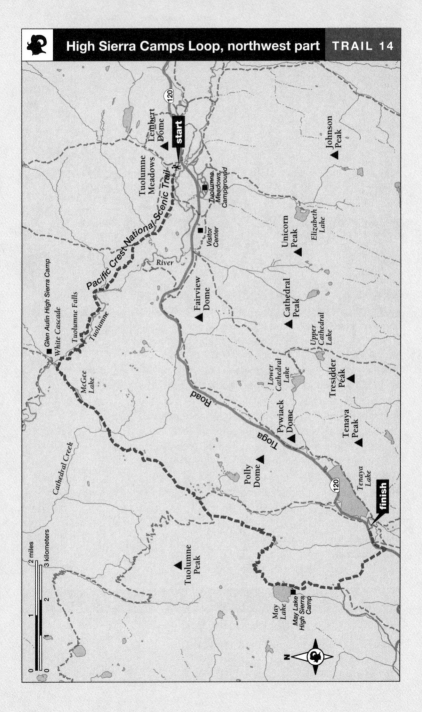

High Sierra Camps Loop, northwest part

The High Sierra Camps Loop hike became very popular years ago, not surprisingly, since the five backcountry camps are spaced about 6 to 10 miles apart, distances that are about right for most backpackers. If you can get reservations to stay at these camps (see "Fees, Camping, and Permits," page 14), then your food and bedding will be provided, which allows you to hike with a light pack. In reality, your chances of getting reservations are poor, so you'll have to settle for staying in the backpacker's camp adjacent to each camp.

I've broken the loop into two parts for two reasons. First, most hikers don't have the luxury of spending six days in the backcountry. Second, by being out fewer days, you will have a lighter pack, since you carry less food. Backpacking in Yosemite, you need to carry your food in a bear canister, which adds another two pounds to your pack's weight. My experience (but perhaps not yours) is that I can fit four days of food in one canister, but not six, so for the entire loop I would need to carry two canisters.

I prefer hiking the loop in a counterclockwise direction, since this way on your first day, when your pack is heaviest and you are perhaps are not in the best of shape, your hike is mostly level and downhill. If you can, you might try day-hiking this part, which takes about as much energy as does the popular Half Dome hike (Trail 34), which hundreds do daily on fair-weather summer weekends. Easy traverses predominate over ups and downs, making this route a great one for serious runners.

TRAIL USE
Dayhike, Backpack,
Run, Horse
LENGTH
17.6 miles/1–3 days
VERTICAL FEET
+2620'/-3000'/±5620'
DIFFICULTY
- 1 2 3 **4** 5 +
TRAIL TYPE
Point-to-Point

FEATURES
Backcountry Permit
Lakes
Streams
Waterfalls
Great Views
Swimming

FACILITIES
Visitor Center
Resort
Store
Visitor Center
Restrooms
Campground
Bus Stop
Picnic Tables
Phone
Water
Horse Staging

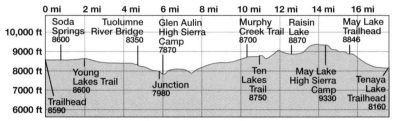

	0 mi	2 mi	4 mi	6 mi	8 mi	10 mi	12 mi	14 mi	16 mi

TRAIL 14 **High Sierra Camps, northwest part Elevation Profile**

Best Time

The best time to hike the loop is when the camps are open, which is around mid-July through mid-September. Before early August, mosquitoes can be quite prevalent, and if you want to avoid them, then hike in mid-August or later. Lakes are near their optimal temperatures from early July through early August, so if you want to minimize mosquitoes and snow and enjoy dips in the lakes, then early August is best. Just you and the rest of the world. As always, you'll have a better chance at getting a wilderness permit and avoiding crowds by hiking Monday through Thursday. If you must go on a weekend, consider hiking out of season, before or after the camps open, ideally, in the second half of September. However, if you are hiking early or late, do plan for the possibility of sudden snowstorms and know what to do if you're caught in one.

Finding the Trail

Drive along the Tioga Road to a dirt road starting west from the base of Lembert Dome, at a spot located at the east end of Tuolumne Meadows and immediately north of the Tuolumne River. Just south of the river is the Tuolumne Meadows Campground, which is the only campground in the area. However, if you are driving east up the Tioga Road, you will also pass the following campgrounds before Tenaya Lake, the first three along spur roads: Tamarack Flat,

White Wolf, Yosemite Creek, and Porcupine Flat.

The route ends at the Tenaya Lake trailhead, along the Tioga Road near the lake's southwest shore. Consider taking a free shuttle bus back to your original trailhead. During the summer season, these buses run about once an hour, plying between Olmsted Point and Tioga Pass and stopping at all the popular trailheads in between. Before starting your hike, check the schedule for the shuttle's last run; you don't want to walk the 8.7 miles back to your original trailhead.

Trail Description

From your parking lot, ▶1 follow a trail west down the Tuolumne River to the backpackers' camp at Glen Aulin High Sierra Camp, the place most hikers spend their first night. This trail begins from the Lembert Dome parking area west of the Tioga Road. First you walk west 0.33 mile along a dirt road to its bend, and then continue west on a gated service road that contours the lodgepole-dotted flank of Tuolumne Meadows. On it you are treated to fine views south across them toward Unicorn Peak, Cathedral Peak, and some of the knobby Echo Peaks. After about 0.25 mile you meet a trail heading northeast to the horse stables, and about 200 yards past this junction you face a split.

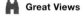 **Great Views**

The left branch heads over to a bridge across the nearby Tuolumne River, which proffers inspiring views. Your road veers right, slightly uphill, and quickly encounters a trail that leads to the still-bubbling, natural Soda Springs. ▶2 You can take this trail west across this vicinity to your road, or take the road, which arcs counterclockwise across the former site of the old Soda Springs Campground.

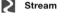 **Stream**

From the effervescent Soda Springs, your west-bound trail undulates through a forest of sparse, small lodgepole pines, and in just under 1.0 mile

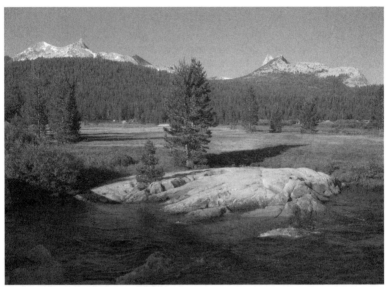

Unicorn Peak and Cathedral Peak *from Tuolumne Meadows (Trails 9, 10, and 14)*

descends to Delaney Creek. You reach the creek about 100 yards after a stock trail from the stables back in the meadows comes in on the right. In early season, look for a log to cross it; later on, boulder-hopping will do. After 0.33 mile you reach the Young Lakes Trail, ▶3 on which those taking Trail 9 branch right, north.

Leaving this trail, you continue westward on your rambling traverse, and after more winding through scattered lodgepoles, it descends some bare granite slabs and enters a flat-floored forest. A mile's pleasant walking since the last junction brings you to the bank of the Tuolumne River, just before three branches of Dingley Creek, near the west end of the huge meadows. From here, the nearly level trail often runs along the river, and in these stretches by the stream there are numerous glacier-smoothed granite slabs on which to take a break—or dip, if the river's current is slow.

Stream

After a mile-long winding traverse, the trail leaves the last slabs to climb briefly up a granite outcrop to get around the river's gorge. You can leave the trail and walk toward a brink, from where you'll see, on the south side of the gorge below you, Little Devils Postpile. Back on the trail you wind down eventually toward a sturdy Tuolumne River bridge, ▶4 and immediately beyond it you can look north up long Cold Canyon to Matterhorn Peak and Whorl Mountain, and, to their right, Mt. Conness. As the river soon approaches nearby Tuolumne Falls, it flows down a series of sparkling rapids separated by large pools and wide sheets of water spread out across slightly inclined granite slopes. Beyond this beautiful stretch of river the trail descends, steeply at times, past Tuolumne Falls and White Cascade to a junction with the trail to May Lake ▶5, your second day's hike.

From here it is only a few minutes' walk to Glen Aulin High Sierra Camp, reached by crossing the river on a bridge below roaring White Cascade. ▶6 During high runoff, you may have to wade just to reach this bridge! From the camp is a short trail to sites in the heavily used Glen Aulin backpackers' camp, complete with bear-proof food-storage boxes, which are found at all the High Sierra Camps. Only 15 yards beyond the spur trail across Conness Creek to Glen Aulin High Sierra Camp is the Tuolumne Canyon Trail, going left.

 Waterfall

Camping

Waterwheel Falls

▶6 If the cascades and waterfalls on the way to Glen Aulin have been impressive, then you ought to continue 3.3 miles down to Water-wheel Falls for an even more spectacular display of dashing waters of the Tuolumne River at high volume. See Trail 10 for details.

OPTIONS

The second day's hike is to the May Lake High Sierra Camp. From the junction immediately south of and above Glen Aulin's bridge across the Tuolumne River, you briefly curve northwest through a notch, and then your duff trail ascends gently southwest, soon crossing and recrossing McGee Lake's northeast-flowing outlet, which dries up by late summer. Where the trail levels off, McGee Lake, long and narrow and bordered on the southwest by a granite cliff, comes into view through the lodgepole trees. The dead snags along the shallow margin, and the fallen limbs and downed trees make fishing difficult, and in late summer the lake may dwindle to a stale pond. Adept campers can find isolated, level spots, some with views, on slopes north of the lake, beneath the east end of Falls Ridge.

Beyond the lake your trail descends along its southwest-flowing outlet for 0.75 mile, and then you cross it. Soon you have a view northwest through the shallow Cathedral Creek canyon to hulking Falls Ridge, which Cathedral Creek has to detour around in order to join the Tuolumne River. After several minutes you reach 20-foot-wide Cathedral Creek, which can be a ford in early season, a boulder-hop later on. Starting a moderate ascent beyond the creek, you soon reach a stand of tall, healthy red firs, and seeing the contrast with the small, over-crowded lodgepole pines earlier on the trail is inescapable.

Higher on the trail, there are good views, and after 3 miles of walking through moderate and dense forest, the panorama seems especially welcome. In the distant northeast stand Sheep Peak, North Peak, and Mt. Conness, encircling the basin of Roosevelt Lake. In the near north, Falls Ridge is a mountain of pinkish granite that contrasts with the white and gray granite of the other peaks. When you look back toward McGee Lake, the route appears to be entirely carpeted with lodgepole pines.

The trail continues up a moderate slope on gravel and granite shelves, through a forest cover of hemlock, red fir, and lodgepole. After arriving at a branch of Cathedral Creek, you cross it, then continue for 0.5 mile to a junction shaded under some tall hemlocks. ▶7 The Murphy Creek Trail departs from this junction to go down to Tenaya Lake. Down this trail, a short 0.5 mile before the lake, a lateral trail departs southwest, parallels the Tioga Road, and ends at a bend in the highway by a trailhead parking area. You'll reach this spot by a longer route.

A half mile from the hemlock-shaded junction, you reach a junction with the Ten Lakes Trail, ▶8 which climbs slopes beneath the very steep east face of Tuolumne Peak. Here you branch left and ascend briefly to a long, narrow, shallow, forested saddle, beyond which large Tenaya Lake is visible in the south. After traversing somewhat open slopes of sagebrush, huckleberry oak, and lupine, you reach a spring, then momentarily come to a series of switchbacks. Progress up the long, gentle gradient of these zigzags is distinguished by the striking views of Mt. Conness, Mt. Dana, and the other peaks on the Sierra crest/Yosemite border. The trail then passes through a little saddle just north of a glacier-smoothed peak, and ahead, suddenly, is another Yosemite landmark, Clouds Rest, rising grandly in the south; you see a part of this largest expanse of bare granite in the park.

Now the trail descends gradually over fairly open granite to a forested flat and bends west above the north shore of Raisin Lake, ▶9 which is one of the warmest "swimming holes" in this section. It also has campsites, including waterless, isolated ones with views, located about 0.25 mile south of the lake. From the lake's vicinity, the trail continues beside a flower-lined runoff streamed under a sparse forest cover of mountain hemlock and western

≋ Lake

▲ Camping

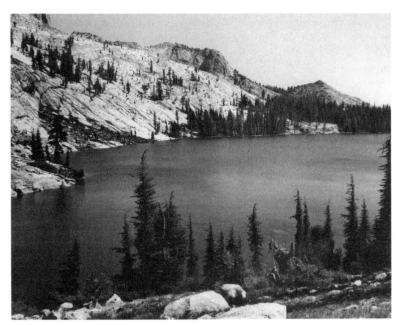

May Lake *from the trail up Mt. Hoffmann (Trail 18)*

white and lodgepole pines, and then swings west to cross three unnamed, seasonal streams.

Finally the trail makes a 0.5-mile-long ascent steeply up to May Lake, across a slope sparsely dotted with red firs, western white pines, and other conifers. Views improve constantly, and presently you have a panorama of the peaks on the Sierra crest from North Peak south to Mt. Gibbs. The Tioga Pass

Mt. Hoffmann

OPTIONS

If you've got the time, you might take the 1.8-mile trail from May Lake ▶10 to the top of Mt. Hoffmann, which is located in the center of Yosemite National Park and offers a 360-degree view of much of the park's lands. Bring a map of the park to identify dozens of features. See Trail 18 for details.

notch is clearly visible. At the top of this climb is a gentle upland where several small meadows are strung along the trail. Corn lilies grow at an almost perceptible rate in early season, while aromatic lupine commands your attention later on. In the west, Mt. Hoffmann dominates. Now you swing south at the northeast corner of May Lake and parallel its east shore to the May Lake High Sierra Camp. ▶10 From May Lake's southeast corner, you'll see a trail striking west, and it has a backpackers' camp that extends westward.

Lake

Camping

You begin the third day's hike, a mere 3.2 miles long and virtually all downhill, by first taking the lake's short trail 1.2 miles south down to the May Lake trailhead. ▶11 Here in Snow Flat, along the old Tioga Road, you follow the road northeast for two minutes to where it is blocked off, then descend the closed stretch of road southeast to the Tioga Road. Cross it and parallel it northeast about 0.75 mile to a fairly large trailhead parking area near the southwest corner of Tenaya Lake. ▶12

🚶 MILESTONES

▶1	0.0	Start at Lembert Dome trailhead
▶2	0.8	Soda Springs
▶3	2.0	Straight at Young Lakes Trail
▶4	4.7	Tuolumne River bridge
▶5	5.8	Right at trail to May Lake
▶6	6.0	Glen Aulin High Sierra Camp
▶7	10.3	Right at Murphy Creek Trail
▶8	10.9	Left at Ten Lakes Trail
▶9	12.6	Raisin Lake
▶10	14.4	May Lake High Sierra Camp
▶11	15.6	May Lake trailhead
▶12	17.6	Tenaya Lake trailhead

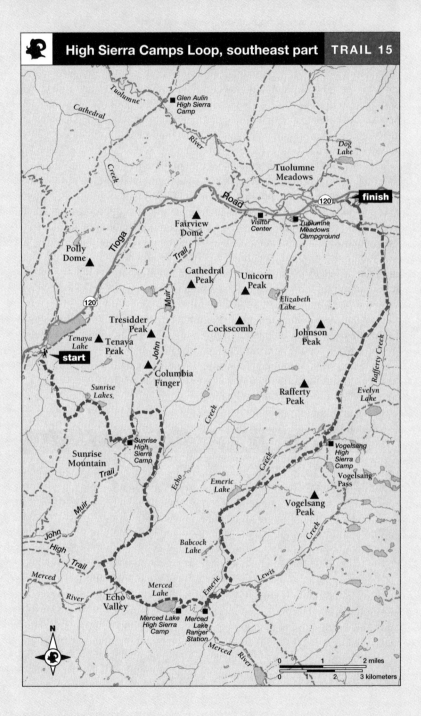

High Sierra Camps Loop, southeast part

The High Sierra Camps Loop hike became very popular years ago, not surprisingly, since the five backcountry camps are spaced about 6 to 10 miles apart, distances that are about right for most backpackers. If you can get reservations to stay at these camps (see "Fees, Camping, and Permits," page 14), then your food and bedding will be provided, which allows you to hike with a light pack. In reality, your chances of getting reservations are poor, so you'll have to settle for staying in the backpacker's camp adjacent to each camp.

I've broken the loop into two parts for two reasons. First, most hikers don't have the luxury of spending six days in the backcountry. Second, by being out fewer days, you will have a lighter pack, since you carry less food. Backpacking in Yosemite, you need to carry your food in a bear canister, which adds another 2 pounds to your pack's weight. My experience (but perhaps not yours) is that I can fit four days of food in one canister, but not six, so for the entire loop I would need to carry two canisters.

I prefer hiking the loop in a counterclockwise direction, since this way on your first day, when your pack is heaviest and you are perhaps are not in the best of shape, your hike is along the shortest stretch, 5.8 miles to Sunrise High Sierra Camp. This stretch offers reasons to pause, first with views and then with two trailside lakes. If you are short on time but are a strong backpacker, you could cut out a day by spending your first night at Merced Lake High Sierra Camp, a lengthy 16.1 miles, but the 10.3 miles past Sunrise High Sierra Camp are

TRAIL USE
Backpack, Horse
LENGTH
33.0 miles, 2–4 days
VERTICAL FEET
+5930'/-5550'/±11,480'
DIFFICULTY
- 1 2 3 4 **5** +
TRAIL TYPE
Point-to-Point

FEATURES
Backcountry Permit
Lakes
Streams
Wildflowers
Great Views
Camping
Swimming

FACILITIES
Restrooms
Bus Stop
Picnic Tables

relatively easy, having only about 600 feet of gain and about 2700 feet of loss.

Alternatively, you might try dayhiking this part, a whopping 33 miles in length (only super-athletes can do the entire 50.6-mile loop in a day). Actually, you can shorten the second part to 32 miles by ending short, at the trailhead near Tuolumne Meadows Lodge rather than the one at the base of Lembert Dome. When I was in my 20s and 30s, I could dayhike this route in about 12 to 15 hours, depending largely on how many lakes I chose to dip into.

Best Time

The best time to hike the loop is when the camps are open, which is around mid-July through mid-September. Before early August, mosquitoes can be quite prevalent, and if you want to avoid them, then hike in mid-August or later. Lakes are near their optimal temperatures from early July through early August, so if you want to minimize mosquitoes and snow and enjoy dips in the lakes, then early August is best. Just you and the rest of the world. As always, you'll have a better chance at getting a wilderness permit and avoiding crowds by hiking Monday through Thursday. If you must go on a weekend, consider hiking out of season, before or after the camps open, ideally, in the second half of September. However, if you are hiking early or late, do plan for the possibility of sudden snowstorms and know what to do if you're caught in one.

Finding the Trail

The trail starts on the Tioga Road at the Tenaya Lake trailhead parking area, at a highway bend near the lake's southwest shore, located 30.5 miles northeast of Crane Flat and 8.5 miles southwest of the Tuolumne Meadows Campground, which is the only campground in the area. However, if you are driving east up the Tioga Road, you will also pass the following campgrounds, the first three along spur roads: Tamarack Flat, White Wolf, Yosemite Creek, and Porcupine Flat.

If you are intent on making the complete hike, then you will park a second vehicle in the trailhead parking area at the base of Lembert Dome, 8.7 miles northeast up the Tioga Road. Alternatively, you could cut your hike short by 0.8 mile and park in the trailhead parking area near the east end of the spur road to Tuolumne Meadows Lodge.

Consider taking a free shuttle bus from either of these two possible Tuolumne Meadows trailheads back to your original trailhead. During the summer season, these buses run about once an hour, plying between Olmsted Point and Tioga Pass and stopping at all the popular trailheads in between. Before starting your hike, check the schedule for the shuttle's last run; you don't want to walk back to your original trailhead.

> At 180 feet, Tenaya Lake is the park's deepest, and it has only been filled with a few feet of sediments since the last glacier retreated by about 15,000 years ago.

Trail Description

From the trailhead parking area near the southwest corner of Tenaya Lake, ▶1 take a trail that heads east, and you soon cross the usually flowing outlet of Tenaya Lake. Just beyond this crossing you reach a trail junction. The trail left goes northeast to start a loop around the lake, and then it continues another 7 miles to the Cathedral Lakes Trail in Tuolumne Meadows.

≋ **Lake**

You veer right on a trail that heads south for 0.25 mile along Tenaya Creek. Over the next 0.5 mile your trail ascends southeast in sparse forest over a little rise and drops to a ford of Mildred Lake's outlet, which, like the other streams between Tenaya Lake and the Sunrise Trail junction, can dry up in late season. Beyond the Mildred Lake stream the

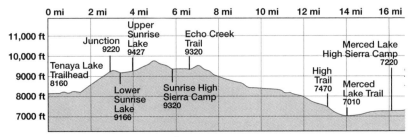

TRAIL 15 High Sierra Camps, southeast part Elevation Profile

trail undulates and winds generally south, passing several pocket meadows browsed by mule deer. The trail then begins to climb in earnest, through a thinning cover of lodgepole pine and occasional red fir, western white pine, and mountain hemlock. As your trail rises above Tenaya Canyon, you pass several vantage points from which you can look back upon its polished granite walls, though you never see Tenaya Lake. To the east the canyon is bounded by Tenaya Peak; in the northwest are the cliffs of Mt. Hoffmann and Tuolumne Peak.

 Great Views

Now on switchbacks, you see the Tioga Road across the canyon and can even hear vehicles, but these annoyances are infinitesimal compared to the pleasures of polished granite expanses all around. These switchbacks are mercifully shaded, and where they become steepest, requiring a great output of energy, they give back the beauty of the finest flower displays on this trail, including lupine, penstemon, paintbrush, larkspur, buttercup, and sunflowers such as aster and senecio. Finally the switchbacks end, and the trail levels as it arrives at a junction on a shallow, forested saddle. ▶2

Steep

Wildflowers

The trail ahead goes to Clouds Rest and beyond (Trail 17), but you turn left, and over 0.5 mile you first contour east, cross a low gap and descend north to lower Sunrise Lake. ▶3 Climbing from this lake and its small campsites, you reach a crest in several minutes, and from it you could descend cross-

Lake

18 mi	20 mi	22 mi	24 mi	26 mi	28 mi	30 mi	32 mi

Fletcher Creek Trail 8110

Babcock Lake Trail 8890

Scissors Junction 7220

Vogelsang High Sierra Camp 10,140

Trail to Tuolumne Meadows 8670

Spur to Tuolumne Meadows Lodge 9490

Lewis Creek Trail 7310

Tuolumne Pass 9490

Pacific Crest Trail 8720

Trailhead at base of Lembert Dome 9490

country an equally short distance north to more isolated, island-dotted middle Sunrise Lake. Your loop trail, however, veers east and gains a very noticeable 150 feet in elevation as it climbs to upper Sunrise Lake, the largest and most popular lake of the trio. ►4 Campsites are plentiful along its north shore, away from the trail.

 Lake

Camping

With 1.7 miles remaining to your day's goal, you leave this lake and climb south up a gully, cross it, then soon climb up a second gully to the east side of a broad gap, from which you see the Clark Range head-on, piercing the southern sky. From the gap, which is sparsely clothed with mountain hemlocks, whitebark pines, and western white pines, you descend south into denser cover, veer east, and then veer north to make a steep descent to a backpackers' camp. By walking briefly north from it you'll reach Sunrise High Sierra Camp. ►5 An overnight stay at either camp gives you an inspiring sunrise over Matthes Crest and the Cathedral Range.

Camping

You begin the second day's hike by starting from the camp and treading the John Muir Trail 0.8 mile, first east and then north to the Echo Creek Trail, ►6 on which you will immediately ford Long Meadow's creek on boulders. This trail, which takes you 6.5 miles to the Merced Lake Trail, quickly switchbacks up to the top of a forested ridge, about 200 feet above the meadow. It then descends through dense hemlock-and-lodgepole forest to a tributary of Echo

Creek. Cross this, descend along it for 0.33 mile, recross, then momentarily reach the west bank of Echo Creek's Cathedral Fork, about 1.5 miles beyond Long Meadow.

From your trail beside the Cathedral Fork you have fine views of the creek's water gliding down a series of granite slabs, and then the trail veers away from the creek and descends gently above it for more than a mile. Even in late season these shaded slopes are watered by numerous rills, which are bordered by still-blooming flowers. On this downgrade the trail crosses the Long Meadow creek, which has found an escape from that meadow through a gap between two small domes high above your trail. The route then levels out in a mile-long flat section of this valley, where the wet ground yields wildflowers all summer but also many mosquitoes in the early season. Beyond this flat "park" the trail descends more-open slopes, and eventually you can see across the valley the steep course of Echo Creek plunging down to its rendezvous with its western Cathedral Fork. By the Cathedral Fork your trail levels off and passes good campsites immediately before you take a bridge over Echo Creek.

Beyond the bridge, your trail leads down the forested valley and easily fords a tributary stream, staying well above the main creek. This pleasant, shaded descent soon becomes more open and steep, and it encounters fibrous-barked juniper trees and butterscotch-scented Jeffrey pines as it drops to another bridge 1.33 miles from the first one. Beyond it, the trail rises slightly and the creek drops precipitously, so that you are soon far above it. Then the sandy tread swings west and diagonals down a brushy slope. Across it the views are excellent of Echo Valley, which is a wide place in the great Merced River canyon below. On this slope you arrive at a junction with the High Trail, ►7 which goes 3 miles west to a junction with the John Muir Trail.

■ **Stream**

Leaving Merced Lake
via Lewis Creek Trail

Leaving the dense growth of huckleberry oak, chinquapin, greenleaf manzanita, and snow bush behind, start southeast and make a drop 450 feet over 0.7 mile to the Merced Lake Trail junction in Echo Valley. ▶8 There is adequate camping here, but your goal is only 2.3 miles ahead. You go east, immediately bridging Echo Creek, pass through a burned-but-boggy area, then climb east past the Merced River's largely unseen, but enjoyable, pools to Merced Lake's west shore. Don't camp here, but rather continue along the north shore for about 0.5 mile and then 0.25 mile east beyond it to Merced Lake High Sierra Camp. ▶9 This has an adjacent campground, which you reach just before the camp.

While day three isn't the longest, it easily has the most elevation to gain, about 3150 feet. Fortunately, by now you should be well acclimatized, should be somewhat in shape, and should have a lighter pack. You begin with an easy warm-up by hiking a level mile east to the Merced Lake Ranger Station and an adjacent trail junction. ▶10 From it you struggle 1.5 miles in a 1000-foot climb northeast up the Lewis Creek Trail to another trail junction. ▶11

≋ **Lake**

▲ **Camping**

⚑ **Steep**

OPTIONS

▲ Camping

≋ Lake

From the junction you leave the Lewis Creek Trail and branch left on the Fletcher Creek Trail, descending on short switchbacks to a bridge over Lewis Creek. Just 50 yards past the bridge is a good campsite, and then the trail enters more open slopes as it climbs moderately on a cobbled path bordered with proliferating bushes of snow bush and huckleberry oak. Just past a tributary 0.5 mile from Lewis Creek, you have fine views of Fletcher Creek chuting and cascading down from the notch at the base of the granite dome before it leaps off a ledge in free fall. The few solitary pine trees on this otherwise blank dome testify to nature's extraordinary persistence. At the notch your trail levels off and reaches the Babcock Lake Trail, ►12 whose lake for most folks won't be worth the 3-mile round-trip effort.

Onward, the sandy Fletcher Creek Trail ascends steadily through a moderate forest cover, staying just east of Fletcher Creek. After 0.75 mile this route breaks out into the open and begins to rise more steeply via rocky switchbacks. From these one can see nearby in the north the outlet stream of Emeric Lake—though not the lake itself, which is behind a dome just to the right of the outlet's notch.

Emeric Lake

OPTIONS

If you wish to camp at Emeric Lake—and it's a fine place—leave the trail here for a shortcut route to it. First cross Fletcher Creek at a safe spot (do not attempt this in high water, and then climb along the outlet creek's west side and camp above the lake's northwest shore. The next morning circle the head of the lake and find a trail at the base of the low granite ridge at the northeast corner of the lake. Follow this trail 0.5 mile northeast to a scissors junction in Fletcher Creek valley.

If you don't take the optional route, then take the equally long main route, which continues up the Fletcher Creek Trail into a long meadow guarded in the west by a highly polished knoll and presided over in the east by huge Vogelsang Peak. When you come to the scissors junction ▶13 near Emeric Lake, veer right and hike 2.3 miles northeast up to the Vogelsang High Sierra Camp. ▶14

⚠ **Camping**

Day four, your last day, is the easiest, being one of the shortest legs, and almost all of it is downhill or level. You begin by dropping slightly as you traverse 0.8 mile north across slopes to Tuolumne Pass. ▶15 From it is a large, linear meadow, and descending about 1.5 miles north through it, you have views north to the Sierra crest between Tioga Pass and Mt. Conness and views behind to cliff-bound, dark-banded Fletcher Peak and Vogelsang Peak to the right of it. Where you leave the meadow, you have a 3.7-mile descent on the Rafferty Creek Trail. You go a viewless half mile down to a meadow, which is about a half-mile long, but the trail stays just within the confines of a lodgepole pine forest. Beyond the meadow the trail descends its namesake creek for about 2.3 viewless miles to a junction with the John Muir Trail. ▶16

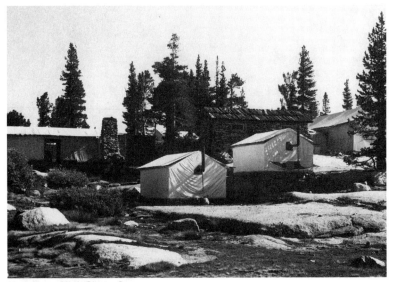

Vogelsang High Sierra Camp

Ahead, the route is almost flat. You traverse 0.66 mile west to a junction, ►17 leave the westbound trail which continues to Tuolumne Campground, and branch north on the route of the John Muir Trail. In about 70 yards you reach two bridges across branches of the Lyell Fork of the Tuolumne River. The meadows above these bridges are among the most delightful in all the Sierra, and anytime you happen to be staying all night at the lodge or nearby, the bridges are a wonderful place to spend the last hour before dinner, something you might consider for your hike out to your trailhead. Mts. Dana and Gibbs glow on the eastern horizon, catching the late sun, while trout dart along the wide Lyell Fork.

Past the second bridge, John Muir Trail leads over a slight rise and descends to a trail junction by the Dana Fork. ►18 Here a trail begins an ascent to the Gaylor Lakes. After a brief walk downstream you bridge the Dana Fork, and find a spur trail that goes

◢ Stream

shortly over to the west end of the parking lot of the Tuolumne Meadows Lodge. ▶19 Rather, you continue downstream 0.33 mile, paralleling the lodge's road, to where you see a large parking lot ▶20 just across the spur road. You can end your hike here and catch a shuttle bus back to the Tenaya Lake trailhead, but if you are a purist and intend to do the entire High Sierra Camps Loop, then continue west to a crossing of the Tioga Road, immediately beyond which is a parking area at the base of Lembert Dome, the starting point for Trail 14. ▶21

🚶 MILESTONES

▶1	0.0	Start at Tenaya Lake trailhead
▶2	2.9	Left at junction on forested saddle
▶3	3.4	Lower Sunrise Lake
▶4	4.0	Upper Sunrise Lake
▶5	5.8	Sunrise High Sierra Camp
▶6	6.6	Right on Echo Creek Trail
▶7	13.1	Straight at High Trail
▶8	13.8	Left on Merced Lake Trail
▶9	16.1	Merced Lake High Sierra Camp
▶10	17.0	Left on Lewis Creek Trail
▶11	18.2	Left on Fletcher Creek Trail
▶12	19.9	Straight at Babcock Lake Trail
▶13	22.1	Right at scissors junction near Emeric Lake
▶14	24.4	Vogelsang High Sierra Camp
▶15	25.2	Tuolumne Pass
▶16	30.4	Left on Pacific Crest Trail
▶17	31.1	Right at trail to Tuolumne Meadows Campground
▶18	31.7	Straight at junction with trail to Gaylor Lakes
▶19	31.8	Straight at junction with trail to Tuolumne Meadows Lodge
▶20	32.1	Straight at spur trail to trailhead parking west of lodge
▶21	33.0	Trailhead parking at base of Lembert Dome

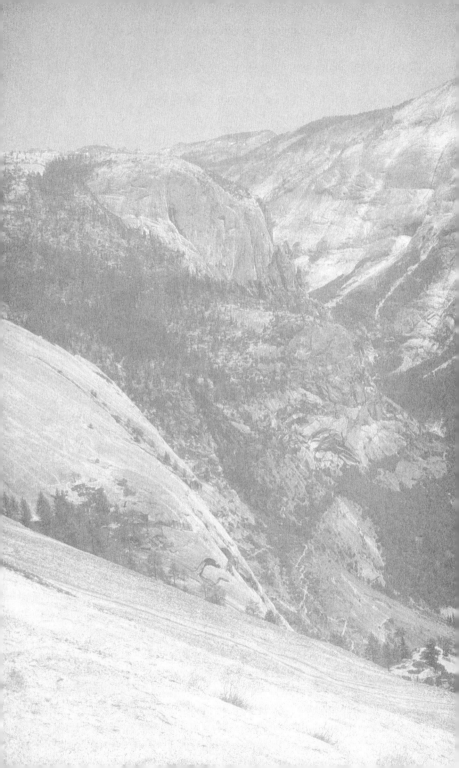

Central Yosemite

Central Yosemite

The most conspicuous and perhaps most photographed feature of the Central Yosemite country is Tenaya Lake, which is skirted by the heavily traveled Tioga Road (also known as Highway 120). If you plan to swim in this chilly lake, do so at the bouldery southwest shore. The sandy beach of the northeast shore is lacking here, but so too are the strong up-canyon winds that were needed to form it. Besides, here you'll find a few small boulder islands worth swimming or wading to—something lacking near the northeast shore. From various points along the lake's shore you may see some protruding tree stumps. There is a myth that during a lengthy former drought this lake dried up, and a forest grew on its floor, then centuries later, when the rains returned, the forest was submerged beneath the lake's water. Actually, rockfalls carry trees into this 180-foot-deep lake, and their heavier ends can become lodged in the lake's sediments. You don't see stumps at other lakes because they lack the three necessary ingredients: steep cliffs, forested slopes, and deep water.

From Tenaya Lake's southwest shore, southeast of the Tioga Road, this chapter's first three trails begin, bound for very different destinations: the three Sunrise Lakes and aptly named Sunrise High Sierra Camp, the summit of Clouds Rest, and an inspiring Tenaya Creek cascade (in early summer).

To view all of Central Yosemite, and indeed, most of the park, make the safe, relatively easy ascent to its highest peak, Mt. Hoffmann. From it you'll see dozens of features identifiable with a topographic map of the park, including May Lake to the peak's east and an assortment of lakes and ponds to the north and west, which are "Lost Lakes," all lying within 3 miles of the Tioga Road. Despite their proximity, only a few cross-country enthusiasts visit them. These are not the Ten Lakes, which are extremely popular and like May Lake are described in this chapter. In my opinion, the best cluster of lakes in the park are in the Ten Lakes Basin. Too many folks visit only the three easily reached lakes, leaving the other four with only moderate to light use.

North Dome is an unmistakable feature rising above the east end of Yosemite Valley, opposite from Half Dome. While one can reach its summit by first climbing vertical Washington Column and then the south route up

Overleaf: *Clouds Rest and Tenaya Canyon from North Dome (Trail 19)*

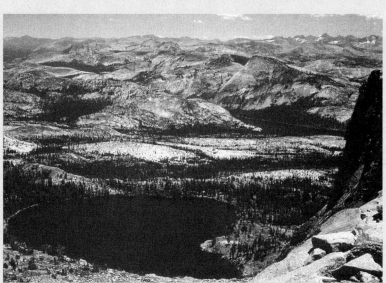
May Lake *from summit of Mt. Hoffmann (Trails 14 and 18)*

the dome (and I've done both), the vast majority of folks prefer taking a relatively short and easy trail heading south from the Tioga Road. As atop Mt. Hoffmann, the summit of North Dome provides panoramic, remunerative views.

Finally, the Central Yosemite chapter ends with two ordinary looking, but relatively rare lakes, Lukens and Harden. Whereas the vast majority of Sierran lakes owe their existence to glaciers excavating basins out of weathered and fractured bedrock, Lukens and Harden lakes owe their existence to water ponded up behind glacial deposits known as lateral moraines. However, in the case of Harden, the deposits are thinner and the lake leaks, so that by midsummer it is quite shallow.

Permits

If you want to reserve a permit, rather than get one in person, see the "Fees, Camping, and Permits" section on page 14.

In person, if you are driving east up Highway 120, get a permit at the Big Oak Flat Information Station, which is immediately past the park's entrance station. You cannot get a permit in the White Wolf area. If you are driving up Highway 140 or Highway 41, get your permit at the Visitor Center in Yosemite Valley, and if you are driving west down Highway 120, stop in Tuolumne Meadows at its wilderness center, mentioned in the previous chapter.

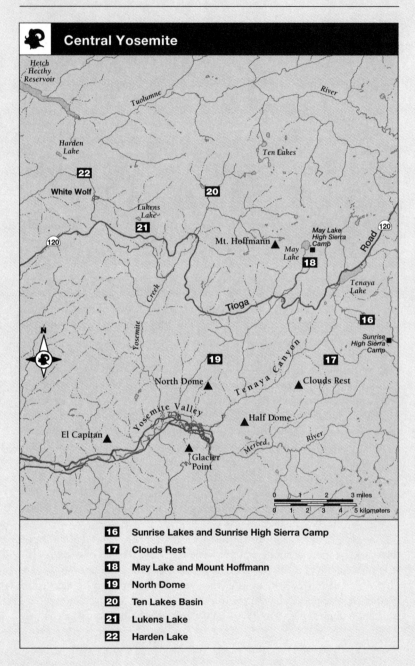

Central Yosemite

Hetch
Hecthy
Reservoir

Tuolumne

River

Harden
Lake

Ten Lakes

22

White Wolf

20

Lukens
Lake

21

Mt. Hoffmann ▲

May Lake
High Sierra
Camp

May
Lake

120

18

120

Tenaya
Lake

Road

Tioga

16

Yosemite Creek

N

Sunrise
High Sierra
Camp

19

Tenaya Canyon

17

North Dome ▲

▲ Clouds Rest

Yosemite Valley

Half Dome ▲

El Capitan ▲

▲ Glacier
Point

Merced

River

| 0 | 1 | 2 | 3 miles |

| 0 | 1 | 2 | 3 | 4 | 5 kilometers |

16	Sunrise Lakes and Sunrise High Sierra Camp
17	Clouds Rest
18	May Lake and Mount Hoffmann
19	North Dome
20	Ten Lakes Basin
21	Lukens Lake
22	Harden Lake

Central Yosemite

TRAIL	Difficulty	Length	Type	USES & ACCESS	TERRAIN	FLORA & FAUNA	OTHER
16	3	11.6	↗	🥾 🚶 🐎	〰 🌊	✳	⋔ ⛺ ⚊
17	4	14.0	↗	🥾 🚶 🐎	⛰ △ 🌊	✳	⋔ ⛺
18	2/3	2.4	↗	🥾 🚶 🐎 👫	⛰ △ 🌊		⋔ ⛺ ⚊
19	3	9.2	↗	🥾 🚶	△ 🌊	✳	⋔ ⛺ ⚊
20	4	12.6	↗	🥾 🚶 🐎	⛰ 〰 🌊	✳	⋔ ⛺ ⚊ 🛁
21	1	2.2	↗	🚶 🏃 👫	〰	✳	⚊
22	2	5.6	↗	🥾 🚶 🐎 🏃 👫	〰	🍁 ✳	⛺ ⚊

USES & ACCESS	TYPE	TERRAIN	FLORA & FAUNA	FEATURES
🚶 Dayhiking	↻ Loop	🏔 Canyon	🍁 Autumn Colors	⋔ Great Views
🥾 Backpacking	↗ Out & Back	⛰ Mountain	✳ Wildflowers	⛺ Camping
🐎 Horses	↘ Point-to-Point	△ Summit	🌲 Giant Sequoias	⚊ Swimming
🏃 Running		🌊 Stream		🛁 Secluded
🚴 Biking	DIFFICULTY	🏞 Waterfall		🪜 Steep
♿ Handicap Access	- 1 2 3 4 5 +	〰 Lake		
👫 Child Friendly	less more			

Maps

For Central Yosemite, here are the USGS 7.5-minute (1:24,000 scale) topographic quadrangles that you will need, listed in the order that you will need them as you hike along your route.

Trails 16 and 17: Tenaya Lake
Trail 18: May Lake, Yosemite Falls
Trail 19: Yosemite Falls
Trail 20: Yosemite Falls, Ten Lakes
Trail 21: Yosemite Falls
Trail 22: Tamarack Flat, Hetch Hetchy Reservoir

Central Yosemite

TRAIL 16

Dayhike, Backpack, Horse

11.6 miles, Out & Back

Difficulty: 1 2 **3** 4 5

Sunrise Lakes and Sunrise High Sierra Camp 153

Considerable climbing at fairly high elevations would normally make this hike a moderate one, but its distance is so short for a backpack trip that it is rated easy. Some hikers go only as far as upper Sunrise Lake. However, if you camp near Sunrise High Sierra Camp you are rewarded with a beautiful sunrise—the reason for the camp's being situated where it is.

TRAIL 17

Dayhike, Backpack, Horse

14.0 miles, Out & Back

Difficulty: 1 2 3 **4** 5

Clouds Rest 159

Although Clouds Rest is higher than Half Dome, it is easier and safer to climb, and it provides far better views of the park than does popular, often overcrowded Half Dome. Except for its last 300 yards, the Clouds Rest Trail lacks the terrifying, potentially lethal drop-offs found along Half Dome's shoulder and back side, thereby making it a good trail for acrophobic photographers.

TRAIL 18

Dayhike, Backpack, Horse

2.4 miles, Out & Back

Difficulty: 1 **2** 3 4 5

May Lake and Mount Hoffmann 165

May Lake is a very popular destination because it is such a short hike. Dayhikers can reach it in under a half hour, and all but the slowest backpackers in under an hour. At 1.2 miles distance, May Lake has the most easily accessible campsites in the park, and so it is ideal for novice backpackers or for those with young children. Additionally, these are good base-camp sites for an ascent of Mt. Hoffmann.

North Dome 169

North Dome, which looks so inaccessible from the Yosemite Valley floor, can be reached in a couple of hours by this route. From the dome you get perhaps the best views of the expansive faces of Half Dome and Clouds Rest, as well as excellent views of Yosemite Valley. Along this hike you can also visit one of Yosemite's few known natural arches, and also visit Indian Rock, which provides a 360-degree panorama.

TRAIL 19

Dayhike, Backpack
9.2 miles,
Out & Back
Difficulty: 1 2 **3** 4 5

Ten Lakes Basin 175

The Ten Lakes Basin is extremely popular with weekend backpackers, for with only a few hours' hiking effort you can attain any of its seven major lakes. The three most accessible receive moderate-to-heavy use, but the other four, off the beaten track, are worth the effort for those who want relatively secluded camping.

TRAIL 20

Dayhike, Backpack,
Horse
12.6 miles, Out & Back
Difficulty: 1 2 3 **4** 5

Lukens Lake 183

This is the shorter approach to Lukens Lake, about one half the length of the trail east from White Wolf. At 2.2 miles round trip, it is a great one to introduce children to an off-road High Sierran lake. No overnight camping is allowed.

TRAIL 21

Dayhike, Run
2.2 miles, Out & Back
Difficulty: **1** 2 3 4 5

Harden Lake 187

Only about an hour's hike from White Wolf Campground, this lake attracts quite a number of summer visitors, virtually all of them dayhikers. From mid-June through July this shallow lake can be fine for swimming, but the lake lies in a leaky basin, and by mid-August it usually has dwindled to an oversized wading pool. Don't expect to catch any fish, since the lake becomes far too shallow by late summer to support any.

TRAIL 22

Dayhike, Backpack,
Run, Horse
5.6 miles,
Out & Back
Difficulty: 1 **2** 3 4 5

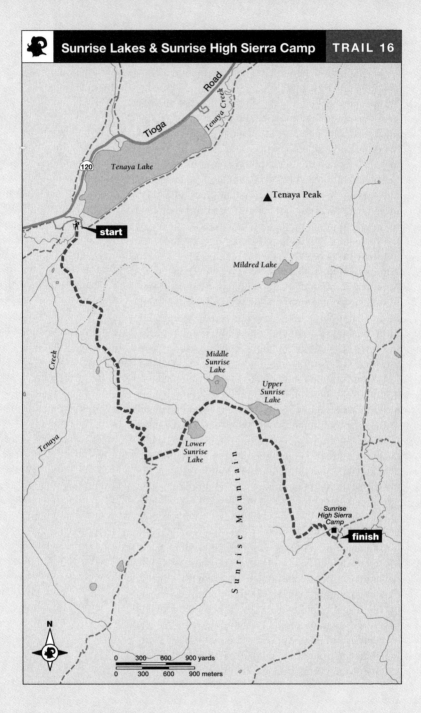

Sunrise Lakes and Sunrise High Sierra Camp

Considerable climbing at fairly high elevations would normally make this hike a moderate one, but its distance is so short for a backpack trip that it is rated easy. Some hikers go only as far as upper Sunrise Lake, only an 8-mile round trip and a good, moderate dayhike, although many are capable of doing the whole route in under a day. However, if you camp near Sunrise High Sierra Camp you are rewarded with a beautiful sunrise—the reason for the camp's being situated where it is.

Best Time

Because of fairly high elevations, the trail can have snow patches even into mid-July, the soonest you'll want to start. Lakes are near their optimal temperatures from early July through early August, so if you want to minimize mosquitoes and snow and enjoy dips in the lakes, then early August is best. To avoid crowds, backpack in mid- and late September. You can even go in early and mid-October, although then be prepared for cool days and subfreezing nights.

Finding the Trail

The trail begins on the Tioga Road at the Tenaya Lake trailhead parking area, at a highway bend near the lake's southwest shore, located 30.5 miles northeast of Crane Flat and 8.5 miles southwest of the Tuolumne Meadows Campground. If you are driving east up the Tioga Road, you will pass the following campgrounds, the first three along spur

TRAIL USE
Dayhike, Backpack, Horse

LENGTH
11.6 miles, 4–8 hours

VERTICAL FEET
+1890'/-710'/±5200'

DIFFICULTY
- 1 2 **3** 4 5 +

TRAIL TYPE
Out & Back

FEATURES
Backcountry Permit
Lakes
Streams
Wildflowers
Great Views
Camping
Swimming

FACILITIES
Restrooms
Bus Stop
Picnic Tables

153

roads: Tamarack Flat, White Wolf, Yosemite Creek, and Porcupine Flat.

Trail Description

From the trailhead parking area near the southwest corner of Tenaya Lake, ▶1 take a trail that heads east, and you soon cross the usually flowing outlet of Tenaya Lake. Just beyond this crossing you reach a trail junction. The trail left goes northeast to start a loop around the lake, and then it continues another 7 miles to the Cathedral Lakes Trail in Tuolumne Meadows.

You veer right on a trail that heads south for 0.25 mile along Tenaya Creek. Over the next 0.5 mile your trail ascends southeast in sparse forest over a little rise and drops to a ford of Mildred Lake's outlet, which, like the other streams between Tenaya Lake and the Sunrise Trail junction, can dry up in late season. Beyond the Mildred Lake stream the trail undulates and winds generally south, passing several pocket meadows browsed by mule deer. The trail then begins to climb in earnest, through a thinning cover of lodgepole pine and occasional red fir, western white pine, and mountain hemlock. As your trail rises above Tenaya Canyon, you pass several vantage points from which you can look back upon its polished granite walls, though you never see Tenaya Lake. To the east the canyon is bounded by Tenaya Peak; in the northwest are the cliffs of Mt. Hoffmann and Tuolumne Peak.

Great Views

Now on switchbacks, you see the Tioga Road across the canyon and can even hear vehicles, but these annoyances are infinitesimal compared to the pleasures of polished granite expanses all around. These switchbacks are mercifully shaded, and where they become steepest, requiring a great output of energy, they give back the beauty of the finest flower displays on this trail, including lupine, penstemon, paintbrush, larkspur, buttercup, and sunflowers such as aster and senecio. Finally the switchbacks end and the trail levels as it arrives at a junction on a shallow, forested saddle. ►2

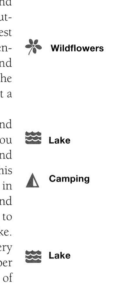 **Wildflowers**

The trail ahead goes to Clouds Rest and beyond (Trail 17), but you turn left, and over 0.5 mile you first contour east, cross a low gap and descend north to lower Sunrise Lake. ►3 Climbing from this lake and its small campsites, you reach a crest in several minutes, and from it you could descend cross-country an equally short distance north to more isolated, island-dotted middle Sunrise Lake. Your loop trail, however, veers east and gains a very noticeable 150 feet in elevation as it climbs to upper Sunrise Lake, the largest and most popular lake of

Lake

Camping

Lake

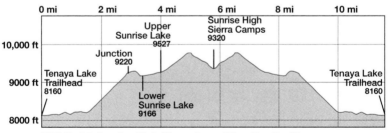

TRAIL 16 Sunrise High Sierra Camp Elevation Profile

Camping

Camping

the trio. ►4 Campsites are plentiful along its north shore, away from the trail.

With 1.7 miles remaining to your day's goal, you leave this lake and climb south up a gully, cross it, then soon climb up a second gully to the east side of a broad gap, from which you see the Clark Range head-on, piercing the southern sky. From the gap, which is sparsely clothed with mountain hemlocks, whitebark pines, and western white pines, you descend south into denser cover, veer east, and then veer north to make a steep descent to a backpackers' camp. By walking briefly north from it you'll reach Sunrise High Sierra Camp. ►5 An overnight stay at either camp gives you an inspiring sunrise over Matthes Crest and the Cathedral Range.

🚶	**MILESTONES**

►1	0.0	Start at Tenaya Lake trailhead
►2	2.9	Left at junction on forested saddle
►3	3.4	Lower Sunrise Lake
►4	4.0	Upper Sunrise Lake
►5	5.8	Sunrise High Sierra Camp

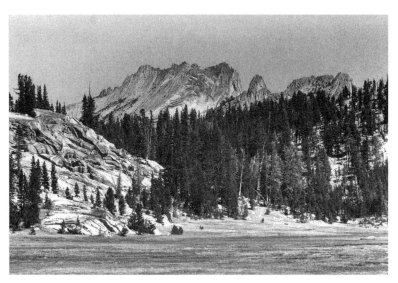

Matthes Crest *from Sunrise Meadow*

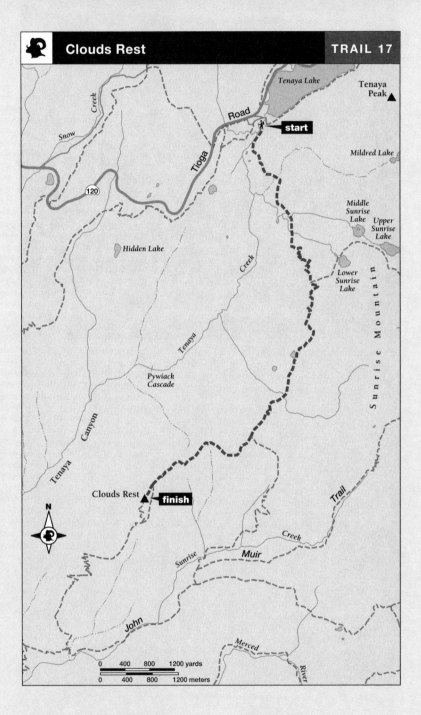

Tenaya Lake

Tenaya Peak ▲

Road

start

Mildred Lake

Tioga

120

Middle Sunrise Lake

Upper Sunrise Lake

Hidden Lake

Creek

Lower Sunrise Lake

Sunrise Mountain

Snow

Creek

Tenaya

Pywiack Cascade

Clouds Rest ▲ finish

Trail

N

Creek

Muir

Sunrise

Canyon

Tenaya

John

Merced

River

| 0 | 400 | 800 | 1200 yards |
| 0 | 400 | 800 | 1200 meters |

Clouds Rest

Although Clouds Rest is higher than Half Dome, it is easier and safer to climb, and it provides far better views of the park than does popular, often overcrowded Half Dome. Except for its last 300 yards, the Clouds Rest Trail lacks the terrifying, potentially lethal drop-offs found along Half Dome's shoulder and back side, thereby making it a good trail for acrophobic photographers. If you're an avid photographer, you'll want to start this trek at the crack of dawn in order to reach this summit before shadows become poor for photography. All hikers should strive to reach this summit by noon or thereabouts, for lightning storms are a real possibility in the mid-to-late afternoon.

Best Time

The optimal time is late July through early September; mid- and late July if you like wildflowers. Mosquitoes, who pollinate some flowers, are plentiful through July. Still, they are common mostly on parts of the lower half of the route, so if you don't dally, you can avoid most of them (and deal with some snow patches) in early July, when there may be fewer hikers. As always, the crowds disappear after Labor Day, and if you like hiking in cooler weather, you often can take this trail through mid- and late October.

Finding the Trail

The trail begins on the Tioga Road at the Tenaya Lake trailhead parking area, at a highway bend near

TRAIL USE
Dayhike, Backpack, Horse

LENGTH
14.0 miles; 5–8 hours

VERTICAL FEET
+2480'/-710'/±6380'

DIFFICULTY
- 1 2 3 **4** 5 +

TRAIL TYPE
Out & Back

FEATURES
Backcountry Permit
Streams
Wildflowers
Summit
Great Views
Camping

FACILITIES
Restrooms
Bus Stop
Picnic Tables

the lake's southwest shore, located 30.5 miles northeast of Crane Flat and 8.5 miles southwest of the Tuolumne Meadows Campground. If you are driving east up the Tioga Road, you will pass the following campgrounds, the first three along spur roads: Tamarack Flat, White Wolf, Yosemite Creek, and Porcupine Flat.

Trail Description

From the trailhead parking area near the southwest corner of Tenaya Lake, ▶1 take a trail that heads east, and you soon cross the usually flowing outlet of Tenaya Lake. Just beyond this crossing you reach a trail junction. The trail left goes northeast to start a loop around the lake, and then it continues another 7 miles to the Cathedral Lakes Trail in Tuolumne Meadows.

≋ **Lake**

You veer right on a trail that heads south for 0.25 mile along Tenaya Creek. Over the next 0.5 mile your trail ascends southeast in sparse forest over a little rise and drops to a ford of Mildred Lake's outlet, which, like the other streams between Tenaya Lake and the Sunrise Trail junction, can dry up in late season. Beyond the Mildred Lake stream the trail undulates and winds generally south, passing several pocket meadows browsed by mule deer. The trail then begins to climb in earnest, through a thinning cover of lodgepole pine and occasional red fir,

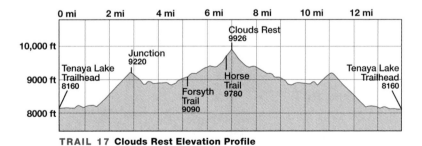

TRAIL 17 Clouds Rest Elevation Profile

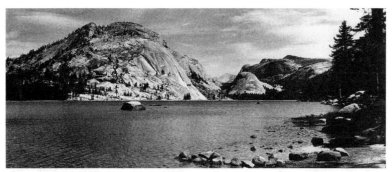

Tenaya Lake, *Polly Dome and Pywiack Dome*

western white pine, and mountain hemlock. As your trail rises above Tenaya Canyon, you pass several vantage points from which you can look back upon its polished granite walls, though you never see Tenaya Lake. To the east the canyon is bounded by Tenaya Peak; in the northwest are the cliffs of Mt. Hoffmann and Tuolumne Peak.

 Great Views

Now on switchbacks, you sees the Tioga Road across the canyon and can even hear vehicles, but these annoyances are infinitesimal compared to the pleasures of polished granite expanses all around. These switchbacks are mercifully shaded, and where they become steepest, requiring a great output of energy, they give back the beauty of the finest flower displays on this trail, including lupine, penstemon, paintbrush, larkspur, buttercup, and sunflowers such as aster and senecio. Finally the switchbacks end and the trail levels as it arrives at a junction on a shallow, forested saddle. ▶2 Here the High Sierra Camps Loop veers left, bound for Sunrise High Sierra Camp (Trail 16).

Wildflowers

Now with all the hard climbing behind you, descend south, bound for Clouds Rest. Your trail switchbacks for a relatively minor descent to a shady, sometimes damp flat, then climbs up to a block-strewn ridge that sprouts dense clumps of chinquapin and aspen. Beyond it the trail descends

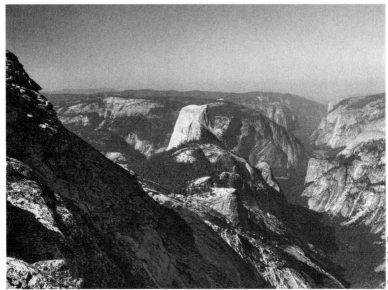

Half Dome and Tenaya Canyon *from Clouds Rest*

briefly to a tree-fringed pond—adequate for nearby camping—then wanders south for 0.5 mile before veering west to cross three creeklets, which will be your last usually reliable sources of water. After you cross the first creeklet, follow the trail briefly downstream, then veer left to cross the second creeklet before climbing up to the third. Beyond it the trail rapidly eases its gradient and soon reaches the Forsyth Trail junction. ▶3 This trail, which is not worth taking, forks left, but you keep right and, for about a mile, ascend the Clouds Rest Trail west to a forested, gravelly crest and then follow it down to a shallow saddle. The final ascent begins here. After a moderate ascent of 0.25 mile, you emerge from the forest cover to get your first excellent views of Tenaya Canyon and the country west and north of it. After another 0.25 mile along the crest you come to a junction with a horse trail. ►4 If you're riding a horse from Tenaya Lake to Yosemite Valley via the Clouds Rest Trail—the most scenic of the possible routes to the valley—you'll want to take this trail after first walking to the summit.

 Great Views

Clouds Rest foot trail now becomes exposed, and you scramble a few feet up to the narrow and potentially dangerous crest. One wishes there was a hand railing in spots. Acrophobics and klutzes should not continue, but they can get some spectacular views of Tenaya Canyon, Half Dome, and Yosemite Valley that are nearly identical with those seen from the summit. Spreading below is the expansive 4500-foot-high face of Clouds Rest—the largest granite face in the park. Those who follow the now steeper, narrow, almost trailless crest 300 yards to the summit ►5 are further rewarded with views of the Clark Range and the Merced River Canyon. Growing on the rocky summit are a few knee-high Jeffrey pines and whitebark pines, plus assorted bushes and wildflowers.

 Caution

 Great Views

🚶	**MILESTONES**
►1	0.0 Start at Tenaya Lake trailhead
►2	2.9 Straight at junction on forested saddle
►3	5.2 Straight at Forsyth Trail
►4	6.8 Straight at horse trail
►5	7.0 Clouds Rest summit

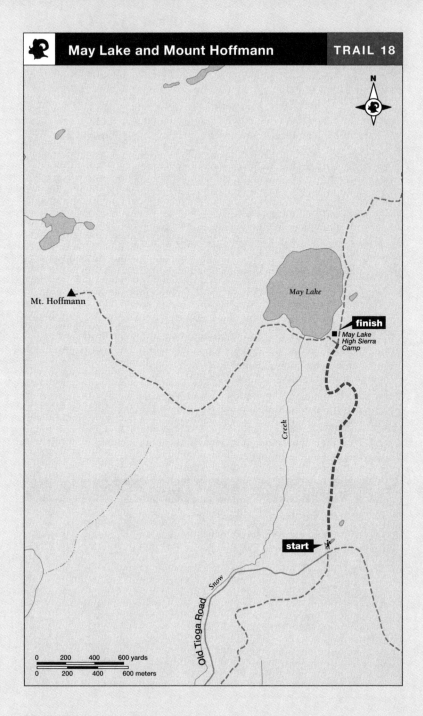

Mt. Hoffmann

May Lake

finish

May Lake
High Sierra
Camp

Creek

start

Snow

Old Tioga Road

| 0 | 200 | 400 | 600 yards |
| 0 | 200 | 400 | 600 meters |

May Lake and Mt. Hoffmann

May Lake is a very popular destination because it is such a short hike. Dayhikers can reach it in under a half hour, and all but the slowest backpackers in under an hour. At 1.2 miles distance, May Lake has the most easily accessible campsites in the park, and so is ideal for novice backpackers or for those with young children. Additionally, these are good base-camp sites for an ascent of Mt. Hoffmann, although strong hikers can reach that summit in about an hour. Mt. Hoffmann, centrally located in Yosemite National Park, provides the best all-around views of this park's varied landscapes. The 3.0-mile hike up to it is offered as a side trip, and if you do it, you will have a total ascent and descent of about 4200 feet.

TRAIL USE
Dayhike, Backpack, Horse
LENGTH
2.4 miles, 1–2 hours
VERTICAL FEET
+530'/-30'/±1120'
DIFFICULTY
- 1 **2 3** 4 5 +
TRAIL TYPE
Out & Back

FEATURES
Backcountry Permit
Child Friendly
Lake
Summit
Great Views
Camping

FACILITIES
Restrooms

Best Time

Snow lingers long at the trailhead's Snow Flat, so August is the best month. Mosquitoes are prevalent before then, but usually only on the first part of the hike. From September through mid-October also are good times, since the crowds are gone, but so too is virtually all the snow, and so the surrounding terrain is less photogenic. For best photography with patches of snow, fight the mosquitoes on the first stretch and hike around mid-July.

Finding the Trail

From Crane Flat drive northeast 27 miles up Tioga Road to the old Tioga Road, this junction being 3.7 miles west of the trailhead parking area by the southwest shore of Tenaya Lake. Driving up the

Tioga Road, you will pass the following campgrounds, the first three along spur roads: Tamarack Flat, White Wolf, Yosemite Creek, and Porcupine Flat. At 3.2 miles past Porcupine Flat Campground, take the old Tioga Road, which is signed for May Lake, 1.75 miles northeast up to an obvious trailhead parking area.

Trail Description

The trail begins by the southwest side of a small pond on Snow Flat ▶1 in a moderately dense stand of hemlock, red fir, and western white and lodgepole pines. To the northwest is the peak that is at the geographic center of the park, Mt. Hoffmann. In a little vale to the east of the trail, water lies late in the season, permitting corn lilies to bloom into August and mosquitoes to thrive just as long. Your sandy trail ascends gently through forest cover, where you recognize western white pines by their long, narrow cones and checkerboard bark pattern, and red firs by the color of their bark and by their cones, which grow upright on the branches near the tops of these trees, unlike the hanging cones of pines and hemlocks.

The initial ascent leads up open granite slabs dotted with lodgepoles. Then, as you switchback west up a short, steep slope, you have fine views of Cathedral Peak in the east, Mt. Clark in the southeast, and Clouds Rest and Half Dome in the south. Near the top of the slope, the forest cover thickens and the western white pines become larger and more handsome. Just beyond the crest, you find

---

🚶 **MILESTONES**

▶1   0.0 Start at Snow Flat trailhead
▶2   1.2 May Lake

yourself in a flat beneath a half-dozen superb, large hemlocks by deep, chilly May Lake and a nearby High Sierra Camp. ▶2 Like at other High Sierra Camps, you'll find bear-proof food-storage boxes. Swimming is not allowed, but you may try your luck at catching the lake's brook or rainbow trout while contemplating the lake's beautiful backdrop of the east slopes of massive Mt. Hoffmann.

≋ **Lake**

▲ **Camping**

Mt. Hoffmann

OPTIONS

Perhaps more hikers ascend Mt. Hoffmann than any other 10,000+ peak in the park, with only Mt. Dana (Trail 5) challenging its popularity. As with any high-peak ascent, wear dark glasses and lots of sunscreen, for there is one-third less air on the summit, and the ultraviolet rays come on strong. Also, avoid altitude sickness, which is brought on by overexerting yourself, particularly after a large meal. If you are not in shape, camp overnight at May Lake to get partly acclimatized, then climb the peak the next day. Take it easy, for the route is short. However, abandon your attempt if a thunderstorm is approaching.

From May Lake's southeast corner, ▶2 you'll see a trail striking west. On it you pass a backpackers' camp that extends westward, and then you traverse across metasedimentary rocks cropping out above the lake's southwest shore. You now follow the trail south, first through a small gap, then through a boulder-strewn wildflower garden. You might lose the trail here, but the route south—up a shallow gully to a small, linear meadow—is quite obvious. From the meadow's south end, near a saddle, the trail goes 100 yards southwest and then climbs northwest up to the lower end of the broad, sloping, lupine-decked summit area. Numerous summits exist, but the western summit is the highest, at 10,850 feet, and you have an easy, safe scramble to its top. Using a topo map of the park, you can identify almost every major peak in it, since most are visible from here. When you return, don't be tempted to take any short cuts, since other routes are potentially dangerous.

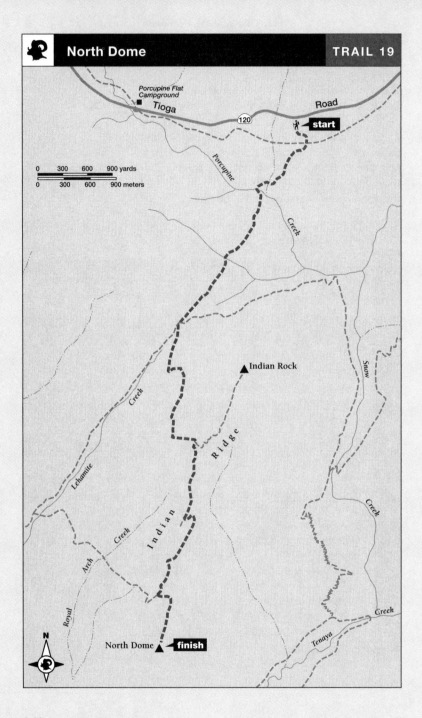

North Dome   TRAIL 19

Porcupine Flat
Campground
Tioga
120
Road

start

0   300   600   900 yards
0   300   600   900 meters

Porcupine

Creek

Indian Rock

Ridge

Snow

Creek

Creek

Lehamite

Creek

Indian

Creek

Arch

Royal

Creek

North Dome   finish

Tenaya

Creek

N

North Dome

North Dome, which looks so inaccessible from the Yosemite Valley floor, can be reached in a couple of hours by this route. From the dome you get perhaps the best views of the expansive faces of Half Dome and Clouds Rest, as well as excellent views of Yosemite Valley. Along this hike you can also visit one of Yosemite's few known natural arches. (Another one is, surprisingly, underwater, near Tuolumne Meadows Lodge.) Additionally, you can visit Indian Rock, which provides a 360-degree panorama of the valley's eastern uplands.

Best Time

Of trails above 8000 feet, this is one of the first to become mostly snow-free, and so you can take it as soon as early July. However, on the shady first 1.8 miles, mosquitoes may be prevalent through mid-July, decreasing afterward. If you do not care for mosquitoes, then hike from late July onward. The Tioga Road in this stretch usually is open through mid-October, and dayhiking until then is great. I prefer September after Labor Day, when trail use is light and temperatures are just about right, neither too hot nor too cold.

Finding the Trail

From Crane Flat drive northeast 23.7 miles up the Tioga Road to the Porcupine Flat Campground, then an additional 1.1 miles to a closed road, on your right. If you're westbound, the trailhead is 2.1 miles west of the May Lake turnoff. Driving up the Tioga

TRAIL USE
Dayhike, Backpack
LENGTH
9.2 miles, 3–6 hours
VERTICAL FEET
+680'/-1270'/±3900'
DIFFICULTY
- 1 2 **3** 4 5 +
TRAIL TYPE
Out & Back

FEATURES
Backcountry Permit
Streams
Wildflowers
Summit
Great Views
Camping
Swimming

FACILITIES
Restrooms

Stream

Road, you will pass the following campgrounds, the first three located along spur roads: Tamarack Flat, White Wolf, Yosemite Creek, and Porcupine Flat.

Trail Description

Through 1976 you could drive to primitive Porcupine Creek Campground, its road beginning at the west end of the trailhead parking strip. You could start there, where it is blocked off, or preferably start from a trailhead sign near the trailhead's outhouse. ▶1 From there a trail descends shortly to the nearby closed road. On it you descend 0.66 mile to Porcupine Creek. Porcupine Creek Campground, which closed in 1977, was alongside Porcupine Creek, which in early season can be a wet ford if you don't find a log to cross it. ▶2 From its west bank your trail makes a rolling traverse for a little over a mile to a junction atop a shady saddle dominated by red firs. ▶3 Through most of summer you may encounter creeks along this traverse, but the route ahead is dry, so carry water.

Just 20 yards beyond the crest of the saddle, the trail to North Dome reaches another junction, and here a trail forking right descends 1.6 miles down along Lehamite Creek to Yosemite Valley's north rim trail, up which you could ascend for an alternate route back to your trailhead. You fork left and traverse 0.33 mile to a spur ridge with a large boulder on it, then contour 0.33 mile, and drop to a gully before climbing steeply to a junction located only yards short of a second red-fir saddle. ▶4

OPTIONS

Indian Rock

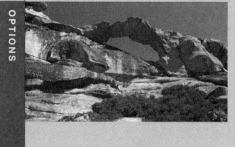

▶4 Veering left is a trail signed for Indian Rock. The trail actually climbs very steeply 0.25 mile up brushy slopes to a delicate arch, not a rock. About 1.5 feet thick at the thinnest part of its span, this 20-foot arch came into existence when the highly fractured rock beneath it broke away. After investigating this curious feature, which is quite easily reached from the northwest, you can return to the main route or continue north 0.5 mile up Indian Ridge to its north end, Indian Rock. This summit was one of the key points on the 1864 Yosemite Valley boundary. The summit area actually is two small—and I do mean small!—summits of nearly equal elevation. If you are uncomfortable with scrambling up short cliffs unroped, don't attempt either.

From the junction by the saddle the main trail descends briefly south, then follows Indian Ridge proper south, traversing across two low, broad ridge knolls before veering east off the now-descending ridge. While most folks take the trail, some merely walk down the view-blessed ridge. After about a 250-foot elevation loss, the trail heads southwest across ridge, from where the ridge-descenders join the trail.

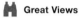 **Great Views**

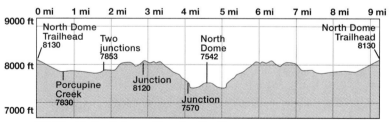

TRAIL 19 North Dome Elevation Profile

From the pine-shaded junction, ►5 all will turn left and take the half-mile spur trail out to the bald, rounded summit of North Dome. ►6 Be careful on the first part of this trail, for a slip on loose gravel could send you sliding down a dangerously steep slope. From the North Dome summit area, you can probably see more of Yosemite Valley and its adjacent uplands than can be seen from any other summit except Half Dome. (The views from about 200 yards south of and below the summit area are even better.) Rising from the floor of Tenaya Canyon is the enormous 4000-foot-high face of Clouds Rest, and to the south and west of it stands mighty Half

 Caution

	MILESTONES
►1	0.0 Start at North Dome trailhead
►2	0.7 Porcupine Creek
►3	1.8 Two close-spaced junctions, left at second
►4	2.9 Straight at junction
►5	4.1 Left at pine-shaded junction
►6	4.6 Summit of North Dome

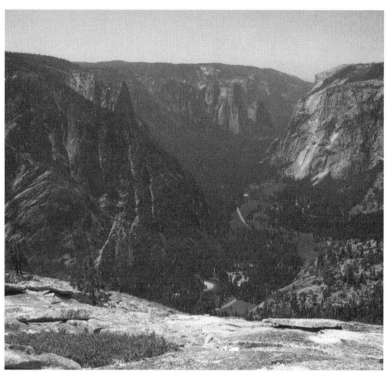

The view west from North Dome *includes Sentinel Rock (left) and El Capitan (right)*

Dome, perhaps Yosemite's best-remembered feature. Continuing your clockwise scan, you next recognize Mt. Starr King, a steep-sided dome above Little Yosemite Valley. West of this unseen valley is Panorama Cliff, and then Illilouette Fall. Glacier Point stands west of the fall's gorge, and above and right of the point, Sentinel Dome bulges up into the sky. Looking down Yosemite Valley you see Sentinel Rock, with its near-vertical north face. Opposite the rock stand the Three Brothers, and beyond them protrudes the brow of El Capitan, opposite the Cathedral Rocks.

Great Views

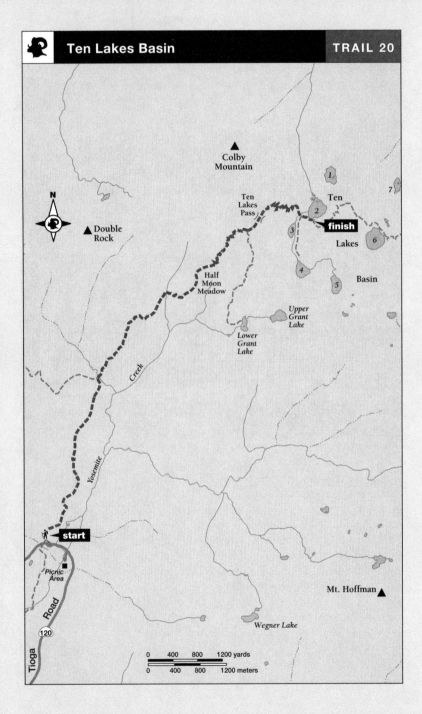

Colby
Mountain

1

7

Ten

2

Ten
Lakes
Pass

finish

3

N

Double
Rock

Lakes

6

Half
Moon
Meadow

4

5

Basin

Upper
Grant
Lake

Lower
Grant
Lake

Creek

Yosemite

start

Picnic
Area

Mt. Hoffman

Road

120

Tioga

Wegner Lake

| 0 | 400 | 800 | 1200 yards |
| 0 | 400 | 800 | 1200 meters |

Ten Lakes Basin

The Ten Lakes Basin is extremely popular with weekend backpackers, for with only a few hours' hiking effort you can attain any of its seven major lakes. The three most accessible receive moderate-to-heavy use, but the other four, off the beaten track, are worth the effort for those who want relatively secluded camping. These lakes plus the two Grant Lakes are situated at about 8950 to 9400 feet, making them subalpine. Still, at least the three lowest of the Ten Lakes Basin warm sufficiently for enjoyable midsummer swimming.

Best Time

Should you like swimming, visit these lakes from mid-July through early August. Be aware that mosquitoes tend to be prevalent at all lakes through July. The lakes are pleasant destinations through September, after the crowds leave, but nights and mornings will be chilly.

Finding the Trail

From Crane Flat drive northeast 19.66 miles up the Tioga Road to the trailhead parking area, on both sides of the highway, immediately before the highway bridges signed Yosemite Creek. Driving up the Tioga Road, you will pass the following campgrounds, all along spur roads: Tamarack Flat, White Wolf, and Yosemite Creek. There is a picnic area about 0.25 mile east of the trailhead parking area, and to the east is Porcupine Flat Campground.

TRAIL USE
Dayhike, Backpack, Horse
LENGTH
12.6 miles, 6 hours–2 days
VERTICAL FEET
+2330'/-880'/±6420'
DIFFICULTY
- 1 2 3 **4** 5 +
TRAIL TYPE
Out & Back

FEATURES
Backcountry Permit
Lakes
Streams
Wildflowers
Camping
Swimming
Secluded

FACILITIES
Restrooms
Picnic Tables

Trail Description

Ten Lakes Basin has only seven lakes; the two Grant Lakes plus another lake, all outside the basin, bring the total to ten.

▶ Stream

✳ Wildflowers

From the west end of the highway's north parking lot ▶1 a spur trail goes 90 yards northwest to the main trail, the Ten Lakes Trail. On it you hike up-canyon, first through a lodgepole-pine flat, then soon diverge from unseen Yosemite Creek and encounter Jeffrey pines, huckleberry oaks, and western junipers as you climb moderately but relatively briefly up to drier granitic slopes. The climb gives you views of Yosemite Creek canyon, Mt. Hoffmann, and the county-line crest north of it. Soon after these views the trail levels, enters a forest, and then, about 2.25 miles into your hike, reaches a creekside junction with a trail to White Wolf. ▶2 Its road, lodge, and campground lie 5.6 miles away.

From the junction you boulder-hop the creek and leave a nearby campsite to begin a moderate climb up a well-forested moraine left after the retreat of a large glacier about 15,000 years ago. Your climbing in a forest of red fir and western white pine ends atop a moraine, behind which lies crescentic, seasonally wet Half Moon Meadow. ▶3 The trail cuts across the meadow's relatively dry north edge, and at its northeast corner, about 4.5 miles from the trail-head, lies a campsite. The next stretch of ascent is steep and dry, so rest here and perhaps get a drink from the nearby creek.

Roughly three dozen short, steep switchbacks guide you about 0.75 mile up, almost to the Tuolumne/Mariposa county-line crest, from which you veer away to a junction with the Grant Lakes Trail, ▶4 a poorly designed trail heading 1.2 miles to lower Grant Lake, 6.5 miles from the trailhead.

From the trail junction, the Ten Lakes Trail climbs gently across a gravelly slope that can be covered in midsummer with large, deliciously scented lupines. These taper off just before you cross the county-line crest, Ten Lakes Pass. ▶5 Leaving the Merced River drainage, you enter the Tuolumne River drainage as you descend briefly north to a shallow saddle. Just beyond it is a small summit and to the left of it is flat-topped Colby Mountain, which crowns the west rim of the Ten Lakes Basin.

As you start a descent from the shallow saddle, a panorama of steep-sided, glaciated Ten Lakes Basin opens all around you, and three of the western lakes are clearly evident. On your descent of short switchbacks into Ten Lakes Basin, the trail veers north far enough for you to get partial views down into the upper part of the Grand Canyon of the Tuolumne River, which is so deep that you can't see the canyon bottom. Beyond the canyon you see park lands north to the Sierran crest.

The descent, which started close to some wind-blown whitebark pines growing on the county-line crest, ends at a creek that flows from Lake 3 to Lake 2. The presence here of hemlock and lodgepole together with lakeside red heather and Labrador tea indicates prime mosquito country—at least before August—and until then use a tent. Camping is quite enjoyable by early August, when the lakes are at their warmest temperatures, and also during September, after most hikers have left. It is then that the dwarf bilberry makes its thumb-size presence known by turning to a blazing crimson color.

 Lake

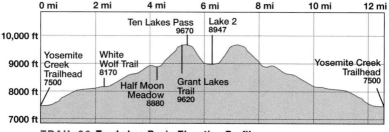

TRAIL 20 Ten Lakes Basin Elevation Profile

Ten Lakes Orientation

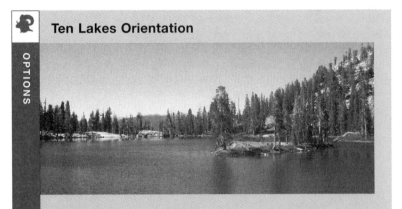

Ten Lakes Basin has seven prominent lakes that appear on the park's topographic map, and for the sake of easy reference, I refer to them by number, starting with the northwesternmost, **Lake 1** (above). I also give distances from the trailhead. Lake 1 (6.8 miles) is situated just west of and below Grand Mountain, a misnamed ridge. To its south is **Lake 2** (6.3 miles; right), ▶6 which, being the first lake one reaches as well as being the largest of the western lakes (just north of and below the trail), is the most popular. (The elevation changes mentioned at the start of this trip are to Lake 2; all other lakes involve additional elevation changes.) Not much south of and above the trail is **Lake 3** (6.3 miles), followed by **Lake 4** (6.8 miles). Continuing counterclockwise you head east up to **Lake 5** (7.3 miles), then northeast down to large, eastern **Lake 6** (7.7 miles), also popular because it is along the trail. North of the trail and considerably below it is **Lake 7** (8.0 miles). The popular Lakes 2 and 6 are also the largest, being, respectively, 21 and 24 acres in area. Lake 3 receives moderate use; Lake 1, lighter use; and Lakes 4, 5, and 7, very little use. All lakes have adjacent barren slopes or cliffs, making all photogenic.

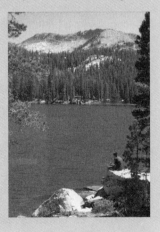

From a boulder-hop or log cross of the creek, you go just 80 yards east on the main trail to a use-trail branching south to Lakes 3 and 4, which will be described later. First, you are about 100 yards above **Lake 2**. To reach it, just head downslope to the lake. ►6 Several ample campsites exist on the broad, low ridge above the lake's west shore; more can be found along its west shore. East along its south shore are obvious diving rocks. From mid-July to mid-August, expect afternoon water temperatures to reach the mid- to high 60s. The northwest corner of the lake is almost cut off from the main part, and there are bedrock benches and small rock islands, and here is the warmest swimming, although it's mostly wadeable. This is a great lake for basking on rocks, but given its popularity, a poor one for fishing.

Just east of the outlet at the lake's north tip you may see a primitive trail climbing north-to-northeast toward Lake 1. This dies out amidst bedrock, along which you may find more than one ducked route. To reach **Lake 1**, just maintain a north-northeast bearing up to a minor gap in the crest, about 100 feet above Lake 2. (If you're heading north downward, you're on your way to a treacherous drop into the Grand Canyon of the Tuolumne River.) From the crest Lake 1 is in plain view, and you drop about 70 feet elevation to reach it in a couple of minutes. Lake 1 has a beautiful backdrop by the east cliff above it (the west side of Grand Mountain). Small camps exist on a bench beside the north shore, and from its edge you have tree-filtered views across the Grand Canyon. Lake 1 competes with Lake 7 as the warmest lake. Afternoon water temperatures can reach 70 degrees or more. You can dive into the lake from its northeast shore or from a linear island along the east shore, near good basking rocks.

From here you can reach **Lake 7**, about 0.6 mile to the east as the nutcracker flies, but walking you'll take about 1 mile. From the lake's southeast corner

You can expect Lake 2 to have as many campers as are at the other six lakes combined.

 Lake

 Caution

 Lake

head south up to the top of a minor ridge, then east up steep but safe treed slopes to a broad crest, then descend more or less due east 0.5 mile to the west shore of Lake 7. An easier way to reach it is from the main trail between Lakes 2 and 6. From the junction between Lakes 2 and 3, this trail climbs about 500 feet to a divide south of Grand Mountain, then drops southeast en route to Lake 6. Where the trail levels out just before Lake 6, just head downslope. Don't try to follow the outlet creek of Lake 6, since the slopes get steep along one stretch. Keep to its west, and where the gradient nearly flattens to zero, head east-northeast about 0.25 mile to Lake 7. This may be the least-visited lake. It is grass lined and may be the most mosquito prone. It is shallow and warm, good for swimming from basking slabs by its northeast shore. This lake rivals Lake 2 for camping area: there is about an acre of nearly flat land beyond the north shore, east of the outlet creek.

From the junction just above popular Lake 2, a fair number of hikers take the mile-long trail east up and then down and then up to Lake 6. Its northwest shore has quite a lot of flat land along it, a large camping area that can hold a couple dozen campers. It tends to be a bit cooler than Lake 2, but probably has better fishing, due to cooler water plus fewer anglers. From the west shore of this lake you have an easy cross-country hike southwest 0.5 mile to chilly Lake 5. (See directions in reverse just below.)

Back at the junction just above Lake 2, about 80 yards beyond the creek crossing, go just 0.1 mile south up a use-trail to reach the north end of Lake 3. Lakes 3, 4, and 5 are best for fishing, since they are coldest. **Lake 3** may have the most dramatic backdrop, since an impressive crest looms high above it. It also has good camping above its north shore, as well as small sites along its east shore. The

≋ Lake

≋ Lake

▲ Camping

use-trail continues south along the lake's east shore, then more or less follows the creek connecting Lakes 3 and 4. This part of the trail receives less use than the section below, and it becomes somewhat obscure about the last 200 yards before reaching **Lake 4**. Also dramatic, this lake is nestled in a very confining cirque. This lake probably is not popular because it is about 0.5 mile off the main trail, and this is seems for the better, given the minimal camping possibilities.

Lake

To reach **Lake 5** you go cross-country. I prefer heading more or less east directly upslope rather than following the winding creek, which saves about 0.25 mile of walking. Like Lake 4, Lake 5 is chilly and hemmed in. And like Lake 7, it is virtually unused, and so it may have great fishing. Look for minimal-sized campsites on gentler slopes high above the northeast shore. From this lake you make a relatively easy cross-country jaunt over to Lake 6. From the outlet you head north about 0.25 mile up to a lakelet, then about 250 yards northeast to a minor gap in the lower part of a northwest-trending ridge, then descend 0.25 mile northeast to the northwest shore of Lake 6, a large, eastern trailside lake.

Lake

Lake

🚶 **MILESTONES**

►1 0.0 Start at Yosemite Creek trailhead
►2 2.3 Straight at junction with trail to White Wolf
►3 4.3 Half Moon Meadow
►4 5.2 Straight at Grant Lakes Trail
►5 5.4 Ten Lakes Pass
►6 6.3 Lake 2

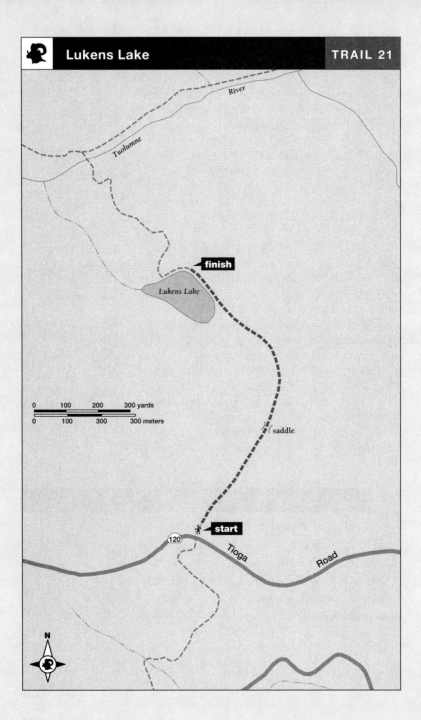

Lukens Lake

TRAIL 21

River

Tuolumne

finish

Lukens Lake

| 0 | 100 | 200 | 300 yards |
| 0 | 100 | 300 | 300 meters |

saddle

120 start

Tioga Road

N

Lukens Lake

This is the shorter approach to Lukens Lake, about one half the length of the trail east from White Wolf. No overnight camping is allowed.

Best Time

Should you like swimming, visit this lake from mid-July through early August. Be aware that mosquitoes tend to be prevalent through July, when wildflowers are at their best. Perhaps more come to fish than to swim, and then this lake is desirable through August and September. Being such an easy hike, this is a great one to introduce children to an off-road High Sierran lake.

Finding the Trail

From Crane Flat drive northeast 14.5 miles up the Tioga Road to the White Wolf turnoff, then continue an additional 1.9 miles to a paved turnout on the highway's south side. Driving up the Tioga Road, you will pass the following campgrounds, all along spur roads: Tamarack Flat, White Wolf, and Yosemite Creek. East beyond the road's crossing of Yosemite Creek is Porcupine Flat Campground.

Trail Description

From the Tioga Road turnout, ▶1 located in a shady gully near a curve in the highway, look for a signed trailhead on the north side of the road. Among red firs and western white pines, make an easy climb north to a viewless saddle, which the mighty

---

TRAIL USE
Dayhike, Run
LENGTH
2.2 miles, 1–2 hours
VERTICAL FEET
+170'/-130'/±600'
DIFFICULTY
- **1** 2 3 4 5 +
TRAIL TYPE
Out & Back

FEATURES
Child Friendly
Lake
Wildflowers
Swimming

FACILITIES
None

Lukens Lake was
named for Theodore
Parker Lukens, a
southern California
conservationist and
contemporary of
John Muir.

◢● Swimming

Tuolumne River glaciers failed to top. On the fairly open bedrock slope ascending west from the saddle are scattered rocks, collectively a lag deposit, a feature rare in this area.

Leaving the saddle, ►2 you make an equally easy descent to the southeast end of a sedge-dominated meadow that also contains conspicuous corn lilies and, as usual, willows. From this meadow's corner the main trail strikes 0.2 mile northwest toward the north shore of Lukens Lake ►3, while a lesser trail—one of use—strikes west toward its south shore. Most folks stick to the main trail and continue to the lake's north shore.

Like Harden Lake (next hike), it is one of the Sierra's rare moraine-dammed lakes. Unlike Harden, Lukens has trout—rainbow, brook, and brown—and it tends to have a grassy bottom, not a bouldery one. Also unlike Harden, the moraine dam here is sufficiently thick to prevent serious leakage, so Lukens's water level does not drop dramatically, as does Harden's. This makes Lukens Lake a good swimming lake, especially with its grassy bottom. No toe-stubbing here.

🚶 MILESTONES

►1	0.0	Start at Lukens Lake trailhead
►2	0.4	Saddle
►3	1.1	Lukens Lake

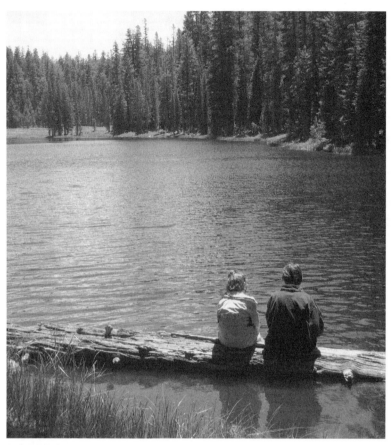

Lukens Lake

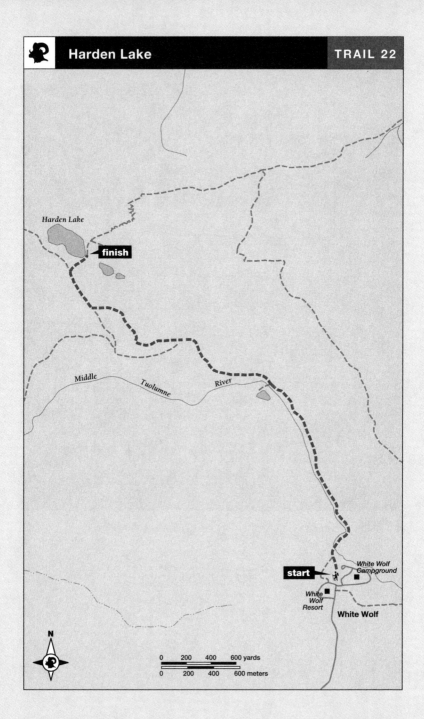

Harden Lake

TRAIL 22

Harden Lake

finish

Middle Tuolumne River

start

White Wolf Campground

White Wolf Resort

White Wolf

N

0   200   400   600 yards
0   200   400   600 meters

Harden Lake

Only about an hour's hike from White Wolf Campground, this lake attracts quite a number of summer visitors, virtually all of them dayhikers, although one could camp near Harden Lake. From mid-June through July this shallow lake can be fine for swimming, but the lake lies in a leaky basin, and by mid-August it usually has dwindled to an oversized wading pool. Don't expect to catch any fish, since the lake becomes far too shallow by late summer to support any.

Best Time

For warm swimming at this relatively low lake, at 7484 feet elevation, visit it from mid-June through July. Be forewarned that mosquitoes may be prevalent along the route before early July, although usually are not much of a problem by the lake. Whereas you could hike to the lake even through much of October, it isn't worth the effort, since later on you won't see a lake. September does provide great fall colors, particularly with the aspens and bracken ferns, but no lake. Joggers may find September and October best, due to cooler temperatures.

Finding the Trail

From Crane Flat drive northeast 14.5 miles up the Tioga Road to the White Wolf turnoff and follow that road down to where it is closed to motor vehicles, just past the entrance to White Wolf Campground. Other campgrounds worth considering are Tamarack Flat, along a spur road, and

TRAIL USE
Dayhike, Backpack,
Run, Horse
LENGTH
5.6 miles, 2–4 hours
VERTICAL FEET
+90'/-480'/±1140'
DIFFICULTY
- 1 **2** 3 4 5 +
TRAIL TYPE
Out & Back

FEATURES
Backcountry Permit
Child Friendly
Lake
Streams
Wildflowers
Camping
Swimming
Autumn Colors

FACILITIES
Resort
Restrooms
Campground
Phone
Water
Horse Staging

Except when Harden Lake is at its highest level, it is usually shallow enough to wade across. Bathers, if they are careless, could scrape their feet on the lake's many submerged glacier-transported boulders.

Yosemite Creek, also along a spur road. East beyond the Tioga Road's crossing of Yosemite Creek is Porcupine Flat Campground.

Trail Description

Your route, a closed road, ▶1 bridges the infant Middle Tuolumne River in under 0.5 mile, then parallels its sometimes splashing course down unglaciated granitic terrain, which sustains a healthy stand of lodgepole pines. After 1.2 miles of easy descent along your road, you come to a closed spur road that goes to a sewage-treatment pond. Over the next 0.6 mile your road first climbs over a low ridge of glacial deposits before dipping into a shady alcove of lodgepole pines and red firs that has a trail junction. ▶2

You take the trail, which branches right and then traverses the slope of a large glacial moraine. The well-drained sediments of this moraine support a different plant community than your generally rocky-road descent, and on this moraine grows a forest of Jeffrey pines together with some firs and aspens. Thousands of bracken ferns seek the forest shade together with chinquapins, the bushes with spiny, seed-bearing spheres. Seeking the sun are snow bushes, which have spine-tipped branches. In 0.75 mile your trail ends at the Harden Lake road. ▶3 This formerly maintained road leaves the main road about 0.5 mile west of your trail junction. The main road parallels the Middle Tuolumne River

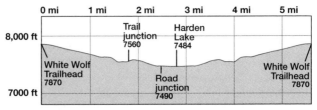

TRAIL 22 Harden Lake Elevation Profile

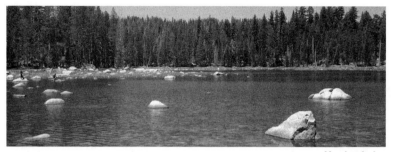

Harden Lake

almost the whole distance of 8 miles to Aspen Valley, which is a private inholding that once was the west entrance to Yosemite National Park. Today, that gently graded road is a pleasant riverside stroll for those looking for a lightly used creekside excursion or for distance running.

Those on the last part of the Harden Lake road walk across relatively flat glacial sediments, passing a seasonally flowery meadow midway along this short traverse to a gravelly junction with a trail to Pate Valley. You branch right, northeast, on the trail, and in a minute's time arrive near the southwest corner of Harden Lake. ▶4

≋ **Lake**

Seasonal Harden Lake has a rather uncommon origin, for it occupies a small depression that formed between two lateral moraines. Most Sierran lakes have existed for only 13,000–16,000 years, but Harden could have originated earlier. This warm, shallow, 9-acre lake has no surface inlet or outlet, and not long after adjacent snow patches melt, the lake's level begins to drop, making it too shallow for trout.

⌁• **Swimming**

🚶 **MILESTONES**

▶1   0.0   Start at White Wolf trailhead
▶2   1.8   Right on to trail
▶3   2.5   Right on Harden Lake road
▶4   2.8   Harden Lake

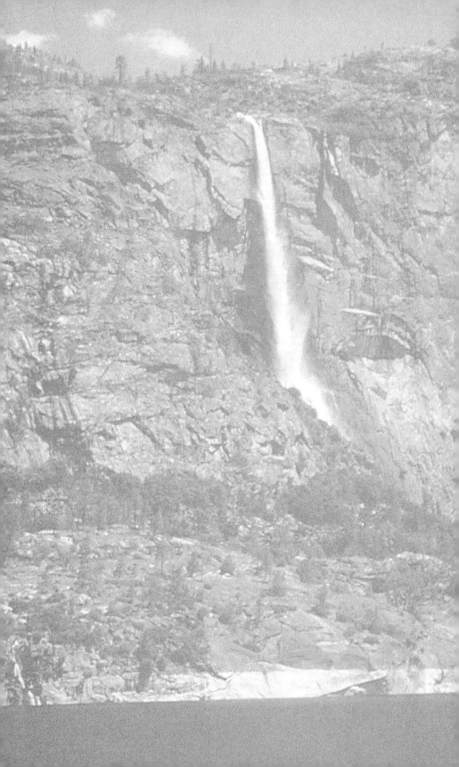

Northwest Yosemite

Northwest Yosemite

Of all this guide's chapters, this is the only one that lacks a prominent, nearby peak, such as Mt. Hoffmann or Mt. Dana, or summit, such as Clouds Rest or Half Dome. It is chiefly a heavily forested uplands landscape of rolling, gentle topography clothed in mostly viewless pines and firs. However, along this land's southern perimeter, the slopes end in steep-walled cliffs that make up the north wall of Yosemite Valley. Lacking alpine scenery, the backcountry trails in this section should get only light-to-moderate use. However, all but Trail 27 are heavily used. Why? Because there are several prized goals. The first, Kibbie Lake, lies just within the park and is reached by a hike through the southernmost sliver of Emigrant Wilderness. The northwest and west lands of the park contain dozens of lakes and ponds, these lightly visited simply because of the several days' effort required to reach them and then return to a trailhead.

Two popular lakes are Laurel Lake and Lake Vernon, and backpackers in good shape can visit both in a weekend. These are mid-sized lakes, each with abundant campsites. These are reached by starting across a dam that has flooded Hetch Hetchy Valley, which is second only to Yosemite Valley as the Sierra's most impressive U-shaped canyon. Along the north slopes of Hetch Hetchy Reservoir is a popular trail that takes you past vernal Tueeulala Falls to perennial Wapama Falls, whose voluminous water roars in May and June and soaks hikers with its spray. Later on, the falls still put on an impressive show. The trail, nearly flat to here, eastward to Rancheria Falls Camp, a popular, spacious backcountry campground beside cascades and pools of Rancheria Creek.

South of Hetch Hetchy Valley the lakes disappear and the forests, except where burned, prevail. On these lands are two groves of giant sequoias, the Tuolumne Grove, just off the start of the Tioga Road at Crane Flat, and the Merced Grove, a few miles west of Crane Flat and south from the Big Oak Flat Road. I've included only the popular Tuolumne Grove because the closed road to it is shorter, and because it has dozens of giant sequoias, some of them very impressive.

Overleaf: *Tueeulala and Wapama falls*

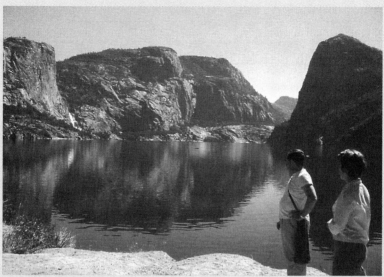

Hetch Hetchy Reservoir *(Trail 25)*

Finally, just as the previous chapter offers an easy route to the summit of North Dome (as opposed to scaling it from the floor of Yosemite Valley) this chapter offers a relatively easy route to the summit of El Capitan. Okay, it is a bit lengthy, especially as a dayhike, but it is a lot easier than scaling the face of "El Cap," as you climbers call it.

Permits

If you want to reserve a permit, rather than get one in person, see the "Fees, Camping, and Permits" section on page 14.

In person, if you're following Trail 23 you should get your permit at the Groveland Ranger District Office on Highway 120 about 8 miles out of Groveland. Also, you can phone them at (209) 962-7825 no more than 24 hours before you start your hike to see if the trailhead quota has been filled. For Trails 24 and 25, use either the Information Station at the park's Big Oak Flat Entrance Station, or use the Hetch Hetchy Entrance Station, by the Mather Ranger Station. The latter is open from about early April through late October. I recommend Trail 25 as a dayhike, and certainly Trail 26, down to the Tuolumne Grove, is day use only. The same goes for Trail 27, which rambles over to the top of El Capitan. However, if you do backpack to it, then you will need a permit, which can be obtained at the Big Oak Flat Entrance Station or down in Yosemite Valley at its Wilderness Center, centrally located in Yosemite Village.

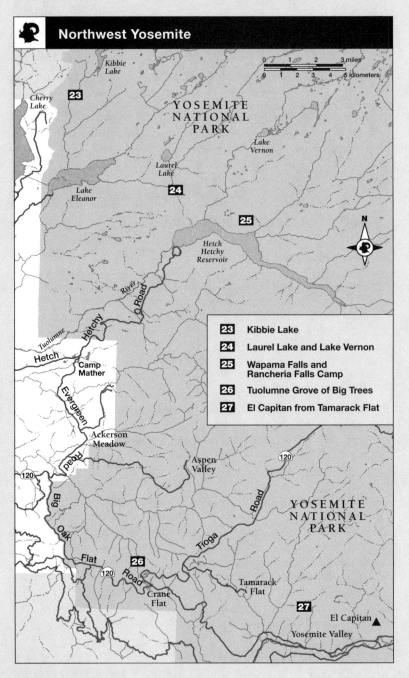

Northwest Yosemite

Kibbie
Lake

Cherry
Lake

23

YOSEMITE
NATIONAL
PARK

0   1   2   3 miles
0 1 2 3 4 5 kilometers

Lake
Vernon

Laurel
Lake

Lake
Eleanor

24

25

N

Hetch
Hetchy
Reservoir

Tuolumne

River

Hetch
Hetchy

Road

Hetch

Camp
Mather

Evergreen

Road

Ackerson
Meadow

Aspen
Valley

120

23 Kibbie Lake

24 Laurel Lake and Lake Vernon

25 Wapama Falls and
       Rancheria Falls Camp

26 Tuolumne Grove of Big Trees

27 El Capitan from Tamarack Flat

120

Big

Oak

Flat

26

120

Road

Crane
Flat

Tioga

Road

YOSEMITE
NATIONAL
PARK

Tamarack
Flat

27

El Capitan ▲

Yosemite Valley

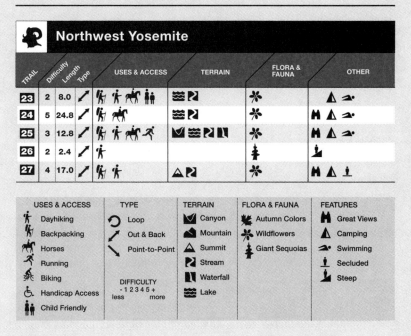

Northwest Yosemite

TRAIL	Difficulty	Length	Type	USES & ACCESS	TERRAIN	FLORA & FAUNA	OTHER
23	2	8.0	↗	🚶🏃🐎👫	≋ ⤴	✳	⛰ ⤳
24	5	24.8	↗	🚶🐎	≋ ⤴	✳	🔭 ⛰ ⤳
25	3	12.8	↗	🚶🏃🐎🏃	◣ ≋ ⤴ ▌	✳	🔭 ⛰ ⤳
26	2	2.4	↗	🚶		🌲	⚓
27	4	17.0	↗	🚶🏃	▲ ⤴	✳	🔭 ⛰ ⚓

USES & ACCESS	TYPE	TERRAIN	FLORA & FAUNA	FEATURES
🚶 Dayhiking	↻ Loop	◣ Canyon	✿ Autumn Colors	🔭 Great Views
🏃 Backpacking	↗ Out & Back	◤ Mountain	✳ Wildflowers	⛰ Camping
🐎 Horses	↘ Point-to-Point	▲ Summit	🌲 Giant Sequoias	⤳ Swimming
🏃 Running		⤴ Stream		⚓ Secluded
🚴 Biking	DIFFICULTY	▌ Waterfall		⬇ Steep
♿ Handicap Access	- 1 2 3 4 5 + less more	≋ Lake		
👫 Child Friendly				

Maps

For the Northwest Yosemite country, here are the USGS 7.5-minute (1:24,000 scale) topographic quadrangles that you will need, listed in the order that you will need them as you hike along your route. Quadrangles in parentheses are for suggested side trips that go off the quadrangles that you need for the principal hike. In addition, most of Trail 27 appears on the USGS Yosemite Valley 1:24,000 topographic map.

    Trail 23: Cherry Lake North, Kibbie Lake
    Trail 24: Lake Eleanor, Kibbie Lake, Tiltill Mountain,
           (Hetch Hetchy Reservoir)
    Trail 25: Lake Eleanor, Hetch Hetchy Reservoir
    Trail 26: Ackerson Mountain
    Trail 27: Tamarack Flat, El Capitan

Northwest Yosemite

Were it not for the long drive to the trailhead, Kibbie Lake would be a popular dayhike. At 4.0 miles distance and only about 700 feet between its trail's high and low points, Kibbie Lake is a good choice for beginning backpackers. Being the lowest natural lake reached by trail in and around the Yosemite National Park environs, it is one of the warmest, and is great for summer swimming. Not only is this the lowest natural lake, it is one of the largest in the park. Therefore, while it can be popular with weekend summer backpackers, there is plenty of shoreline on which to establish secluded camps.

This relatively low-elevation loop, a good early-summer conditioner, visits two fairly large lakes—Laurel and Vernon—both good rainbow-trout fisheries. These two lakes are popular on summer weekends, and most hikers go no farther. At 6490 feet in elevation, Laurel Lake is the lowest of any large natural lake in the park that is reached by trail, and it provides relatively warm swimming. Lake Vernon, at 6564 feet in elevation, is a bit higher; furthermore, you cross a low ridge and then drop 400 feet to the lake. This is a more aesthetic lake, and it has plenty of slabs great for sunbathing, especially for warming up after a swim.

Wapama Falls and Rancheria Falls Camp 213

A stately grove of pines and incense-cedars harboring a spacious camping area near Rancheria Falls marks the terminus of this hike. Its cascades and pools are the goals for some, but also rewarding are inspirational vistas of the awesome cliffs and two waterfalls, Tueeulala and Wapama, seen along the undulating path on the north wall of Hetch Hetchy Reservoir. Since you are traversing above a reservoir, you might think that this is an easy hike. Well, it basically is easy to Wapama Falls, but then you face gains and losses of hundreds of feet. Also, the route, being quite open and at a relatively low elevation, can be quite sunny and hot, and so on a summer's day it is best begun in early morning.

TRAIL 25

Dayhike, Backpack, Run, Horse
12.8 miles, Out & Back
Difficulty: 1 2 **3** 4 5

Tuolumne Grove of Big Trees 219

The Tuolumne Grove has over a dozen trees at least 10 feet in diameter near the base, and although this pales in comparison with the much larger Mariposa Grove's approximately 200 trees of similar or larger size, you'll certainly see fewer tourists and no trams. In the Tuolumne Grove, a few trees reach about 15 feet in diameter, the largest being about 10 feet short of the diameter of the Mariposa Grove's Grizzly Giant.

TRAIL 26

Dayhike
2.4 miles, Out & Back
Difficulty: 1 **2** 3 4 5

El Capitan from Tamarack Flat 223

The vertical walls of 3000-foot-high El Capitan attract rock climbers from all over the world, and more than five dozen extremely difficult routes ascend it. For nonclimbers this hike provides a much easier, safer way to attain El Capitan's summit, which stands only 15 feet above the northside approach.

TRAIL 27

Dayhike, Backpack, Horse
17.0 miles, Out & Back
Difficulty: 1 2 3 **4** 5

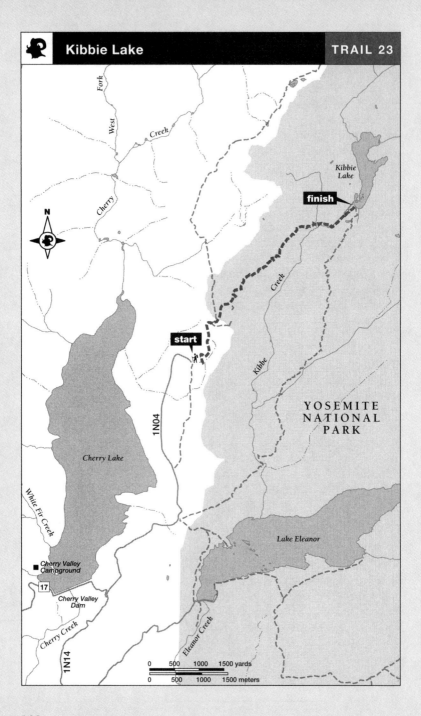

Kibbie Lake

Were it not for the long drive to the trailhead, Kibbie Lake would be a popular dayhike. At 4 miles distance and only about 700 feet between its trail's high and low points, Kibbie Lake is a good choice for beginning backpackers. Being the lowest natural lake reached by trail in and around the Yosemite National Park environs, it is one of the warmest, and is great for swimming from about mid-June through August. Not only is this the lowest natural lake, it is one of the largest in the park, measuring barely under 1 mile in length. Therefore, while it can be popular with weekend summer backpackers, there is plenty of shoreline on which to establish secluded camps.

Best Time

Situated at 6513 feet elevation, Kibbie Lake can be virtually snow-free by the Memorial Day weekend, and some hikers may try to beat the summer crowds by going to it by that weekend or in June. July and August are best, with a minimum of mosquitoes and a maximum of summer temperatures, great for basking and swimming. With September come cooler temperatures but also fewer backpackers, so solitude increases through the weeks of September. With the start of hunting season in late September, you must park down by the reservoir, making the hike not worth the effort unless you want serious solitude.

TRAIL USE
Dayhike, Backpack, Horse

LENGTH
8.0 miles,
3 hours–2 days

VERTICAL FEET
+1000'/-360'/±2720'

DIFFICULTY
- 1 **2** 3 4 5 +

TRAIL TYPE
Out & Back

FEATURES
Backcountry Permit
Child Friendly
Wildflowers
Lakes
Streams
Camping
Swimming
Secluded

FACILITIES
Campground
Horse Staging

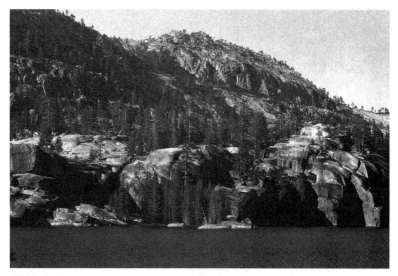

Kibbie Lake

Finding the Trail

From Groveland drive east 13.6 miles on Tioga Road to paved Cherry Road 1N07, also known as Forest Route 17, starting just beyond the highway bridge over South Fork Tuolumne River. (A spur road right, immediately before the bridge, leads briefly down to the popular Rainbow Pool day-use area—a refreshing spot to visit after your hike.) Take F. R. 17 5.3 miles to a junction with paved Hetch Hetchy Road, also known as F. R. 12, and branch left. Still on F. R. 17, go 17.6 miles to Cottonwood Road 1N04. The signed Cherry Dam parking area is just yards east down this road. You'll find the Cherry Valley Campground along a road that traverses over to Cherry Lake's southeast shore.

While you could start your hike from the parking area, most people would prefer to save 4.3 trail miles and a 1200-foot ascent by starting at a newer trailhead. To reach it, drive across Cherry Valley

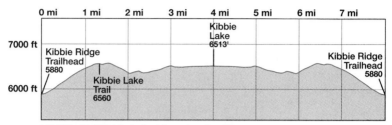

TRAIL 23 Kibbie Lake Elevation Profile

Dam, then continue 0.5 mile beyond it to a **T** junction with Road 1N45Y. Turn left, north, up this good road, then down, in the next 2.0 miles passing a succession of signed trailheads and parking lots for, respectively, Lake Eleanor, Kibbie Creek–Flora Lake, and old Kibbie Ridge trails. Onward, the road climbs alongside Kibbie Ridge, just a short distance below the old trail. Three switchbacks eventually lead up to the trail at a dead-end at 5880 feet.

Trail Description

From the road's end, ▶1 you start on a spur trail that leads east-northeast uphill to the nearby Kibbie Ridge Trail. Just about a minute's walk down this main trail is Shingle Spring, with beautiful dogwoods and nearby camps. However, you take the main route north, gaining about 400 feet in elevation as it first climbs to a descending ridge and then curves east into cooler, forested Deadhorse Gulch. Just past its upper end you reach the main ridge and, in a conifer grove beside a small grass-choked pond, 1.25 miles into your hike, meet the 2.7-mile-long Kibbie Lake Trail. ▶2

Skirting this pond, the Kibbie Lake Trail nears a ridgetop open space, then it quickly enters Yosemite National Park and drops into a small canyon. Next you head north through a sodden bottom land, passing the first lodgepole pines of your trip, which

▲ Camping

 Wildflowers

Kibbie Lake is named
for pioneer H. G.
Kibbie, who
constructed small
cabins in the Lake
Eleanor vicinity, at
Tiltill Meadow, and on
Rancheria Mountain.

▲ Camping

≋ Lake

▲ Camping

➤• Swimming

here, accompanied by white firs, form a dense canopy. Wildflowers thrive in the shadows, enticing the traveler to linger in coolness. Before July, mosquitoes will no doubt urge you on!

The trail leaves the forest, climbing northeast onto granitic slabs mottled by huckleberry oaks to a 6500-foot saddle. The rocky route next descends to cross a tributary of Kibbie Creek under a south-facing dome; then you closely parallel pools on Kibbie Creek. You pass a good camp on the right, and, just yards later, before a poorer trail climbs up to the right of a granitic outcrop to continue over slabs to the west shore of Kibbie Lake, your route angles down to a 30-foot rock-hop of Kibbie Creek. Across the ford, among lodgepoles, is a very good camp. The trail turns upstream, climbing over blasted granitic ledges, the route indicated by rock ducks.

After passing lagoons presaging 106-acre, 6513-foot-high Kibbie Lake, you reach its south shore, where camps are found in a lodgepole-and-Labrador-tea fringe. ▶3 Kibbie Lake is bounded on the west by gently sloping granite, while the east shore is characterized by steep, broken bluffs and polished bosses. Therefore, to find secluded camping, traverse north along the west shore, which offers many opportunities. The relatively warm lake is mostly shallow, with an algae-coated sandy bottom, where distinctively orange-colored California newts may take your bait if a rainbow trout doesn't. Especially along its west shore there are many spots for swimming, sunbathing, and fishing.

🚶 MILESTONES

▶1   0.0   Start at Kibbie Ridge trailhead

▶2   1.3   Kibbie Lake Trail

▶3   4.0   Kibbie Lake

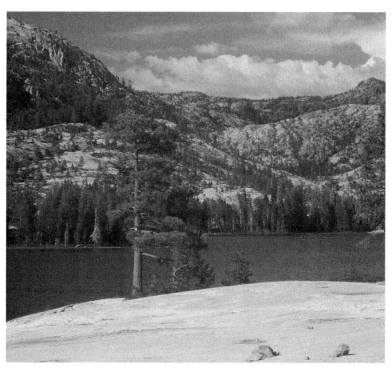

Lake Vernon *(Trail 24)*

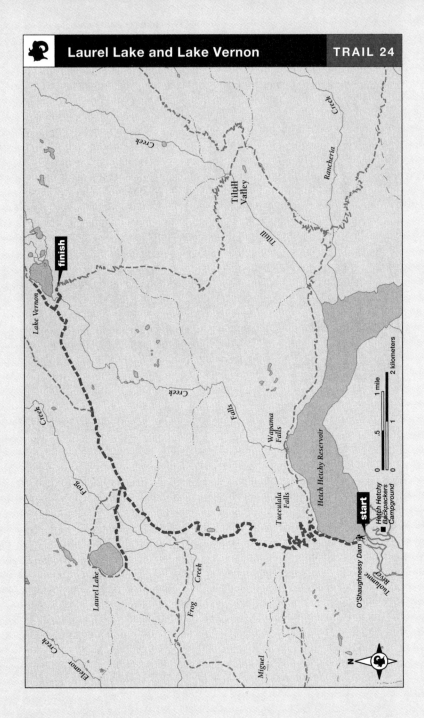

Laurel Lake and Lake Vernon

This relatively low-elevation loop, a good early-summer conditioner, visits two fairly large lakes—Laurel and Vernon—both good rainbow-trout fisheries. If you hike only to Laurel Lake, you go only 8.4 miles, and your total elevation gain and loss will be about 6680 feet. If you hike only to Lake Vernon, you go only 10.6 miles, and the elevation gain and loss will be about 8400 feet. These two lakes are popular on summer weekends, and most hikers go no farther. At 6490 feet in elevation, Laurel Lake is the lowest of any large natural lake in the park that is reached by trail, and it provides relatively warm swimming. Being lower, this conifer-ringed lake lacks the inspiring scenery of the park's higher lakes. But in compensation, there are many campsites above its lengthy shore, these allowing for secluded camping even when others are present. Lake Vernon, at 6564 feet in elevation, is a bit higher; furthermore, you cross a low ridge and then drop 400 feet to the lake. This is a more aesthetic lake, and it has plenty of slabs great for sunbathing, especially for warming up after a swim.

Best Time

The trails up to both lakes are mostly snow-free by late June, but mosquitoes can linger well into July. Generally mid-July through early August is prime time, when lakes are at their maximum temperatures for swimming. Non-swimmers might plan for a September hike, after most of the hikers have left, and for solitude, the first half of October is even better, although nights and mornings can dip below

---

TRAIL USE
Backpack, Horse

LENGTH
24.8 miles, 2–3 days

VERTICAL FEET
+3860'/1100'/±9160'

DIFFICULTY
- 1 2 3 4 **5** +

TRAIL TYPE
Out & Back

FEATURES
Backcountry Permit
Lakes
Streams
Wildflowers
Great Views
Camping
Swimming

FACILITIES
Restrooms
Campground
Water

freezing. An advantage of hiking in these two months is the long ascent, which can be hot in summer, is a lot more bearable.

Finding the Trail

Just 0.6 mile before the Park's boundary below the Big Oak Flat Entrance Station, leave Tioga Road and drive north 7.5 miles on Evergreen Road to its junction with the Hetch Hetchy Road. Turn right and go 1.3 miles to the Hetch Hetchy Entrance Station/Mather Ranger Station. From the station, drive 7.1 miles to a junction branching left for the Hetch Hetchy Backpacker Campground. Backpackers turn here, park in the obvious parking area by the road's start, then walk 0.5 mile on the road to O'Shaughnessy Dam. Dayhikers continue driving 0.7 mile past the junction to the dam, beyond which is its trailhead parking. If you are just dayhiking and want to stay in a relatively nearby campground, the only one is the Dimond O Campground along the Evergreen Road.

Logistics

Because of a perceived threat of terrorists (foreign? local enviros?) wanting to destroy O'Shaughnessy Dam, road use is restricted. Day-use hours are from 7 a.m. to 5 p.m., and the gate at the station is locked at night. Although I was told that the gate is locked around 9 p.m., you ought to play it safe and try to exit past the station by 5 p.m. Should you fall behind schedule and find yourself exiting late and finding the gate is locked, you could try walking 1.3 miles along the road to Camp Mather to seek help, but don't count on getting it.

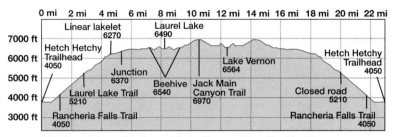

TRAIL 24 Laurel Lake and Lake Vernon Elevation Profile

Trail Description

Backpackers, starting from their parking area, will add 1 mile to their round-trip distance. Summer hikers should start early in the morning, since the switchbacking route up from the reservoir is only partly shaded, and temperatures can reach into the 90s by noon. Carry sufficient water; in late season it's two or more hours before you come to water.

You begin by starting across the top of O'Shaughnessy Dam (3814 feet) at Hetch Hetchy Reservoir. ▶1 On the south wall, the prow of Kolana Rock soars 2000 feet above the reservoir, while to its north, tiered Hetch Hetchy Dome rises about 400 feet higher. In a shaded cleft on the dome's west flank, two-stepped Wapama Falls plunges an aggregate of 1400 feet. In early summer its gossamer companion, Tueeulala Falls, glides down steep slabs farther west.

Across the 600-foot-long dam, you enter a 500-foot-long tunnel blasted through solid granite when the original dam was raised 85 feet in 1938. Emerging from this bat haven, the formerly paved road traverses above the rocky west shore of Hetch Hetchy Reservoir in a pleasant grove of Douglas-fir, gray pine, big-leaf maple, and bay trees. One mile into your route, you reach the Rancheria Falls Trail (Trail 25), branching right, just before your route's first switchback. ▶2

Keeping to the former road, you ascend moderately steep switchbacks and have better views up the reservoir of LeConte Point and the Grand Canyon of the Tuolumne River.

As you ascend, fairly open, lower slopes give way to oak-shaded slopes, then near the top to oak-and-conifer-shaded ones. The last of eight switchbacks swings north into a gully with a trail junction on a small flat, where you leave the closed road. ►3 With one-third of the distance covered and with half of the elevation gain under your belt, you start up a trail through a partly burned conifer forest. In 0.25 mile you reach a mile-high creeklet which, although diminutive, usually flows through the summer. This is your first reliable water, and people have camped hereabouts. Up the trail about 200 yards past the creeklet, and about 3.2 miles from the trailhead, you'll see a shallow gully on your right, which is the start of a relatively easy 1.5-mile-long cross-country route east to the brink of Wapama Falls.

▲ Camping

Unlike the closed road you ascended, which maintains a nearly constant grade, your ascending trail varies, being locally steep, moderate, gentle, or even briefly down. You'll eventually climb 1000 feet above the creeklet before the serious climbing ends. About 0.5 mile beyond the creeklet, your trail curves east and levels off, and you may want to rest. Ahead the trail climbs north, then northwest, and then the serious climbing ends with a curve east to cross a crest of a lateral moraine. On this ascent look for linear deposits, which too are lateral moraines. Once on top, 4.6 miles into your hike, take a break; you deserve it.

Your hike ahead is now relatively easy. After rounding the linear lakelet's ►4 east end, the trail crosses the broad moraine's crest, drops momentarily, and then ascends 0.4 mile through an open white-fir forest to a junction with a southwest-

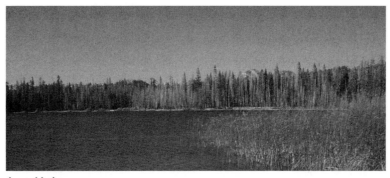

Laurel Lake

descending trail. ▶5 Laurel Lake, though only 0.75 mile northwest of you, is at least 2.5 trail miles away by either trail you can take, and one wonders why a trail was not built directly to it. If you've not found water so far, take the trail southwest 0.25 mile down to reliable Frog Creek. Rather than ascend back up to the junction, you might ascend first along the west side of the creek, then along the west side of the lake's outlet creek.

From your junction, follow the often shady trail northeast, dip to cross a bracken-bordered creeklet, then soon hike alongside a linear meadow, which in season is profuse with wildflowers. The meadow pinches off at a low gap, beyond which you quickly find yourselves in the southwest corner of a triangular meadow. Staying among white firs and lodgepole pines, you parallel the meadow's edge northeast over to its east corner, called the Beehive, the site of an 1880s cattlemen's camp, where there is a trail junction. ▶6 About 20 yards before it, just within the meadow, is a usually reliable spring. Just beyond the junction, among trees, is a spacious campsite.

 Wildflowers

 Camping

With most of your ascent behind you, you turn left and walk northwest 160 yards on the Laurel Lake Trail to reach a trail split. ▶7 Here a path that loops around Laurel Lake's north shore branches north, while a shorter trail to the lake's outlet strikes west. Following this latter route, you keep left and drop easily down into a gully and then broad Frog Creek, which could be a wet ford in early season. Along its north bank you contour west briefly, then ascend steeply to a heavily forested ridge before gently dropping to good camps near Laurel Lake's outlet. ▶8 A brief stint brings you to a junction with the north-shore loop trail, branching northwest to the best campsites (and more-secluded ones beyond). At fairly deep 60-acre Laurel Lake, western azalea grows thickly just back of the locally grassy lakeshore, a fragrant accompaniment to huckleberry and thimbleberry. Fishing is fair for rainbow trout, but swimming, especially in July and early August, can be wonderful.

After your stay at the lake, return to the Beehive junction. ▶9 Now take the eastbound Lake Vernon Trail, which winds 1.5 miles easily up to a moraine-crest junction with the left-branching Jack Main Canyon Trail, just below the slightly higher crest of Moraine Ridge. ▶10 From the junction you descend to an open, granite bench. Now on bedrock, you follow a well-ducked trail down past excellent examples of glacier-smoothed rock—glacier polished and glacier-transported boulders—glacier erratics. Along this section you can look across the far wall of Falls Creek canyon until a nearby minor outlier, 0.5 mile southwest of Lake Vernon, obstructs your view, about 1.25 miles from the last junction. Just after this happens, you angle southeast and follow a winding, ducked route up toward the point, but cross a low ridge just north of it. Now below you lies spreading Lake Vernon on a broad, flat-floored canyon.

 Camping

Lake

Swimming

From this inspirational ridge you descend generally northeast and in 0.33 mile reach a junction
with a spur trail. Leaving a small flat with a few
nearby aspens among Jeffrey pines, this trail shoots
northeast. After 0.25 mile of walking, you'll be close
to the shore of the unseen lake, and you can head
southeast to it. There you'll find a fairly large campsite among lodgepoles. Other campsites lie along
this northwest shore of Lake Vernon. ▶11 The trail
continues past a snow-gauge marker and adjacent
park cabin, then dies out about a mile past the lake,
by a large camp close to where the creek angles from
northeast to north and its gradient increases dramatically.

 Camping

Rather than take the Lake Vernon Trail, you can
take the main trail southeast briefly to a bridge
across Falls Creek, just below the lake, and then
equally briefly northeast around a bedrock slope to
Lake Vernon's southwest shore. Additional campsites are found near it. The lake, mostly shallow and
lying at about 6564 feet, is one of the warmer park
lakes for swimming.

 Lake

Swimming

🚶	**MILESTONES**
▶1	0.0 Start at Hetch Hetchy trailhead
▶2	1.0 Rancheria Falls Trail
▶3	2.8 Right on to trail at small flat
▶4	4.6 Linear lakelet
▶5	5.3 Straight at southwest-descending trail
▶6	7.2 Left at Beehive junction
▶7	7.3 Left at split
▶8	8.2 Laurel Lake
▶9	9.2 Left at Beehive junction
▶10	10.5 Right at Jack Main Canyon Trail junction
▶11	12.4 Lake Vernon
▶12	24.8 Return to Hetch Hetchy trailhead

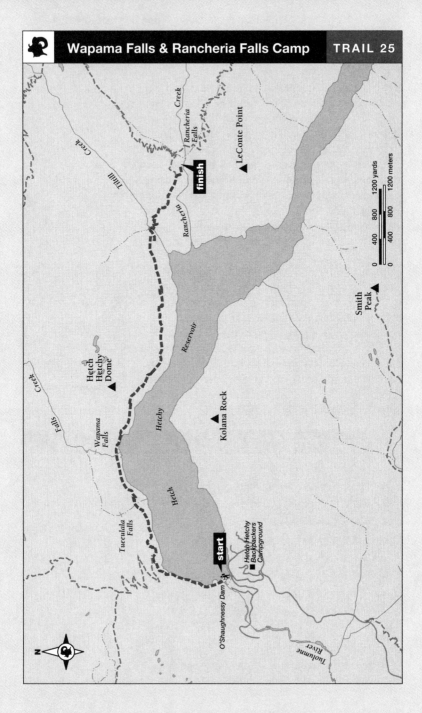

Creek

Rancheria Falls

LeConte Point ◄

finish

Rancheria

Tiltill

Creek

1200 yards

1200 meters

0 400 800

0 400 800

Smith Peak ◄

Reservoir

Hetch Hetchy Dome ◄

Creek

Hetchy

Kolana Rock ◄

Falls

Wapama Falls

Hetch

Tueeulala Falls

start

Hetch Hetchy Backpackers Campground ■

O'Shaughnessy Dam

Tuolumne River

N

Wapama Falls and Rancheria Falls Camp

A stately grove of pines and incense-cedars harboring a spacious camping area near Rancheria Falls marks the terminus of this hike. Its cascades and pools are the goals for some, but also rewarding are inspirational vistas of the awesome cliffs and two waterfalls, Tueeulala and Wapama, seen along the undulating path on the north wall of Hetch Hetchy Reservoir. Since you are traversing above a reservoir, you might think that this is an easy hike. Well, it basically is easy to Wapama Falls, but then you face gains and losses of hundreds of feet. Also, the route, being quite open and at a relatively low elevation, can be quite sunny and hot, and so on a summer's day it is best begun in early morning.

Best Time

The road to the Hetch Hetchy trailhead can open in April, but if you are after the two waterfalls and the wildflowers, May and June are best. After June, Tueeulala Falls quickly fades into oblivion although Wapama Falls remains impressive through about mid-July, then gradually diminishes after that, but it persists throughout the hiking season. The Rancheria Falls camping area is acceptable from May through October, July and August perhaps being the best months, since mosquitoes are gone and after mid-July Rancheria Creek's pools usually are safe to enter.

TRAIL USE
Dayhike, Backpack,
Run, Horse
LENGTH
12.8 miles,
4 hours–2 days
VERTICAL FEET
+1490'/-780'/±4540'
DIFFICULTY
- 1 2 **3** 4 5 +
TRAIL TYPE
Out & Back

FEATURES
Backcountry Permit
Reservoir
Streams
Waterfall
Wildflowers
Great Views
Camping
Swimming

FACILITIES
Restrooms
Campground
Water
Horse Staging

Finding the Trail

Trailside latite tuff
indicates that 9.5
million years ago the
Hetch Hetchy canyon
would have been
almost as deep and
wide as it is today.

Just 0.6 mile before the Park's boundary below the Big Oak Flat Entrance Station, leave Tioga Road and drive north 7.5 miles on Evergreen Road to its junction with the Hetch Hetchy Road. Turn right and go 1.3 miles to the Hetch Hetchy Entrance Station/ Mather Ranger Station. From the station, drive 7.1 miles to a junction branching left for the Hetch Hetchy Backpacker Campground. Backpackers turn here, park in the obvious parking area by the road's start, then walk 0.5 mile on the road to O'Shaughnessy Dam. Dayhikers continue driving 0.7 mile past the junction to the dam, beyond which is its trailhead parking. If you are just dayhiking and want to stay in a relatively nearby campground, the only one is the Dimond O Campground along the Evergreen Road.

Logistics

Because of a perceived threat of terrorists (foreign? local enviros?) wanting to destroy O'Shaughnessy Dam, road use is restricted. Day-use hours are from 7 a.m. to 5 p.m., and the gate at the station is locked at night. Although I was told that the gate is locked around 9 p.m., you ought to play it safe and try to exit past the station by 5 p.m. Should you fall behind schedule and find yourself exiting late and finding the gate is locked, you could try walking 1.3 miles along the road to Camp Mather to seek help, but don't count on getting it.

Trail Description

Backpackers, starting from their parking area, will add 1 mile to their round-trip distance. Summer hikers should start early in the morning, since the switchbacking route up from the reservoir is only partly shaded, and temperatures can reach into the

90s by noon. Carry sufficient water; in late season it's two or more hours before you reach water.

You begin by starting across the top of O'Shaughnessy Dam (3814 feet) at Hetch Hetchy Reservoir. ▶1 On the south wall, the prow of Kolana Rock soars 2000 feet above the reservoir, while to its north, tiered Hetch Hetchy Dome rises about 400 feet higher. In a shaded cleft on the dome's west flank, two-stepped Wapama Falls plunges an aggregate of 1400 feet. In early summer its gossamer companion, Tueeulala Falls, glides down steep slabs farther west.

Across the 600-foot-long dam, you enter a 500-foot-long tunnel blasted through solid granite when the original dam was raised 85 feet in 1938. Emerging from this bat haven, the formerly paved road traverses above the rocky west shore of Hetch Hetchy Reservoir in a pleasant grove of Douglas-fir, gray pine, big-leaf maple, and bay trees. One mile into your route, you reach the Rancheria Falls Trail, branching right, just before your route's first switchback. ▶2

On it you descend gently first south and then east across an exfoliating granitic nose, then switchback once down to a broad, sloping ledge, sparingly shaded by grayish-green foliage of gray pines, and from April through June you may see an assortment of wildflowers in bloom, along with patches of moss-like selaginella, a relative of ferns. You follow this ledge 0.5 mile to a minor stream that descends, until about early summer, as Tueeulala Falls. Beyond it you wind down along the north shore of Hetch Hetchy Reservoir to a bridge over a steep ravine, where your views east to the lake's head expand impressively. On the north wall stands multifaceted Hetch Hetchy Dome, guarding split-level Wapama Falls. Opposite this monolith towers Kolana Rock, which forces a constriction in the 8-mile-long reservoir's tadpole shape.

 Waterfall

Great Views

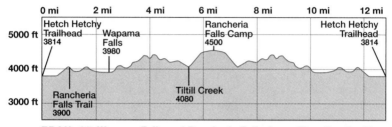

	0 mi	2 mi	4 mi	6 mi	8 mi	10 mi	12 mi
5000 ft	Hetch Hetchy Trailhead 3814	Wapama Falls 3980		Rancheria Falls Camp 4500			Hetch Hetchy Trailhead 3814
4000 ft							
3000 ft	Rancheria Falls Trail 3900			Tiltill Creek 4080			

TRAIL 25 Wapama Falls and Rancheria Falls Camp Elevation Profile

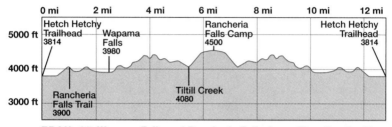 **Waterfall**

Caution

A few minutes of easy traverse east from here end at a steep, dynamited descent through a field of huge talus blocks under a tremendous precipice. Soon, if you're passing this way in early summer, flecks of spray dampen your path, as you come to the first of several bridges below the base of Wapama Falls. ▶3 During some high-runoff years, even these high, sturdy bridges are inundated by seasonally tumultuous Falls Creek.

East of Wapama Falls, your rocky path leads up around the base of a steep bulge of glacier-polished and striated granite under a fly-infested canopy of canyon live oak, bay tree, poison oak, and wild grapevines. After your terrace tapers off, the frequently dynamited trail undulates along a steep hillside in open chaparral of yerba santa and mountain mahogany, switchbacking on occasion to circumvent some cliffy spots. Eventually your path descends to the shaded gorge cut by Tiltill Creek, and you cross two bridges, the second one high above the creek.▶4 You can get water just above this bridge by making a cautious traverse over to a pool at the brink of the creek's fall. When the current's not too strong, the pool is great to dip in on a hot day.

Stream

Beyond the creek your route climbs the gorge's east slope via a set of tight switchbacks to emerge 250 feet higher on a gentle hillside. Where this ascent eases off, you may see, on your right, the start of an old trail that follows a descending ridge just south of Tiltill Creek, ending just above Hetch Hetchy Reservoir. No camping is allowed within 200 feet of its shoreline.

Soon, your way levels off, and you spy Rancheria Creek. By walking a few paces right, you have an excellent vantage point of it. The creek here slides invitingly over broad rock slabs, its pools superb for skinny-dipping when the creek isn't swift. Every step of your way has been on granite, but just 0.2 mile past your vantage point you may note a tiny remnant of a much larger volcanic deposit that was transported to this spot in a south-directed eruption of latite tuff about 9.5 million years ago.

Just 0.1 mile past the volcanic remnant you reach a junction with a short trail to the spacious Rancheria Falls Camp.►5 Rancheria Creek is a moment's walk away, and you can head up and down it in pursuit of cascades and pools. One nearby cascade is a small fall, about 25 feet high, which in high volume shoots over a ledge of resistant, dark, intrusive rock. Fishing below the falls might yield pan-size rainbow trout. Be warned that this popular camping area is often visited by black bears. If you leave them alone, they leave you alone; just don't leave food lying about.

Camping

Waterfall

Caution

🚶	MILESTONES

►1	0.0	Start at Hetch Hetchy trailhead
►2	1.0	Rancheria Falls Trail
►3	2.5	Wapama Falls
►4	5.5	Tiltill Creek
►5	6.4	Rancheria Falls Camp

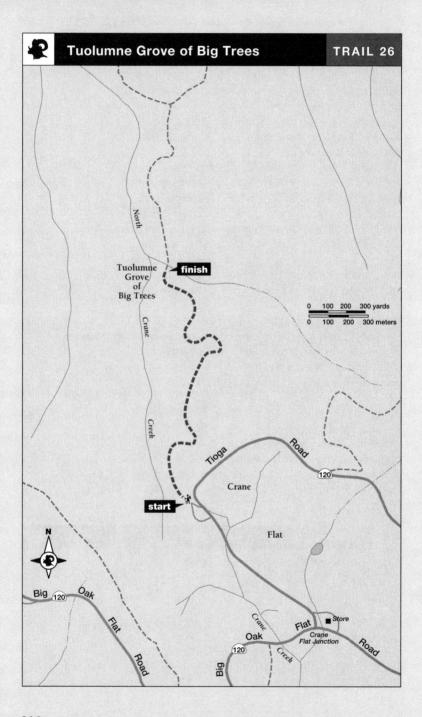

North

Tuolumne
Grove
of
Big Trees

finish

Crane

Creek

| 0 | 100 | 200 | 300 yards |
| 0 | 100 | 200 | 300 meters |

Tioga

Road

120

Crane

start

Flat

N

Big 120 Oak

Crane

Flat

Oak

Big 120

Creek

Flat

Crane
Flat Junction

■ Store

Road

Flat Oak Road

Tuolumne Grove of Big Trees

The Tuolumne Grove has over a dozen trees at least 10 feet in diameter near the base, and although this pales in comparison with the much larger Mariposa Grove's (Trail 44) approximately 200 trees of similar or larger size, you'll certainly see fewer tourists and no trams. In the Tuolumne Grove, a few trees reach about 15 feet in diameter, the largest being about 10 feet short of the diameter of the Mariposa Grove's Grizzly Giant.

TRAIL USE
Dayhike

LENGTH
2.4 miles, 1–2 hours

VERTICAL FEET
+0'/-490'/±980'

DIFFICULTY
- 1 **2** 3 4 5 +

TRAIL TYPE
Out & Back

Best Time

Because the route is through a shady forest, there are no prominent displays of flowers, and so any time from early May through mid-November, when the closed road usually is snow-free, is fine.

FEATURES
Giant Sequoias
Steep

FACILITIES
Store
Campground
Restrooms
Picnic Tables

Finding the Trail

Drive along the Big Oak Flat Road to a junction with the Tioga Road, at Crane Flat, then drive 0.5 mile up the Tioga Road to a large parking area on your left. Two relatively near campgrounds in these park lands are Hodgdon Meadow, near the Big Oak Flat Entrance Station, and Crane Flat, just west of the Crane Flat junction.

Trail Description

In the area covered by this book's map, there are three sequoia groves, Merced, Tuolumne, and Mariposa. What they have in common today are similar elevations, between 5000 and 6000 feet, and perhaps more importantly, some underlying metamorphic bedrock. Metamorphic bedrock weathers to produce soils with more nutrients and more ground-water capacity than soils derived from granitic bedrock, and in times of warmer, drier climates, such as a few thousand years ago, metamorphic soils may have enabled our sequoias to survive.

The route is obvious, an old closed road for hikers only. ▶1 It first curves 0.25 mile over to a gully below the back side of the Yosemite Institute, which provides outdoor education to groups of students and to other groups. The road then takes on a steep gradient as it first descends to a switchback west, then to one north. Just past it, about 0.9 mile into your hike, you enter the Tuolumne Grove, and about 0.2 mile farther down the road, you come to a junction beside an impressive sequoia about 15 feet in diameter. You could continue down the main road, but the alternate road is more desirable. About 130 yards along it you pass through the Tunnel Tree, a dead, charred hulk with a base diameter of 29.5 feet. In its glory, it must have been one of Yosemite's tallest specimens. A tunnel was carved in it back in 1878, before two were carved in the Mariposa Grove. From the Tunnel Tree the alternate road goes 160 yards down to a reunion with the main road. ▶2 Here in the heart of the Tuolumne Grove is a picnic area plus two ends of a self-guiding nature trail that winds through a group of sequoias. Taking this informative trail adds about 0.5 mile to the total length of your hike.

🚶 **MILESTONES**

▶1   0.0 Start at Tuolumne Grove trailhead
▶2   1.2 Tuolumne Grove

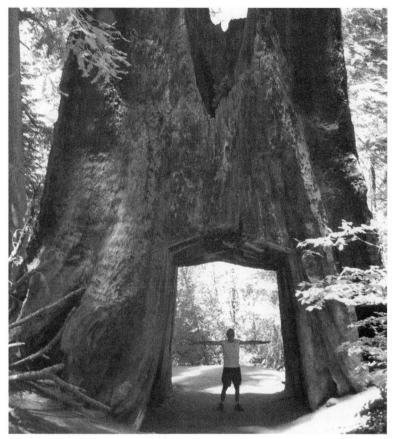

Tunnel Tree

Most folks turn around at the picnic area, if not sooner, but you can descend the main road 0.25 mile beyond it to the lower, northern edge of the grove. If you look to your left you'll see a lone giant sequoia at the far edge of a gently sloping flat, among mature sugar pines and white firs. Beyond it the road descends about 4.5 miles to Hodgdon Meadow Campground, which lies just east of the Big Oak Flat Entrance Station.

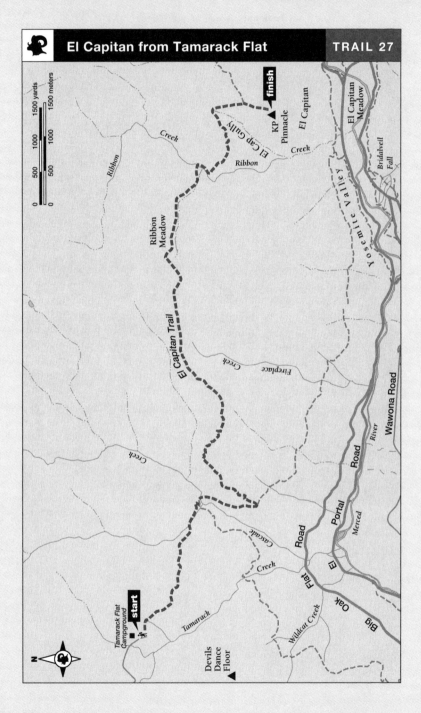

El Capitan from Tamarack Flat

The vertical walls of 3000-foot-high El Capitan attract rock climbers from all over the world, and more than five dozen extremely difficult routes ascend it. For nonclimbers this hike provides a much easier, safer way to attain El Capitan's summit, which stands only 15 feet above the north-side approach. Although the round-trip distance is 17 miles, I nevertheless recommend this trail as a dayhike, for two reasons. First, although the distance is comparable to a round-trip to the top of Half Dome and back, which most aspirants dayhike, it involves only about 70 percent as much elevation gain and loss. And second, the main source of water along this trail is Ribbon Creek, which dries up around midsummer.

Best Time

Despite being mostly snow-free by early July and staying that way usually until mid- or late October, this trail has a shorter hiking season. The reason for this is that the road down to Tamarack Flat Campground is open only from about mid-July to early September, and when the road is closed, the hike is too long to be rewarding for most people.

Finding the Trail

From Crane Flat drive northeast 3.75 miles up the Tioga Road to the Tamarack Flat Campground turnoff, immediately before the Gin Flat scenic turnout. Drive southeast down the old Big Oak Flat

TRAIL USE
Dayhike, Backpack, Horse

LENGTH
17.0 miles, 6 hours–2 days

VERTICAL FEET
+2470'/-1250'/±7440'

DIFFICULTY
- 1 2 3 **4 5** +

TRAIL TYPE
Out & Back

FEATURES
Backcountry Permit
Streams
Wildflowers
Summit
Great Views
Camping
Secluded

FACILITIES
Restrooms
Campground
Water
Horse Staging

Road to the east end of Tamarack Flat Campground,
3.25 miles from the Tioga Road.

Trail Description

From Tamarack Flat Campground ►1 you immediately cross Tamarack Creek and then ascend slopes
on the old (original) Big Oak Flat Road for a 100-
foot elevation gain. Here, white firs become
dominant, and along both sides of the road you'll
see large, partly buried granitic boulders. Just before
you reach a prominent cluster of rocks—ideal for
rock-climbing practice— your road begins a steady
descent to Cascade Creek. At a road switchback just
240 yards before the bridge across this creek, you'll
see a junction with a trail to the new Big Oak Flat
Road. Down at this lower, warmer, drier elevation
you'll find Jeffrey and sugar pines intermingled with
the firs. Along the first 200 yards below its bridge,
►2 Cascade Creek splashes down low cascades into
small pools, and in late season these make nice
swimming holes. Before then the creek is likely to be
too swift for safe frolicking, particularly since the
water-polished rock can be quite slippery. Rooted in
this creek are large-leaved umbrella plants, and
creekside dogwoods, willows, western azaleas and
serviceberries. Some folks go no farther than here,
perhaps having a creekside picnic, under shady, spacious conifers, before returning to the campground.
If you are hiking later than about mid-August, this
may be your last reliable water, so carry enough to
last.

Bound for El Capitan, you continue 0.5 mile
down the old Big Oak Flat Road—now more like a
trail—to a junction with Yosemite Valley's North

Stream

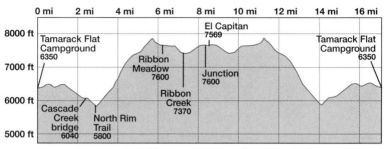

TRAIL 27 El Capitan from Tamarack Flat Elevation Profile

Rim Trail. ▶**3** Or, continue only 200 yards below Cascade Creek to a well-graded, abandoned road, on the left, and follow it 0.25 mile up to the El Capitan Trail. The Park Service ought to also abandon the current trail junction and place it at the junction with the abandoned road. This change would save hikers almost 0.5 mile. From either junction is a major climb of almost 2000 feet.

Starting in a forest of incense-cedar, ponderosa and sugar pines, and white fir, you climb hundreds of feet—steeply at times—up to drier slopes dotted with clusters of greenleaf manzanita and huckleberry oak. Occasionally you see black oaks, but these diminish to shrub height as you climb higher, disappearing altogether by the time you reach a small drop on a ridge. Three miles from the old road, lodgepoles join in the ranks as you make a short descent from it down to a sedge-filled damp meadow, the western outskirts of Ribbon Meadow, ▶**4** which sprouts water-loving wildflowers. The meadow guides you to a crossing of a Ribbon Creek tributary—a wide bog in early summer—and then you parallel it east one mile down to Ribbon Creek. ▶**5**

Wildflowers

Ribbon Meadow, which you traverse on the first part of this descent, is more forest than meadow, and on the bark of lodgepoles you'll see blazes to guide you where the route becomes a little vague. Along the banks of Ribbon Creek are the trail's only acceptable campsites—but waterless when the creek dries up about midsummer. Now only 1.25 miles from your goal, you make a brief climb, an equally brief descent, and then an ascending traverse east to the top of El Capitan Gully.

Your first views of El Capitan and the south wall of Yosemite Valley appear on this traverse to El Capitan Gully, and views continue as you climb south from the gully to a junction with the El Capitan spur trail. ▶6 If you are hiking this trail in late summer, after Ribbon Creek has dried up, you may want to continue on the main trail 0.5 mile northeast to two trickling springs. The trail beyond them is not all that interesting.

Along the short spur trail south to El Capitan's broad, rounded summit, ▶7 you can gaze up-canyon and identify unmistakable Half Dome, at the valley's end; barely protruding Sentinel Dome, above the

▲ Camping

🅷 Great Views

valley's south wall; and fin-shaped Mt. Clark, on the skyline above the dome. Take your time exploring El Capitan's large, domed summit area, but don't stray too far from it. The first 200 yards below it are safe, but then the summit's slopes gradually get steeper and you could slip on loose, weathered crystals, giving yourself a one-way trip to the bottom. Remember that many climbing deaths occur after the triumphant party has reached the summit.

Caution

		MILESTONES
►1	0.0	Start in Tamarack Flat Campground
►2	2.4	Cascade Creek bridge
►3	2.9	Left at North Rim Trail
►4	6.2	Ribbon Meadow
►5	7.2	Ribbon Creek
►6	8.3	Right at El Capitan spur trail
►7	8.5	El Capitan's summit

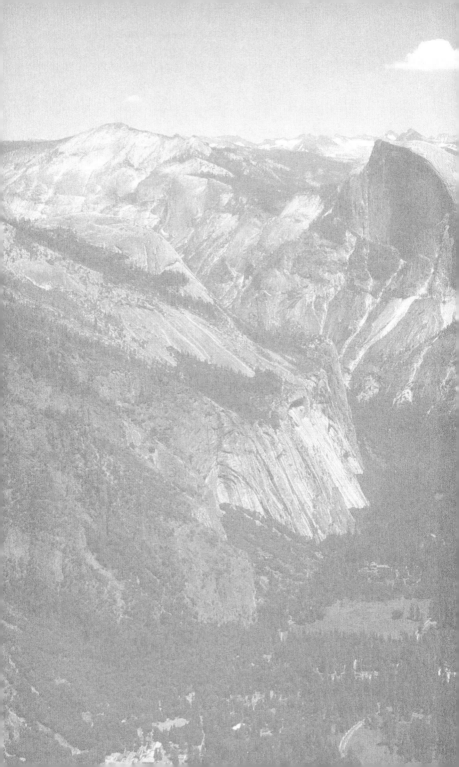

Yosemite Valley

Yosemite Valley

Rightly called "The Incomparable Valley," Yosemite Valley is a magnet that attracts visitors from all over the world. As John Muir noted long ago, the Sierra Nevada has several "Yosemites," though none of them matches Yosemite Valley in grandeur. Hetch Hetchy, to the north, is the foremost example of such a Yosemite. Though some of these Yosemites rival or exceed Yosemite Valley in the depth of their canyons and the steepness of their walls, none has the prize-winning combination of its wide, spacious floor, its world-famous waterfalls, and its unforgettable monoliths—El Capitan and Half Dome.

This hiking section is actually composed of two groups. Trails 28, 29, and 31 are relatively flat, taking you to three tourist destinations: respectively, Bridalveil Fall, Lower Yosemite Fall, and Mirror Lake. The other trails involve climbing, of which Trail 32, to the Vernal Fall Bridge, is the shortest but, nevertheless, steep. On any fair-weather summer day you are likely to meet hundreds of tourists along it. The four others involve strenuous, protracted climbing, and only those in good shape (excellent is better) should attempt them. The first three, to the brink of Upper Yosemite Fall, the top of Nevada Fall, and the summit of Half Dome, can have hundreds of hikers on many summer days. Only along the last, to Merced Lake, do the numbers dwindle to dozens. The plentiful numbers of hikers on all of this chapter's trails attest to the grand views encountered on each. While most hikers ascending the 100-plus switchbacks up the Yosemite Falls Trail go only as far as the upper fall's brink, a few are rewarded with a push to the small summit of Eagle Peak, the highest of the Three Brothers. An even smaller number backpack up to just below its summit in order to view sunset and sunrise over Yosemite Valley.

Overleaf: *Yosemite Valley from Eagle Peak (Trail 30)*

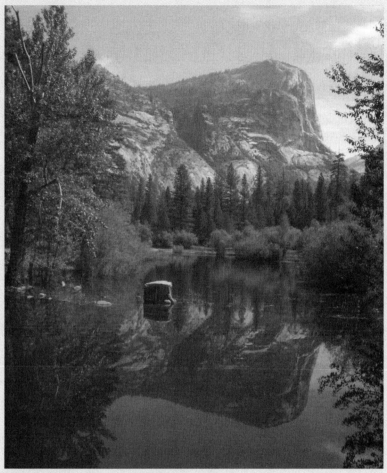

Mirror Lake *and Mt. Watkins (Trail 31)*

Campgrounds

Back in the early days, when visitation was light by today's standards, there were up to 14 campgrounds in the valley.

There are only three regular campgrounds—North, Upper, and Lower Pines—plus two smaller, walk-in campgrounds—Camp 4 and Backpackers. The former is heavily dominated by rock climbers, and the latter is for back-packers who have a wilderness permit and need a place to stay the night before they start their hike. For most visitors, camping in the valley will remain an unfulfilled dream.

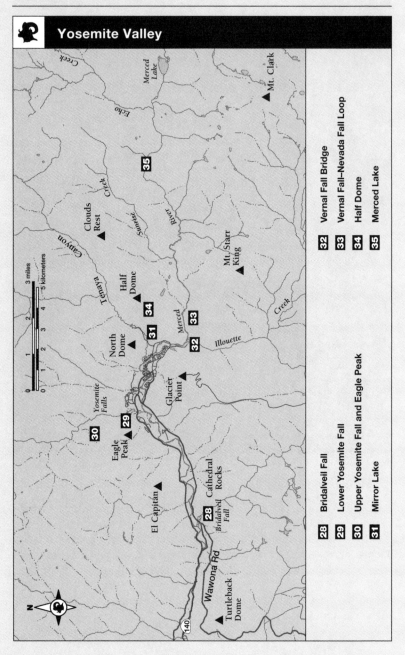

CHAPTER 5

Yosemite Valley

28 Bridalveil Fall

29 Lower Yosemite Fall

30 Upper Yosemite Fall and Eagle Peak

31 Mirror Lake

32 Vernal Fall Bridge

33 Vernal Fall–Nevada Fall Loop

34 Half Dome

35 Merced Lake

Yosemite Valley

TRAIL	Difficulty	Length	Type	USES & ACCESS	TERRAIN	FLORA & FAUNA	OTHER
28	1	0.4	Point-to-Point	Dayhiking, Handicap Access, Child Friendly	Stream, Waterfall		
29	1	1.1	Loop	Dayhiking, Handicap Access, Child Friendly	Stream, Waterfall		
30	4	7.0	Point-to-Point	Backpacking, Dayhiking	Summit, Stream, Waterfall		Great Views, Camping, Steep
31	1	2.0	Point-to-Point	Biking, Dayhiking, Horses, Running, Child Friendly	Canyon, Lake, Stream		Great Views
32	2	2.0	Point-to-Point	Dayhiking	Canyon, Stream, Waterfall		Great Views, Camping, Steep
33	3	6.5	Loop	Dayhiking	Canyon, Stream, Waterfall		Great Views, Camping, Steep
34	5	15.5	Point-to-Point	Backpacking, Dayhiking, Horses	Canyon, Mountain, Summit, Stream, Waterfall		Great Views, Camping, Steep
35	5	28.4	Point-to-Point	Backpacking, Horses	Canyon, Lake, Stream, Waterfall	Wildflowers	Great Views, Camping, Swimming

USES & ACCESS	TYPE	TERRAIN	FLORA & FAUNA	FEATURES
Dayhiking	Loop	Canyon	Autumn Colors	Great Views
Backpacking	Out & Back	Mountain	Wildflowers	Camping
Horses	Point-to-Point	Summit	Giant Sequoias	Swimming
Running		Stream		Secluded
Biking	DIFFICULTY	Waterfall		Steep
Handicap Access	- 1 2 3 4 5 +	Lake		
Child Friendly	less more			

Permits

If you want to reserve a permit, rather than get one in person, see the "Fees, Camping, and Permits" section on page 14. Most of the hikes in this section are dayhikes. For multi-day hikes, get your permit at the Wilderness Center, centrally located in Yosemite Village.

Maps

For the Yosemite Valley, Trails 28 to 34 are on the USGS (1:24,000-scale) Topographic Map of Yosemite Valley, which is readily available in the park. Trail 35 begins on this map, but you will also need the USGS Merced Peak 7.5-minute (1:24,000-scale) topographic quadrangle.

Yosemite Valley

TRAIL 28

Dayhike
0.4 mile, Out & Back
Difficulty: **1** 2 3 4 5

Bridalveil Fall 239

The hike to a view of Bridalveil Fall is one of three extremely popular, wheelchair-accessible trails in the park, the other two being to the base of Lower Yosemite Fall and out to Glacier Point. In May and June, when Bridalveil Fall is at its greatest flow, not only do you have a dramatic view of the fall but also you can be moistened (or even soaked) by its spray.

TRAIL 29

Dayhike
1.1 miles, Loop
Difficulty: **1** 2 3 4 5

Lower Yosemite Fall 243

From Memorial Day to the Labor Day weekend perhaps over a thousand visitors daily make a short pilgrimage north to the base of Lower Yosemite Fall, many (if not most) arriving by tour buses and from out of state. And why not? Yosemite National Park is one of the most famous UNESCO World Heritage Sites; Yosemite Valley is its star attraction, and Lower Yosemite Fall is its most accessible fall. On your hike the vast majority of hikers only go to the bridge view of Lower Yosemite Fall and return the way they came, whereas I describe a slightly longer route, a 1.1-mile loop.

Upper Yosemite Fall & Eagle Peak ..249

Most park visitors walk to the base of Lower Yosemite Fall. This popular trail gets you to the other end—the brink of Upper Yosemite Fall. For some, the hike is quite strenuous, and many ascend only to Columbia Rock, which is a worthy goal in itself. This trail also comes with a steep but scenic optional extension.

TRAIL 30

Hike, Backpack
7.0 miles, Out & Back
Difficulty: 1 2 3 **4** 5

Mirror Lake 257

Once, first cars and then shuttle buses went to Mirror Lake and Indian Caves, but now the paved road is used by cyclists. Most hikers also use it, though paths offer quieter routes to these sites. Be forewarned that Mirror Lake is just a broad stretch of Tenaya Creek, not a true lake. In time of high water it is quite impressive and reflective, but in July the flow diminishes and the "lake's" width greatly decreases

TRAIL 31

Dayhike, Bike,
Run, Horse
2.0 miles,
Out & Back
Difficulty: **1** 2 3 4 5

Vernal Fall Bridge 261

Popular, paved paths go to near the bases of Yosemite and Bridalveil falls, and a paved one goes to this bridge. If you have only one day here, take all three. Although the trail to the bridge is a mere 1.0 mile from the Happy Isles shuttle stop, it is steep and so is intimidating for out-of-shape flatlanders. Perhaps 1000 or more hikers make this ascent on any sunny summer day. In contrast, "only" a few hundred go on to the brink of Nevada Fall.

TRAIL 32

Dayhike
2.0 miles,
Out & Back
Difficulty: 1 **2** 3 4 5

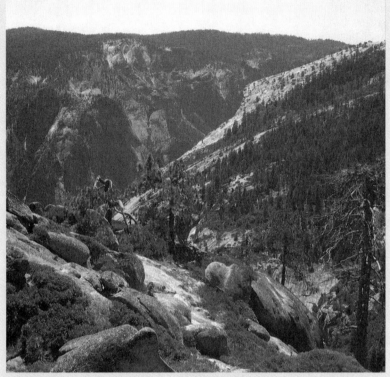

Looking west from Eagle Peak *(Trail 30) toward El Capitan (far right)*

Vernal Fall–Nevada Fall Loop 265

Mile for mile, the very popular semi-loop hike up to the brink of Nevada Fall and back may be the most scenic one in the park. The first part of this loop goes up the famous (or infamous) Mist Trail—a steep, strenuous trail that sprays you with Vernal Fall's mist, which cools you on hot afternoons but makes the mostly bedrock route slippery and dangerous.

TRAIL 33

Dayhike
6.5 miles, Loop
Difficulty: 1 2 **3** 4 5

Half Dome 273

Many a backpacker has spent his or her first night in the "wilderness" of Little Yosemite Valley. Indeed, more backpackers camp in it than in any other Yosemite backcountry area. For many camped in Little Yosemite Valley, their ultimate goal is the summit of Half Dome. On a good summer day, hundreds of hikers attempt this summit, but many turn back, either from exhaustion of from fear. If I as a first-time visitor were allowed to make only one dayhike in the park, I would unquestionably choose this hike—the one that introduced me to Yosemite and fired my desire to "climb every mountain."

TRAIL 34

Dayhike, Backpack, Horse
15.5 miles, Semi-loop
Difficulty: 1 2 3 4 **5**

Merced Lake 285

Best done in three days with overnight stops at Little Yosemite Valley and Merced Lake, this hike is often done in two by energetic weekend hikers. Its route, up a fantastic river canyon, is one of the Sierra's best. Located at an elevation of about 7200 feet, relatively large Merced Lake is about 2000+ feet lower than the popular ones reached from Tuolumne Meadows' trailheads, and therefore it is snow-free sooner.

TRAIL 35

Dayhike, Backpack, Horse
28.4 miles, Out & Back
Difficulty: 1 2 3 4 **5**

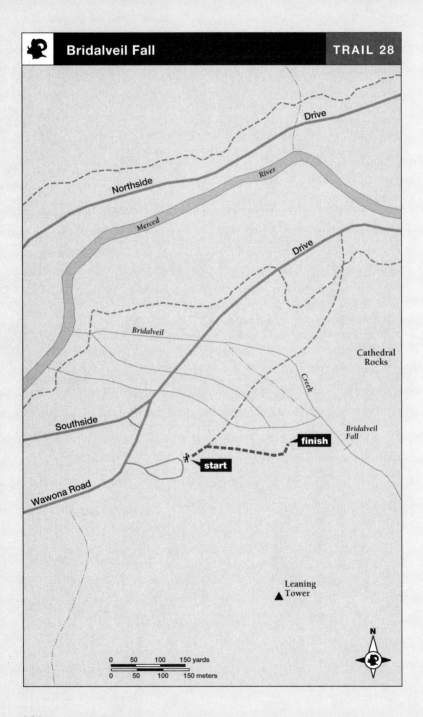

Drive

River

Northside

Merced

Drive

Bridalveil

Cathedral
Rocks

Creek

Bridalveil
Fall

Southside

finish

start

Wawona Road

Leaning
Tower

N

0   50   100   150 yards

0   50   100   150 meters

Bridalveil Fall

The hike to a view of Bridalveil Fall is one of three extremely popular, wheelchair-accessible trails in the park, the other two being to the base of Lower Yosemite Fall (Trail 29) and out to Glacier Point (Trail 39). In May and June, when Bridalveil Fall is at its greatest flow, not only do you have a dramatic view of the fall but also you can be moistened (or even soaked) by its spray.

Best Time

Snowmelt feeding Bridalveil Creek and other Yosemite Valley falls is greatest in May and June, which are the best months to visit all of these falls. If you don't mind visiting a diminished Bridalveil Fall, then you can take the trail from April through November. During the months of December through March the trail can be snowbound and/or icy, making it slippery.

Finding the Trail

The trail starts at Bridalveil Fall parking lot, 120 yards before the descending Wawona Road reaches a junction on the floor of Yosemite Valley.

The valley has only three regular campgrounds—North, Upper, and Lower Pines—plus two smaller, walk-in campgrounds—Camp 4 and Backpackers. The former is heavily dominated by rock climbers, and the latter is for backpackers who have a wilderness permit and need a place to stay the night before they start their hike.

TRAIL USE
Dayhike
LENGTH
0.4 mile, 10–30 minutes
VERTICAL FEET
+80'/-0'/±160'
DIFFICULTY
- **1** 2 3 4 5 +
TRAIL TYPE
Out & Back

FEATURES
Child Friendly
Handicap Access
Streams
Waterfall

FACILITIES
Resort
Store
Visitor Center
Restrooms
Campgrounds
Picnic Tables
Phone
Water

Trail Description

The valley's Miwok Indians named the fall Pohono, "fall of the puffing winds," for at low volume its water is pushed around by gusts of wind.

Caution

Waterfall

Starting from the east end of the Bridalveil Fall parking lot, ▶1 you hike just two or three minutes on a paved trail to a junction with a spur trail. ▶2 On it you veer right and parallel a Bridalveil Creek tributary as you climb an equally short trail up to its end at the Bridalveil Fall viewpoint. ▶3 During May and June, when Bridalveil Fall is at its best, your viewpoint will be drenched in spray, making the last part of the trail very slippery and making photography from this vantage point nearly impossible. If you are dressed for the spray, such as in a T-shirt and shorts, it is exhilarating, not annoying, and of course, kids love the spray. Of Yosemite's other falls, only Vernal Fall leaps free over a dead-vertical cliff, but its flow—the Merced River—is too strong to be greatly affected by the wind. The other major falls drop over cliffs that are less than vertical, and hence the falls partly glide down them.

🚶	MILESTONES
▶1	0.0 Start at Bridalveil parking lot
▶2	0.1 Right on to Bridalveil spur trail
▶3	0.2 Bridalveil Fall viewpoint

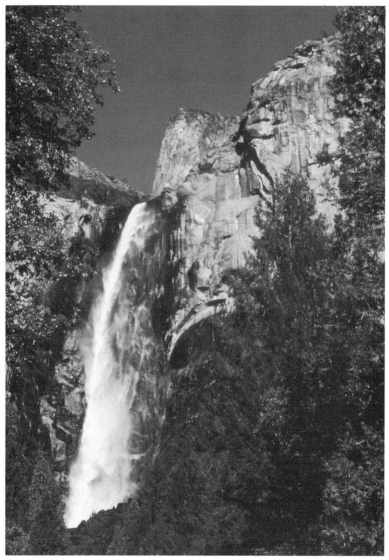

Bridalveil Fall

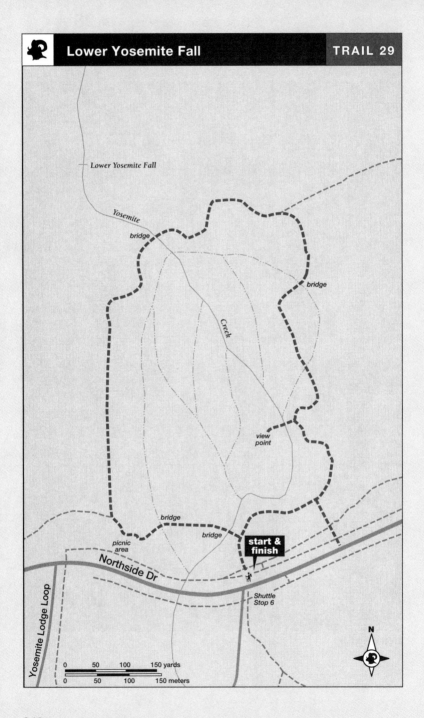

Lower Yosemite Fall

TRAIL 29

Lower Yosemite Fall

Yosemite

bridge

bridge

Creek

view point

bridge

bridge

picnic area

start & finish

Northside Dr

Shuttle Stop 6

Yosemite Lodge Loop

| 0 | 50 | 100 | 150 yards |
| 0 | 50 | 100 | 150 meters |

N

Lower Yosemite Fall

From Memorial Day to the Labor Day weekend per-haps over a thousand visitors daily make a short pilgrimage north to the base of Lower Yosemite Fall, many (if not most) arriving by tour buses and from out of state. And why not? Yosemite National Park is one of the most famous UNESCO World Heritage Sites; Yosemite Valley is its star attraction, and Lower Yosemite Fall is its most accessible fall. On your hike the vast majority of hikers only go to the bridge view of Lower Yosemite Fall and return the way they came, whereas I describe a slightly longer route, a 1.1-mile loop.

Best Time

Snowmelt feeding Yosemite Creek and other Yosemite Valley falls is greatest in May and June, which are the best months to visit all of these falls. By the end of August there may be very little water plunging over Lower Yosemite Fall's brink, and in September and into October, the fall can be com-pletely dry. Once the rains return, followed by snow, the fall is resurrected, and although not nearly at full volume, it can be inspirational from November through April.

Finding the Trail

Take the shuttlebus to stop 6. If you are driving, you might chance to find parking on both sides of Northside Drive just east of stop 6, but don't count on it, especially on weekends.

TRAIL USE
Dayhike
LENGTH
1.1 miles,
30 minutes–1 hour
VERTICAL FEET
+160'/-160'/±320'
DIFFICULTY
- **1** 2 3 4 5 +
TRAIL TYPE
Loop

FEATURES
Child Friendly
Handicap Access
Streams
Waterfalls

FACILITIES
Resort
Store
Visitor Center
Restrooms
Campgrounds
Bus Stop
Picnic Tables
Phone
Water

The valley has only three regular campgrounds—North, Upper, and Lower Pines—plus two smaller, walk-in campgrounds—Camp 4 and Backpackers. The former is heavily dominated by rock climbers, and the latter is for backpackers who have a wilderness permit and need a place to stay the night before they start their hike.

Trail Description

The Lower Yosemite Fall loop trail begins along Northside Drive from shuttle stop 6, which is just east of the Lower Yosemite Fall complex. ▶1 The shorter way to it is a paved path that parallels Northside Drive 0.2 mile west. The recommended slightly longer, quieter way is to start from the west side of the bus stop and take a path 70 yards north to a junction. You'll be finishing your loop on the path heading right, northeast. You head left, west, for 170 yards, bridging two branches of Yosemite Creek on your way to a building with restrooms and, immediately west of it, a drinking fountain and tables. In front of the building is a display that introduces you to this area. More displays lie ahead along your loop.

You are at the southeast edge of the Lower Yosemite Fall complex, and now you arc 80 yards northwest to the start of an arrow-straight path north. Ahead your broad path aims directly toward Lower Yosemite Fall and Upper Yosemite Fall behind it, this view courtesy of many trees felled long ago to present visitors with this Kodak moment. It seems that virtually all visitors try to take a photo of the falls and their family/friends, trying not to include all the others attempting the same task.

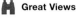 **Great Views**

Ahead, the 0.3-mile path north to the lower fall is obvious, and your photogenic path soon reaches a loop marked periodically with displays. On the path north from the loop you quickly encounter rocks on your left, many the size of cabins and several the size of houses. These broke loose from the cliffs above, and more rockfalls are likely in future years. Soon the paved path begins to climb and curve gently, then moderately (the only part tough in a wheelchair), and after several minutes you arrive a wide bridge ►2 across Yosemite Creek, which offers a seasonally impressive view of Lower Yosemite Fall. In late spring and early summer, visitors are treated to the thunderous roar of the fall, a sound that reverberates in the alcove cut in this rock. During this time the visitor is further treated to the fall's spray as well. But by mid-July Yosemite Falls are somewhat diminished, and by late August the lower fall, like its upper counterpart, is usually reduced to a mist, and even this can be gone by the Labor Day weekend. Dry or not, Lower Yosemite Fall should not be examined at close range, for even if boulder-choked Yosemite Creek is bone-dry, its rocks are water-polished to an ice-like finish.

From the bridge, most folks return the way they came, but keeping to the clockwise loop, you take the paved path briefly northeast toward a cliff, then on a short counterclockwise loop, first southeast then northeast, to traverse around slopes. In this vicinity you may hear or see climbers on one of about a dozen difficult routes up the cliff just north of you. While some routes are short, others ascend to a long, linear ledge known as Sunnyside Bench, about 400 feet above you. After a couple of minutes walking eastward you reach a junction, 0.2 mile

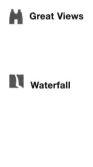

Great Views

Waterfall

Caution

beyond the bridge. ►**3** Here you turn right, take a gently winding, forested path south and slightly down, between two branches of Yosemite Creek for another 0.2 mile to a second junction. ►**4**

For another view of the falls, turn right and walk 100 yards southwest to a dead end above a branch of Yosemite Creek, where you'll find a James Hutchings bench and a John Muir plaque.

Nearly through with your loop, you keep left and wind 150 yards south to the north edge of an informative exhibit area, complete with benches and a fine view of Upper Yosemite Fall. Continuing south through this area will get you to Northside Drive at a spot about 100 yards east of the start of your loop. This is your first way back to shuttle stop 6. ►**5** My preferred way—when Yosemite Creek is flowing briskly—is to branch right at the north edge of the area and take a path that parallels a creek branch west to a junction, from which you retrace your first steps 70 yards south to the west side of the bus stop.

Stream

	MILESTONES	
►**1**	0.0	Start at shuttle stop 6
►**2**	0.5	Bridge at Lower Yosemite Fall
►**3**	0.7	Right at junction
►**4**	0.9	Right at second junction
►**5**	1.1	End at shuttle stop 6

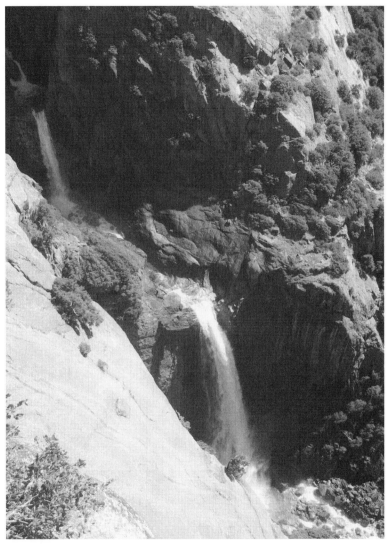

Bird's-eye view of Lower Yosemite Fall *from partway up Trail 30*

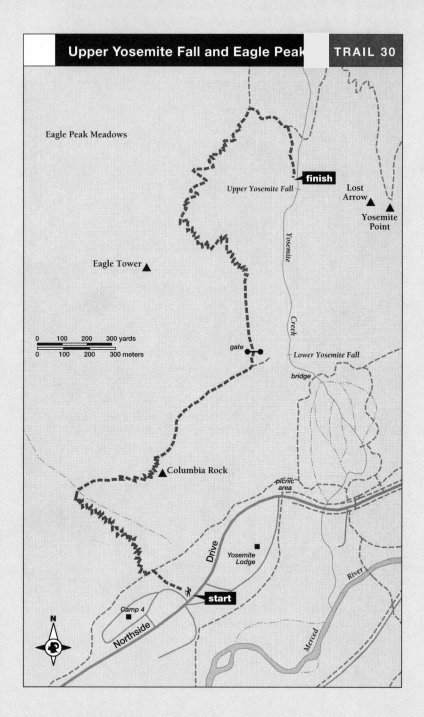

Eagle Peak Meadows

finish

Upper Yosemite Fall

Lost Arrow ▲

Yosemite Point ▲

Eagle Tower ▲

0   100   200   300 yards
0   100   200   300 meters

gate

Yosemite Creek

Lower Yosemite Fall

bridge

▲ Columbia Rock

picnic area

Drive

Yosemite Lodge ■

start

Camp 4 ■

Northside

River

Merced

N

Upper Yosemite Fall and Eagle Peak

Most park visitors walk to the base of Lower Yosemite Fall. This popular trail gets you to the other end—the brink of Upper Yosemite Fall. For some, the hike is quite strenuous, and many ascend only to Columbia Rock, which is a worthy goal in itself.

Strategically located Eagle Peak, highest of the Three Brothers, provides commanding views both up and down Yosemite Valley. The hike to it also provides exciting views, and it is included here as a side trip. Doing this optional extension of Trail 30 will increase your round-trip distance from 7.0 to 12.8 miles and your total elevation gain and descent by about 3000 feet, to 9800 feet.

Best Time

Snowmelt feeding Yosemite Creek and other Yosemite Valley falls is greatest in May and June, which are the best months to visit all of these falls. However, in years of heavy snowfall, the trail may be closed at least in the first part of May. Therefore, June is the best month. If you are backpacking to sites above the falls, then the first half of July may be better, since Upper Yosemite Fall is still impressive, but the upland's mosquito population is greatly diminished. In August not much water plunges over the brink of Upper Yosemite Fall, and in September and into October, the fall can be completely dry.

TRAIL USE
Hike, Backpack
LENGTH
7.0 miles, 3–6 hours
VERTICAL FEET
+3000'/-410'/±6820'
DIFFICULTY
- 1 2 3 **4 5** +
TRAIL TYPE
Out & Back

FEATURES
Backcountry Permit
Streams
Waterfalls
Summit
Great Views
Camping
Steep

FACILITIES
Resort
Store
Visitor Center
Restrooms
Campgrounds
Bus Stop

Finding the Trail

Take the shuttlebus to stop 7. This is where the bus, heading west on Northside Drive past the Lower Yosemite Fall complex (stop 6), turns right onto a road to start a loop through the grounds of Yosemite Lodge. From that road junction walk over to the nearby entrance to Camp 4 Walk-In Campground, on the opposite side of Northside Drive.

In addition to this campground, which is heavily dominated by rock climbers, the valley has only three regular campgrounds—North, Upper, and Lower Pines—plus Backpackers Walk-In. This is for backpackers who have a wilderness permit and need a place to stay the night before they start their hike.

Trail Description

From beside Northside Drive, ▶1 you begin on a north-heading trail that separates Camp 4 Walk-In Campground from its adjacent parking lot, and in about 200 yards reach the northside valley floor trail. By walking west on it about 25 yards, you reach the start of the Yosemite Falls Trail. You leave conifers behind as you start up nearly four dozen short switchbacks. Under the shade of canyon live oaks, which dominate talus slopes like the one you're on, your so-far viewless ascent finally reaches a usually dry wash that provides you with framed views of Leidig Meadow and the valley's central features.

With more than one-fourth of the elevation gain below you, you pass more oaks and an occasional bay tree as you now switchback east to a panoramic viewpoint, Columbia Rock, which at 5031 feet elevation is just over 1000 feet above the valley floor. ▶2 At its safety railing you can study the valley's geometry from Half Dome and the Quarter Domes west to the Cathedral Spires. Several steep, gravelly

M Great Views

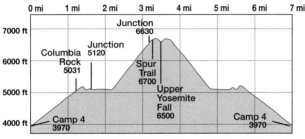

TRAIL 30 Upper Yosemite Fall Elevation Profile

switchbacks climb from the viewpoint, and then the trail traverses northeast, drops slightly, passes an enormous Douglas-fir and then drops some more before it bends north for a sudden dramatic view of Upper Yosemite Fall. Here, at a minor low spot in the trail, is a cryptic junction. ▶3

 Waterfall

Next the main trail quickly switchbacks to take you down to an adjacent gate, ▶4 which is closed in times of potential danger, such as when covered with snow or when rockfall may be imminent. Your climb up a long, steep trough ends among white firs and Jeffery pines, about 135 switchbacks above the valley floor. Here, in a gully beside a seasonal creeklet, your come to a junction, and your trail turns right, while the trail to Eagle Peak continues ahead. ▶5 Your trail makes a brief climb east out of the gully and reaches a broad crest and a spur trail ▶6

 Caution

View All of the Fall

From the cryptic junction ▶3, a 50-yard-long trail descends to a railing with an incredible view. Here you look almost directly down on Lower Yosemite Fall and can trace Yosemite Creek up past its cascades to Upper Yosemite Fall. There is no other trail spot in the valley where you can see the entire falls' sequence. Be forewarned, however, that the trail is somewhat exposed, and a careless step could result in a fatal slip over the brink of a cliff.

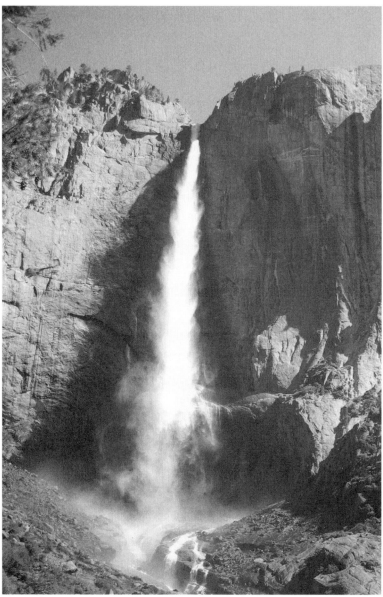

Upper Yosemite Fall

heading south to Upper Yosemite Fall. If you are backpacking to this vicinity, continue east just a bit farther to a conspicuous use-trail that goes 200-plus yards north to a large camping area near the west bank of Yosemite Creek. You can find relatively isolated campsites by going either west or north of this area.

Camping

Those bound for the fall, keep to the crest as you follow the spur trail south almost to the valley's rim; then at a juniper you veer east and descend more steps to a fenced-in viewpoint. If you're acrophobic you should not attempt the last part of this descent, even though it has a hand railing, for it is possible, though unlikely, that you could slip on loose gravel or smooth bedrock and tumble over the brink. Beside the lip of Upper Yosemite Fall ►7 you see and hear it plunge all the way down its 1430-foot drop to the rocks below.

Waterfall

After returning up the crest you can briefly take a trail east down to a bridge over Yosemite Creek and obtain water. However, be careful! Occasionally people wading in the creek's icy water slip on the glass-smooth creek bottom and are swiftly carried over the fall's brink. From the creek's bridge you could continue eastward 0.75 mile up a trail to Yosemite Point, a highly scenic goal.

Caution

Great Views

🚶	**MILESTONES**	
►1	0.0	Start at entrance to Camp 4 Walk-In Campground
►2	1.2	Columbia Rock
►3	1.6	Straight or right at cryptic junction
►4	1.7	Gate
►5	3.2	Right at junction
►6	3.3	Right at spur trail
►7	3.5	Upper Yosemite Fall

Eagle Peak

Should you wish to climb to the very rewarding summit of Eagle Peak, first return to the junction in the gully west of the fall, ▶5 from which most people descend 3.2 miles back down to the valley floor. Bound for Eagle Peak, about 2.9 miles distant and about 1160 feet above your junction, you now commence a shady trek 0.6 mile north, climbing out of the gully, descending into a second one, and climbing out of a third to a minor-divide junction.

Leaving the Yosemite Creek environs, you momentarily cross Eagle Peak Creek and then climb more than 300 feet, at first steeply, before leveling off in a bouldery area—part of a moraine that was left by a glacier that descended from the west slopes of Mt. Hoffmann. Now you turn south, generally leaving Jeffrey pines and white firs for lodgepole pines and red firs as you climb to Eagle Peak Meadows, whose north edge is blocked by another moraine.

Beyond the sometimes boggy meadow you cross the headwaters of Eagle Peak Creek and in a few minutes reach a hillside junction, 1.7 miles from the last junction. From it an old trail climbs and drops along a 1.8-mile course to the El Capitan spur trail. To reach the summit of that monolith, it is easier to start from Tamarack Flat Campground (Trail 27). From the junction you branch left for a moderate 0.6-mile ascent to the diminutive summit of **Eagle Peak**. From the summit you have far-ranging views, which extend all the way to the Sierra crest along the park's east boundary. Below, central Yosemite Valley spreads out like a map, and if you've brought along a detailed map of this Valley, you should be able to identify most of its major landmarks plus dozens of minor features. After your stay atop Eagle Peak, return directly to your trailhead, a distance of 6.1 miles.

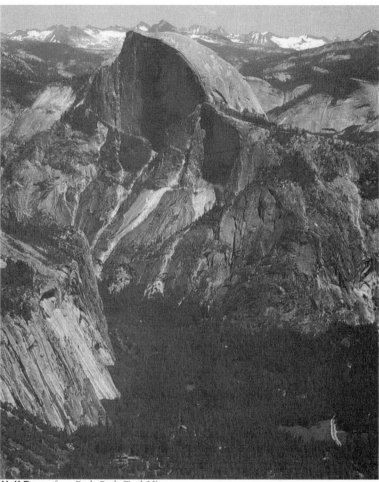

Half Dome *from Eagle Peak (Trail 30)*

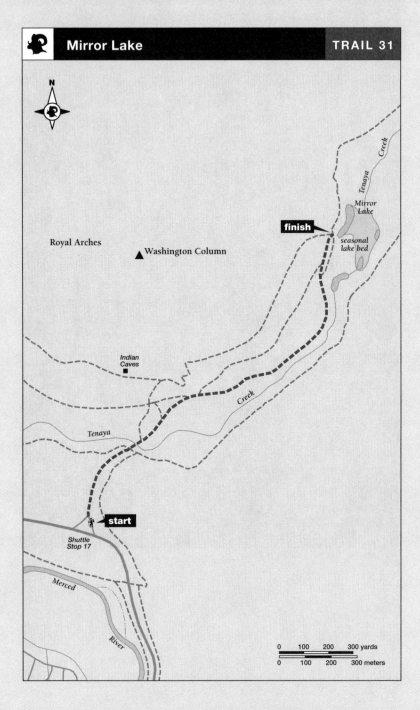

N

Royal Arches

▲ Washington Column

Mirror
Lake

finish

seasonal
lake bed

Tenaya Creek

Indian
Caves
■

Creek

Tenaya

start

Shuttle
Stop 17

Merced

River

| 0 | 100 | 200 | 300 yards |
| 0 | 100 | 200 | 300 meters |

Mirror Lake

Once, first cars and then shuttle buses went to Mirror Lake and Indian Caves, but now the paved road is used by cyclists. Most hikers also use it, though paths offer quieter routes to these sites. Be forewarned that Mirror Lake is just a broad stretch of Tenaya Creek, not a true lake. In time of high water, typically in May and June, it is quite impressive and reflective, but in July the flow diminishes and the "lake's" width greatly decreases, exposing widening stream banks. By late summer the creek can entirely dry up.

Best Time

To see the reflections in Mirror Lake, you need to visit during the time of maximum runoff, which is about early May through late June. Most visitors, however, visit it later, when the "lake" is merely a wide stretch of Tenaya Creek.

Finding the Trail

Take a shuttlebus to stop 17, which is 0.25 mile east of stop 18 beside Clarks Bridge, by the entrance to the Yosemite stables.

The valley has only three regular campgrounds—North, Upper, and Lower Pines—plus two smaller, walk-in campgrounds—Camp 4 and Backpackers. The former is heavily dominated by rock climbers, and the latter is for backpackers who have a wilderness permit and need a place to stay the night before they start their hike.

TRAIL USE
Dayhike, Bike, Run, Horse
LENGTH
2.0 miles,
30 minutes–2 hours
VERTICAL FEET
+140'/-20'/±320'
DIFFICULTY
- **1** 2 3 4 5 +
TRAIL TYPE
Out & Back

FEATURES
Child Friendly
Streams
Great Views

FACILITIES
Resort
Store
Visitor Center
Restrooms
Campgrounds
Bus Stop
Phone
Water
Horse Staging

Trail Description

The shortest route to Mirror Lake is along the paved bike path from shuttle stop 17 north to the lake. At shuttle stop 17 the low ridge you see just south of the shuttlebus stop is the valley's "Medial Moraine." Not formed by the converging Tenaya Canyon and Merced Canyon glaciers, this actually is a recessional moraine left by the retreating Merced Canyon glacier.

The bike path starts north from stop 17, ▶1 from which you'll see an adjacent outhouse plus a path immediately branching right. This momentarily reaches a trail that connects the Happy Isles environs to the Mirror Lake environs. It is slightly longer but quieter, more for the nature lovers, and it skirts an area of giant rockfall boulders that testify to the instability of Half Dome.

On the virtually level bike path you walk, bike, or jog 0.3 mile, first north then northeast to Tenaya Creek Bridge. ▶2 Standing on the Tenaya Creek Bridge, you can get a good idea of the status of Mirror Lake. If Tenaya Creek is a raging torrent descending toward you, Mirror Lake will be worth the visit, but if there is only slow water or no water at all, you're likely to be in for a disappointment.

Immediately before the bridge a trail heads east about 0.8 mile to Mirror Lake. Just a couple of minutes past the bridge you reach a bike-path junction. ▶3

Stream

Indian Caves

OPTIONS

▶3 West from the junction, you can take the bike path, or a horse trail immediately north of it, about 100 yards to enter the Indian Caves area. In the past this area was a favorite, with its several caves located among dozens of house-size boulders.

Those bound for Mirror Lake curve right and make an easy traverse east over to Tenaya Creek. The last part of the path up to the seasonal lake is a moderate ascent up alongside the creek, and those on rental bikes have to park them at the start of this ascent. After about 0.25 mile you reach a shallow pond, if indeed it is a pond at all. Formerly it was deeper and until the mid-1990s was a popular summertime swimming hole. But it is paralleling the evolution of adjacent Mirror Lake, reverting to just a broad stretch of Tenaya Creek. From the north side of the former swimming hole and just beyond an outhouse, a nature trail loops over to the southwest edge of former Mirror Lake, while the main trail continues briefly north to the lake's northwest edge, ▶4 at which photographers gather to take seasonally reflective photos. To get the mirrored reflection of Mt. Watkins, take this hike in times of high water and take the broad path to its end. Also from this path's end, a former parking area, there is a horse trail that you can take southwest to Indian Caves or northeast up lower Tenaya Creek canyon.

 Great Views

≋ **Lake**

▶ **Stream**

🚶	**MILESTONES**	
▶1	0.0	Start at shuttle stop 17
▶2	0.2	Tenaya Creek Bridge
▶3	0.3	Right at bike path junction
▶4	1.0	Mirror Lake

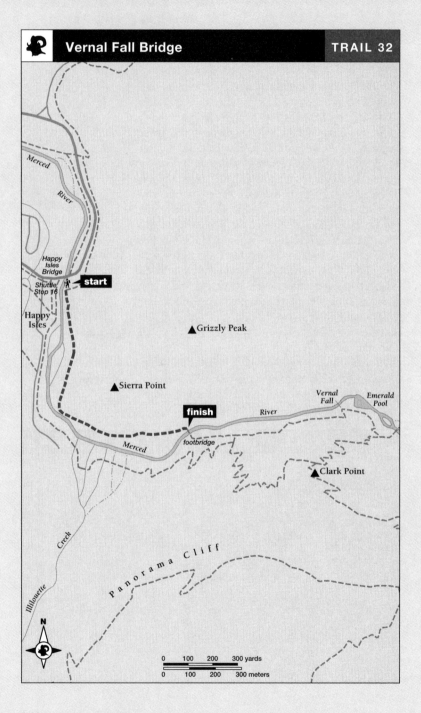

Merced

River

Happy
Isles
Bridge

Shuttle
Stop 16

start

Happy
Isles

▲Grizzly Peak

▲Sierra Point

Vernal
Fall

Emerald
Pool

finish

River

footbridge

Merced

▲Clark Point

Creek

Panorama Cliff

Illilouette

N

0	100	200	300 yards
0	100	200	300 meters

Vernal Fall Bridge

Popular, paved paths go to near the bases of Yosemite and Bridalveil falls, and a paved one goes to this bridge. If you have only one day here, take all three. Although the trail to the bridge is a mere 1.0 mile from the Happy Isles shuttle stop, it is steep and so is intimidating for out-of-shape flatlanders. Perhaps 1000 or more hikers make this ascent on any sunny summer day. In contrast, "only" a few hundred go on to the brink of Nevada Fall.

Best Time

Because the Merced River flows year round, you could take the trail up the Bridalveil Fall view almost any time of year, except when the Park Service might close it, such as during a bad snow storm. Ideally, May through July are best because so much water then leaps over the brink of the fall. Still, April and August also are worth considering. By September the discharge of the river has greatly abated, but still the fall is photogenic.

Finding the Trail

Take a shuttle bus to stop 16, at Happy Isles, immediately west of a bridge across the Merced River.

The valley has only three regular campgrounds—North, Upper, and Lower Pines—plus two smaller, walk-in campgrounds—Camp 4 and Backpackers. The former is heavily dominated by rock climbers, and the latter is for backpackers who have a wilderness permit and need a place to stay the night before they start their hike.

TRAIL USE
Dayhike
LENGTH
2.0 miles,
30 minutes–2 hours
VERTICAL FEET
+430'/-30'/±920'
DIFFICULTY
- 1 **2** 3 4 5 +
TRAIL TYPE
Out & Back

FEATURES
Streams
Waterfall
Steep

FACILITIES
Resort
Store
Visitor Center
Restrooms
Campgrounds
Bus Stop
Picnic Tables
Phone
Water

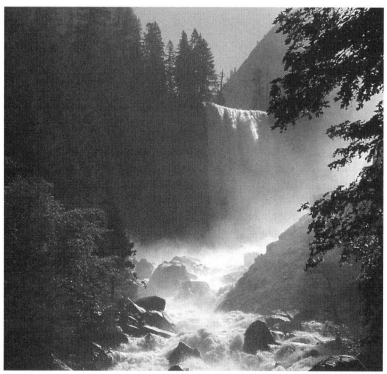

Vernal Fall

Trail Description

From the shuttle stop ▶1 you walk briefly east across an adjacent bridge and head south, soon reaching the start of the famous John Muir Trail, which heads about 210 miles southward to the summit of Mt. Whitney. After a few minutes you reach a small spring-fed cistern with questionably pure water.

Beyond it the climb south steepens, and before bending east you get a glance back at Upper Yosemite Fall, partly blocked by the Glacier Point Apron.

Note the canyon wall south of the apron, which has a series of oblique-angle cliffs—all of them remarkably similar in orientation since they've fractured along the same series of joint planes. At the canyon's end Illilouette Fall plunges 370 feet over a vertical, joint-controlled cliff. Just east of the fall is a large scar that marks the site of a major rock fall that broke loose during the winter of 1968–69.

Climbing east, you head up a canyon whose floor in times past was buried by as much as 1800 feet of glacier ice. Hiking beneath the unstable, highly fractured south wall of Sierra Point, you cross a talus slope—an accumulation of rock fall boulders. More rock falls may occur. Entering forest shade once more, you ascend a steep stretch of trail before making a quick drop to the Vernal Fall bridge. ▶2 From it you see Vernal Fall, a broad curtain of water plunging 320 feet over a vertical cliff before cascading toward you. Looming above the fall are two glacier-resistant masses, Mt. Broderick (left) and Liberty Cap (right). Just beyond the bridge are restrooms and an emergency telephone (for events such as heart attacks or slips on dangerous rocks).

A few yards before the spring-fed cistern, a treacherous trail once climbed to Sierra Point, but was closed in 1977 due to the high frequency of accidents.

Great Views

Waterfall

🚶	MILESTONES	
▶1	0.0	Start at shuttle-bus stop 16
▶2	1.0	Vernal Fall bridge

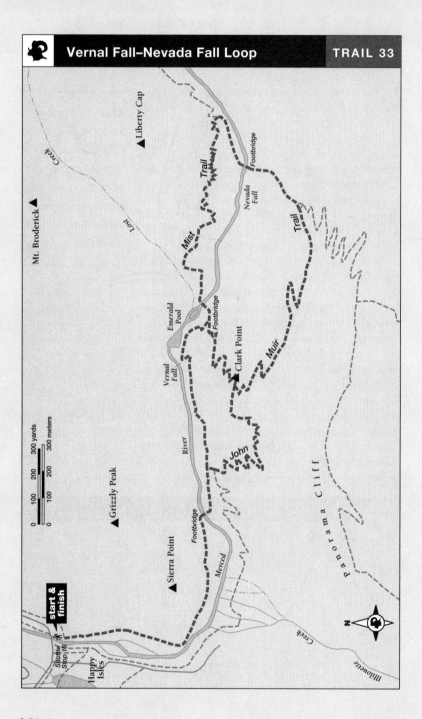

Vernal Fall–Nevada Fall Loop

Mile for mile, the very popular semi-loop hike up to the brink of Nevada Fall and back may be the most scenic one in the park. The first part of this loop goes up the famous (or infamous) Mist Trail—a steep, strenuous trail that sprays you with Vernal Fall's mist, which cools you on hot afternoons but makes the mostly bedrock route slippery and dangerous. Take rain gear or, if it is a warm day, strip down to swimwear, since you can dry out on slabs above the fall. For best photos start after 10 a.m.

Best Time

To visit Vernal and Nevada falls in all their glory, it is best to go during the time of the Merced River's maximum runoff, which usually is in May and June. In some years this semi-loop trail may not open until late May or early June, so unless you know in advance that the trail is open, don't go in May. During July there still is plenty of water coming over the falls, but they diminish considerably by August and continue to diminish until sufficient precipitation comes, usually in November, when the trail likely will be closed.

Finding the Trail

Take a shuttle bus to stop 16, at Happy Isles, immediately west of a bridge across the Merced River.

The valley has only three regular campgrounds—North, Upper, and Lower Pines—plus two smaller, walk-in campgrounds—Camp 4 and Backpackers. The former is heavily dominated by

TRAIL USE
Dayhike
LENGTH
6.5 miles, 3–6 hours
VERTICAL FEET
+2100'/-2100'/±4200'
DIFFICULTY
- 1 2 **3** 4 5 +
TRAIL TYPE
Loop

FEATURES
Streams
Waterfalls
Great Views
Steep

FACILITIES
Resort
Store
Visitor Center
Restrooms
Campgrounds
Bus Stop
Picnic Tables
Phone
Water

rock climbers, and the latter is for backpackers who have a wilderness permit and need a place to stay the night before they start their hike.

Trail Description

From the shuttle stop ►1 you walk briefly east across an adjacent bridge and head south, soon reaching the start of the famous John Muir Trail, which heads about 210 miles southward to the summit of Mt. Whitney. After a few minutes you reach a small spring-fed cistern with questionably pure water. Beyond it the climb south steepens, and before bending east you get a glance back at Upper Yosemite Fall, partly blocked by the Glacier Point Apron.

Note the canyon wall south of the apron, which has a series of oblique-angle cliffs—all of them remarkably similar in orientation since they've fractured along the same series of joint planes. At the canyon's end Illilouette Fall plunges 370 feet over a vertical, joint-controlled cliff. Just east of the fall is a large scar that marks the site of a major rock fall that broke loose during the winter of 1968–69.

Climbing east, you head up a canyon whose floor in times past was buried by as much as 1800 feet of glacier ice. Hiking beneath the unstable, highly fractured south wall of Sierra Point, you cross a talus slope—an accumulation of rock fall boulders. More rockfalls may occur. Entering forest shade once more, you ascend a steep stretch of trail before making a quick drop to the Vernal Fall bridge. ►2 From it you see Vernal Fall, a broad curtain of water plunging 320 feet over a vertical cliff before cascading toward you. Looming above the fall are two glacier-resistant masses, Mt. Broderick (left) and Liberty Cap (right). Just beyond the bridge are restrooms and an emergency telephone (heart attacks, slips on dangerous rocks).

 Caution

Waterfall

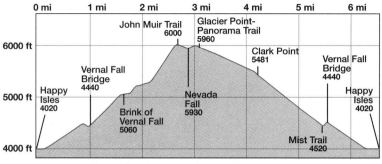

TRAIL 33 Vernal Fall–Nevada Fall Loop Elevation Profile

About 200 yards beyond the bridge you come to the start of your loop. ▶3 Here the Mist Trail continues upriver, while the John Muir Trail starts a switchbacking ascent to the right. This is the route taken by those with horses or other pack stock. You'll go up the Mist Trail and down the John Muir Trail. You can, of course go up or down either, but by starting the loop up the Mist Trail, you stand less chance of an accident. Hikers are more apt to slip or to twist an ankle descending than ascending, and the Mist Trail route to Nevada Fall has ample opportunities for mishaps.

 Caution

Dressed for the upcoming mist, which can really soak you in May or June, start up the Mist Trail and soon, rounding a bend, receive your first spray. If you're climbing this trail on a sunny day, you may see one, if not two, rainbows come alive in the fall's spray. The spray increases as you advance toward the fall, but you get a brief respite behind a large boulder. Beyond it, complete your 300-plus steps, most of them wet, which guide you up through a verdant, spray-drenched garden. The last few dozen steps are under the shelter of trees; then, reaching an alcove beneath an ominous overhang, you scurry left up a last set of stairs. These, protected by a railing, guide one to the top of a vertical cliff. Pausing

Waterfall

Caution

here you can study your route, the nearby fall, and the river gorge. The railing ends near the brink of Vernal Fall, ►4 but unfortunately, people venture beyond it, and sometimes people are swept over the fall. Just above it is Emerald Pool, and due to the danger of its treacherous current, wading and swimming are forbidden.

Plunging into the upper end of chilly Emerald Pool is churning Silver Apron, and a bridge spanning its narrow gorge is your immediate goal. At times the trail has been vague in this area, due to use-paths, but the correct route leaves the river near the pool's far (east) end, and you'll find outhouses here. After a brief climb south, the trail angles east to a nearby junction. ►5 From it a view-blessed trail climbs almost 0.5 mile to Clark Point, where it meets the John Muir Trail. You, however, stay low and curve left over to the Silver Apron bridge. ►6 Beyond it you have a short, moderate climb up to a broad bench. Then, spurred onward by the sight and sound of plummeting Nevada Fall, you climb eastward, to soon commence a series of more than two dozen short switchbacks. As you ascend them, Nevada Fall slips out of view, but you can see towering Liberty Cap. The climb ends at the top of a joint-controlled gully where, on brushy slopes, you once again meet the John Muir Trail, with outhouses just up it. ►7 From this junction you head southwest toward nearby Nevada Fall. ►8

 Waterfall

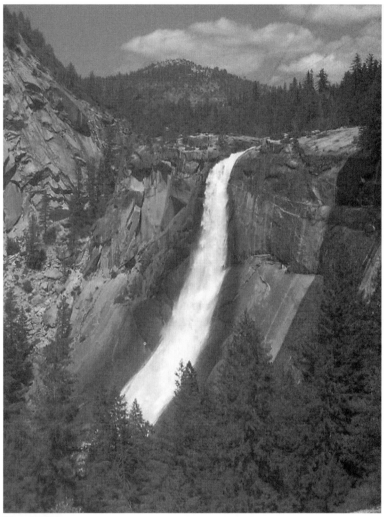

Nevada Fall

From the Nevada Fall bridge you strike southwest, immediately passing more glacier polish and erratic boulders, and shortly end a gentle ascent just beyond a seeping spring, at a junction with the Glacier Point–Panorama Trail (Trail 41). ►9 Now you begin a descent to Happy Isles along the John Muir Trail. This starts with a high traverse that provides an ever-changing panorama of domelike Liberty Cap and broad-topped Mt. Broderick—both once overridden by glaciers. As you progress west, Half Dome becomes prominent, its hulking mass vying for your attention. Eventually you descend to Clark Point, ►10 where you meet a scenic connecting trail that switchbacks down to Emerald Pool. If you enjoyed the Mist Trail, you can visit it again by first descending this lateral, but remember to be careful while descending the Mist Trail.

 Great Views

Backpackers, packers, and those wishing to keep dry continue down the John Muir Trail, which curves south into a gully, switchbacks down to the base of spreading Panorama Cliff, then switchbacks down a talus slope. Largely shaded by canyon live oaks and Douglas-firs, it reaches a junction with a horse trail (no hikers allowed) that descends to the valley's stables. Continue a brief minute more to a junction with the Mist Trail, ▶11 turn left, and quickly reach the Vernal Fall bridge, ▶12 from which you retrace your steps down to Happy Isles. ▶13

🚶 MILESTONES

▶1	0.0	Start at shuttle stop 16
▶2	1.0	Vernal Fall bridge
▶3	1.1	Straight on Mist Trail
▶4	1.6	Brink of Vernal Fall
▶5	1.7	Left at junction
▶6	1.8	Silver Apron bridge
▶7	2.7	Right on John Muir Trail
▶8	2.9	Nevada Fall
▶9	3.1	Glacier Point–Panorama Trail
▶10	4.2	Clark Point
▶11	5.4	Mist Trail
▶12	5.5	Vernal Fall bridge
▶13	6.5	Happy Isles

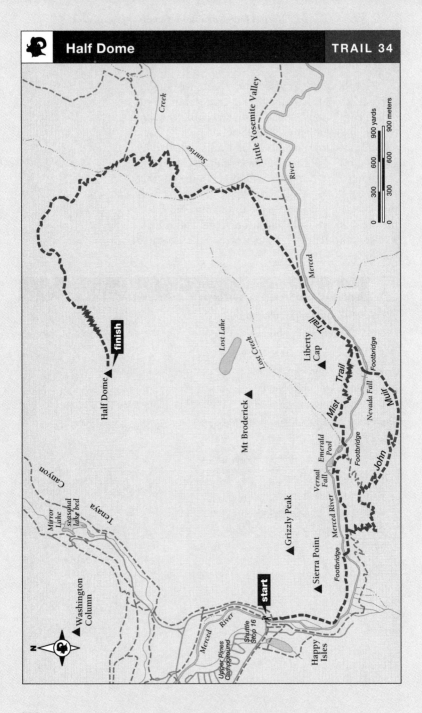

900 yards

900 meters

Little Yosemite Valley

Creek

Sunrise

River

Merced

finish

Half Dome ▲

Lost Lake

Lost Creek

Liberty Cap ▲

Trail

Footbridge

Mist

Nevada Fall

Trail

Mt Broderick ▲

Muir

Emerald Pool

Vernal Fall

Footbridge

John

Merced River

Footbridge

Canyon

Tenaya

Grizzly Peak ▲

Mirror Lake

seasonal lake bed

Sierra Point ▲

Footbridge

Washington Column ▲

N

start

Merced River

Shuttle Stop 16

Upper Pines Campground

Happy Isles

Half Dome

Many a backpacker has spent his or her first night in the "wilderness" of Little Yosemite Valley. Indeed, more backpackers camp in it than in any other Yosemite backcountry area. Perhaps too, more bears visit it than any other backcountry area. During the summer this area is patrolled by rangers stationed near the backpackers camp. If you hike only this far, your entire semi-loop route up the Mist Trail and down the John Muir Trail will be just 8.7 miles long, and the total ups and downs will be a mere 4800 feet. If you ascend and descend only along the Mist Trail, your round-trip distance is 7.4 miles; if entirely along the John Muir Trail, it is 9.6 miles.

For many camped in Little Yosemite Valley, their ultimate goal is the summit of Half Dome. On a good summer day, hundreds of hikers attempt this summit, but many turn back, either from exhaustion of from fear. If I as a first-time visitor were allowed to make only one dayhike in the park, I would unquestionably choose this hike—the one that introduced me to Yosemite and fired my desire to "climb every mountain."

However, Half Dome is certainly not for acrophobics, klutzes, those out of shape, or those who have bad knees. The hike up Half Dome's shoulder and its cables is exposed and potentially life-threatening. Far too many "innocents abroad" attempt to make this climb, even in threatening thunderstorms. Do not attempt to climb the dome's shoulder and its cables if weather is threatening, for the exposed rock becomes very slippery and a lightning strike is possible. Occasionally people die on this route; more fall and are injured. Do not take it lightly, and

TRAIL USE
Dayhike, Backpack, Horse
LENGTH
15.5 miles; 6–12 hours
VERTICAL FEET
+5400'/-5400'/±10,800'
DIFFICULTY
- 1 2 3 4 **5** +
TRAIL TYPE
Semi-loop

FEATURES
Backcountry Permit
Streams
Waterfalls
Summit
Great Views
Camping
Steep

FACILITIES
Resort
Store
Visitor Center
Restrooms
Campgrounds
Bus Stop
Picnic Tables
Phone
Water
Horse Staging
Patrol Cabin

although I've seen kids as young as 8 on the cables, I discourage anyone under the age of 12. Call me a cautious parent.

The preferred route between the Vernal Fall bridge and Nevada Fall ascends the Mist Trail and descends the John Muir Trail, for a total of 15.5 miles, exposing you to the maximum amount of scenery. If you ascend and descend only along the Mist Trail, your round-trip distance is 14.4 miles; if entirely along the John Muir Trail, it is 16.6 miles.

Best Time

Half Dome's hiking season is limited to when its cables are in place, which depends a lot on the amount of snowfall and on the presence or absence of stormy weather. Cables may be placed as early as early May or as late as late June, and they may be removed any time in October. Therefore, if you're hiking before July or after September, be sure to inquire if the cables are up. Earlier is better for viewing Vernal and Nevada falls, but later is better for cooler temperatures and less chance of a thunderstorm (generally most prevalent in July).

Finding the Trail

Take a shuttle bus to stop 16, at Happy Isles, immediately west of a bridge across the Merced River.

The valley has only three regular campgrounds—North, Upper, and Lower Pines—plus two smaller, walk-in campgrounds—Camp 4 and Backpackers. The former is heavily dominated by rock climbers, and the latter is for backpackers who have a wilderness permit and need a place to stay the night before they start their hike.

Trail Description

From the shuttle stop ▶1 you walk briefly east across an adjacent bridge and head south, soon reaching the start of the famous John Muir Trail, which heads about 210 miles southward to the summit of Mt. Whitney. After a few minutes you reach a small spring-fed cistern with questionably pure water. Beyond it the climb south steepens, and before bending east you get a glance back at Upper Yosemite Fall, partly blocked by the Glacier Point Apron.

Note the canyon wall south of the apron, which has a series of oblique-angle cliffs—all of them remarkably similar in orientation since they've fractured along the same series of joint planes. At the canyon's end Illilouette Fall plunges 370 feet over a vertical, joint controlled cliff. Just east of the fall is a large scar that marks the site of a major rockfall that broke loose during the winter of 1968–69.

Great Views

Climbing east, you head up a canyon whose floor in times past was buried by as much as 1800 feet of glacier ice. Hiking beneath the unstable, highly fractured south wall of Sierra Point, you cross a talus slope—an accumulation of rockfall boulders. More rockfalls may occur. Entering forest shade once more, you ascend a steep stretch of trail before making a quick drop to the Vernal Fall bridge. ▶2 From it you see Vernal Fall, a broad curtain of water plunging 320 feet over a vertical cliff before cascading toward you. Looming above the fall are two glacier-resistant masses, Mt. Broderick (left) and Liberty Cap (right). Just beyond the bridge are restrooms and an emergency telephone (for such events as heart attacks, slips on dangerous rocks).

Waterfall

About 200 yards beyond the bridge you come to the start of your loop. ▶3 Here the Mist Trail continues upriver, while the John Muir Trail starts a

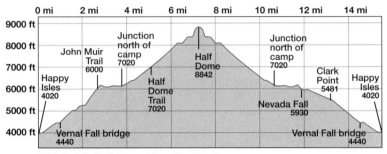

TRAIL 34 **Half Dome Elevation Profile**

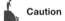
Caution

switchbacking ascent to the right. This is the route taken by those with horses or other pack stock. You'll go up the Mist Trail and down the John Muir Trail. You can, of course go up or down either, but by starting the loop up the Mist Trail, you stand less chance of an accident. Hikers are more apt to slip or to twist an ankle descending than ascending, and the Mist Trail route to Nevada Fall has ample opportunities for mishaps.

Dressed for the upcoming mist, which can really soak you in May or June, start up the Mist Trail and soon, rounding a bend, receive your first spray. If you're climbing this trail on a sunny day, you may see one, if not two, rainbows come alive in the fall's spray. The spray increases as you advance toward the fall, but you get a brief respite behind a large boulder. Beyond it, complete your 300-plus steps, most of them wet, which guide you up through a verdant, spray-drenched garden. The last few dozen steps are under the shelter of trees; then, reaching an alcove beneath an ominous overhang, you scurry left up a last set of stairs. These, protected by a railing, guide one to the top of a vertical cliff. Pausing here you can study your route, the nearby fall, and the river gorge. The railing ends near the brink of

Waterfall

Vernal Fall, ►4 but unfortunately, people venture beyond it, and sometimes are swept over the fall. Just above it is Emerald Pool, and due to the danger of its treacherous current, wading and swimming are forbidden.

 Caution

Plunging into the upper end of chilly Emerald Pool is churning Silver Apron, and a bridge spanning its narrow gorge is your immediate goal. At times the trail has been vague in this area, due to use-paths, but the correct route leaves the river near the pool's far (east) end, and you'll find outhouses here. After a brief climb south, the trail angles east to a nearby junction. ►5 From it a view-blessed trail climbs almost 0.5 mile to Clark Point, where it meets the John Muir Trail. You, however, stay low and curve left over to the Silver Apron bridge. ►6 Beyond it you have a short, moderate climb up to a broad bench. Then, spurred onward by the sight and sound of plummeting Nevada Fall, you climb eastward, to soon commence a series of more than two dozen short switchbacks. As you ascend them, Nevada Fall slips out of view, but you can see towering Liberty Cap. The climb ends at the top of a joint-controlled gully where, on brushy slopes, you once again meet the John Muir Trail, with outhouses just up it. ►7

From this junction you climb up a gully that is generally overgrown with scrubby huckleberry oaks. From its top you quickly descend into forest cover and reach a fairly large "swimming hole" on the Merced River. Though chilly, it is far enough above the river's rapids to provide a short, refreshing dip. A longer stay would make you numb. Beneath lodgepole and Jeffrey pines, white firs, and incense-cedars you continue northeast along the river's azalea-lined bank, then quickly encounter a trail fork. ►8

Swimming

Alternate Trip to Little Yosemite Valley

►8 If you are backpacking first to Little Yosemite Valley, then you should take the right fork, which parallels the Merced River upstream to the valley's large backpackers camp with bear-proof storage boxes. Just beyond it are outhouses, and the a spur trail northeast over to a rangers' camp. Just ahead of that is a junction with the left-fork route.

Those bound for Half Dome generally take the left fork after first obtaining enough water from the Merced River, which is your last reliable source. This trail is 0.1 mile shorter than the right-fork route, but it climbs and then descends the low east ridge of Liberty Cap, negating its advantage over the level right-fork route, and it reaches a junction north of backpackers camp. ►9

From the junction north of backpackers camp you've not yet expended half the energy required to reach Half Dome's summit. After 1.3 miles of forested ascent you leave the John Muir Trail and keep left, starting up the Half Dome Trail. ►10 After about 0.7 mile the trail bends west just before reaching a saddle, which is worth the minor effort for a viewful rest stop. In the next 0.5 mile, the trail first climbs through a forest of red firs and Jeffrey pines instead of white firs and incense-cedars. Half Dome's northeast face comes into view before the trail tops a crest. Here you get a fine view of Clouds Rest and its satellites, the Quarter Domes, these accessible by a somewhat brushy cross-country ascent from the previously mentioned saddle. Between them and you, previous glaciers once spilled into Tenaya Canyon. The shoulder of Half Dome, west of and above you, never was glaciated. Those on horseback need to end here, if not a bit sooner, under forest cover.

Great Views

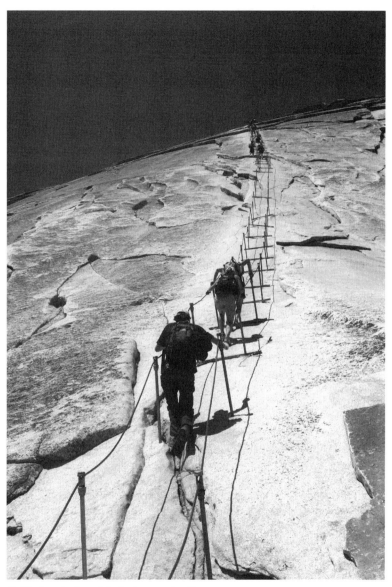

Cable handrails *aid the final ascent of Half Dome.*

You now have a 0.3-mile traverse, which reveals more views, including Tenaya Canyon, Mt. Watkins, Mt. Hoffmann, and much of the upper Merced River basin. This traverse ends all too soon at the base of Half Dome's intimidating shoulder.

Great Views

Almost two dozen very short switchbacks guide you up the view-blessed ridge of the dome's shoulder. For too long the real danger on this steep section was loose gravel, which could prove fatal if you fell off the trail—or were pushed off it due to heavy traffic—at one or more exposed spots, but in 2005 it was extensively reworked to make it safer. Topping the shoulder, you are confronted with the dome's even more intimidating pair of cables, which definitely cause some hikers to retreat.

Steep

The ascent starts out gently enough, but it too quickly steepens almost to a 45-degree angle. On this stretch, first-timers often slow to a snail's pace, clenching both cables with sweaty hands. Looking down, you can see that you don't want to fall. In recent years hikers have used gloves for the cables and then left them for others. Perhaps fresh gloves may be better than sweaty hands, but old, well-used gloves seem just as slippery. Remember that even when thunderstorms are miles away, static electricity can build up here. Out of a seemingly fair-weather sky a charge can bolt down the cable, throwing your arms off it—or worse. If your hair starts standing on end, beat a hasty retreat.

Caution

The rarefied air certainly hinders your progress as you ascend, but eventually an easing gradient gives new incentive and soon you are scrambling up to the broad summit of Half Dome, an area about the size of 17 football fields. ▶11 With caution most hikers proceed to the dome's high point (8842 feet), located at the north end, from where they can view the dome's overhanging northwest point. Stouthearted souls peer over the lip of this point for an adrenaline-charged view down the dome's 2000-foot-high northwest face, perhaps seeing climbers ascending it. In the past a few folks liked to camp overnight to view the sunrise, but in 1993 camping was banned.

From the broad summit of this monolith, which began to form in the late days of the dinosaurs, you have a 360-degree panorama. You can look down Yosemite Valley to the bald brow of El Capitan and up Tenaya Canyon past Clouds Rest to Cathedral Peak, the Sierra crest, and Mt. Hoffmann. Mt. Starr King—a dome that rises only 250 feet above you—dominates the Illilouette Creek basin to the south, while the Clark Range cuts the sky to the southeast. Looking due east across Moraine Dome's summit, you see Mt. Florence, whose broad form hides the park's highest peak, Mt. Lyell, behind it.

Great Views

To return, backtrack 4.5 miles to the junction northeast of Nevada Fall, at the top of the Mist Trail, Milestone 7 on your ascent. ▶12 From here the John Muir Trail traverses southwest toward nearby Nevada Fall. ▶13

Nevada Fall viewpoint

OPTIONS

▶13 Just a few yards before the Nevada Fall bridge you can strike northwest to find a short spur trail that drops to a viewpoint beside the fall's brink. This viewpoint's railing is seen from the fall's bridge, thereby giving you an idea where the trail ends. Don't stray along the cliff's edge and, as said earlier, respect the river—people have been swept over this fall too.

From the Nevada Fall bridge you strike south-west, immediately passing more glacier polish and erratic boulders, and shortly end a gentle ascent just beyond a seeping spring, at a junction with the Glacier Point–Panorama Trail (Trail 41). ▶14 Now you begin a descent to Happy Isles along the John Muir Trail. This starts with a high traverse that provides an ever-changing panorama of domelike Liberty Cap and broad-topped Mt. Broderick—both overridden by glaciers. As you progress west, Half Dome becomes prominent, its hulking mass vying for your attention. Eventually you descend to Clark Point, ▶15 where you meet a scenic connecting trail that switchbacks down to Emerald Pool. If you enjoyed the Mist Trail, you can visit it again by first descending this lateral, but remember to be careful while descending the Mist Trail.

Backpackers, packers, and those wishing to keep dry continue down the John Muir Trail, which curves south into a gully, switchbacks down to the base of spreading Panorama Cliff, then switchbacks down a talus slope. Largely shaded by canyon live oaks and Douglas-firs, it reaches a junction with a horse trail (no hikers allowed) that descends to the valley's stables. Continue a brief minute more to a junction with the Mist Trail, ▶16 turn left, and quickly reach the Vernal Fall bridge, ▶17 from which you retrace your steps down to Happy Isles. ▶18

🚶 MILESTONES

►1   0.0 Start at shuttle stop 16

►2   1.0 Vernal Fall bridge

►3   1.1 Straight on Mist Trail

►4   1.6 Brink of Vernal Fall

►5   1.7 Left at junction

►6   1.8 Silver Apron bridge

►7   2.7 Left on John Muir Trail

►8   3.3 Left at trail fork

►9   3.8 Left at junction north of backpackers camp

►10 5.1 Left on Half Dome Trail

►11 7.2 Summit of Half Dome

►12 11.7 Straight at junction northeast of Nevada Fall

►13 11.9 Nevada Fall

►14 12.1 Glacier Point–Panorama Trail

►15 13.2 Clark Point

►16 14.4 Mist Trail

►17 14.5 Vernal Fall bridge

►18 15.5 Happy Isles

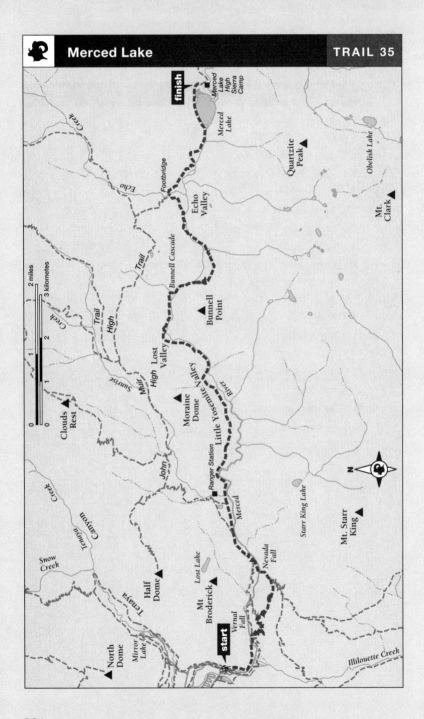

Merced Lake

TRAIL 35

finish

Merced Lake High Sierra Camp

Merced Lake

Quartzite Peak

Obelisk Lake

Echo Creek

Footbridge

Echo Valley

Mt. Clark

Bunnell Cascade

Bunnell Point

High Trail

Sunrise Creek

High Trail

Lost Valley

Muir High Trail

Moraine Dome

Little Yosemite Valley

Clouds Rest

Ranger Station

2 miles
3 kilometres

Merced River

John Muir Trail

Tenaya Creek

Canyon

Snow Creek

Half Dome

Lost Lake

Mt Broderick

Starr King Lake

Mt. Starr King

Nevada Fall

North Dome

Mirror Lake

Tenaya

Vernal Fall

start

Illilouette Creek

N

Merced Lake

Best done in three days with overnight stops at Little Yosemite Valley and Merced Lake, this hike is often done in two by energetic weekend hikers. Its route, up a fantastic river canyon, is one of the Sierra's best. Located at an elevation of about 7200 feet, relatively large Merced Lake is about 2000+ feet lower than the popular ones reached from Tuolumne Meadows' trailheads, and therefore it is snowfree sooner.

Best Time

Some folks make this hike in June, when Vernal and Nevada falls are spectacular, but mosquitoes up at Merced Lake are ubiquitous. Early July is better, but you'll definitely want a tent. By late July, the lake's environs are relatively mosquito-free, and the lake is about as warm as it is going to get. This deep lake stays tolerably "warm" through mid-August, then begins to chill. Anglers and the relatively recluse may find September best, after the crowds have left. The nights and morning temperatures are nippy, but the afternoon ones are about perfect.

Finding the Trail

Take a shuttle bus to stop 16, at Happy Isles, immediately west of a bridge across the Merced River.

The valley has only three regular campgrounds—North, Upper, and Lower Pines—plus two smaller, walk-in campgrounds—Camp 4 and Backpackers. The former is heavily dominated by rock climbers, and the latter is for backpackers who

TRAIL USE
Backpack, Horse
LENGTH
28.4 miles, 2–3 days
VERTICAL FEET
+4480'/-4480'/±8960'
DIFFICULTY
- 1 2 3 4 **5** +
TRAIL TYPE
Out & Back

FEATURES
Backcountry Permit
Lake
Streams
Waterfalls
Wildflowers
Great Views
Camping
Swimming

FACILITIES
Resort
Store
Visitor Center
Restrooms
Campgrounds
Bus Stop
Picnic Tables
Phone
Water
Horse Staging
Patrol Cabin

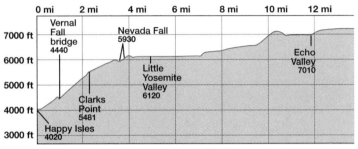

TRAIL 35 Merced Lake Elevation Profile

have a wilderness permit. For Trail 35, you probably will want to stay the night here before you start your hike.

Logistics

This trip's mileage is based on starting from the Happy Isles shuttle stop and ascending the John Muir Trail. If you have a vehicle, you have to leave it at the backpackers' trailhead parking lot just east of the last cabins of Curry Village; then you'll have to walk a bit farther.

Curry Village to Happy Isles

OPTIONS

If you start from the trailhead parking lot just east of **Curry Village**, you can take the paved, roadside path 0.5 mile east to the shuttle stop, but a quieter route begins from the southeast edge of the trailhead parking lot. This rolls southeast, staying about 100–150 yards from the unseen shuttle-bus road. In 0.4 mile it intersects a southbound stock trail that links the valley stables to the John Muir Trail. Beyond this intersection you head east on planks across a boggy area, and although mosquitoes may be bothersome in late spring and early summer, the bog then produces its best wildflowers. At a huge, lone boulder by the bog's east side, your trail angles southeast toward the hub of the Happy Isles area, and you head briefly north to its shuttle stop, ▶1 0.6 mile from the trailhead parking lot.

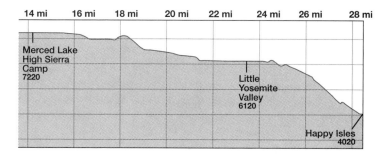

Trail Description

From the Happy Isles shuttle stop ►1 you walk briefly east across an adjacent bridge and head south, soon reaching the start of the famous John Muir Trail, which heads about 210 miles southward to the summit of Mt. Whitney. After a few minutes you reach a small spring-fed cistern with questionably pure water. Beyond it the climb south steepens, and before bending east you get a glance back at Upper Yosemite Fall, partly blocked by the Glacier Point Apron.

Entering forest shade once more, you ascend a steep stretch of trail before making a quick drop to the Vernal Fall bridge. ►2 From it you see Vernal Fall, a broad curtain of water plunging 320 feet over a vertical cliff before cascading toward you. Looming above the fall are two glacier-resistant masses, Mt. Broderick (left) and Liberty Cap (right). Just beyond the bridge are restrooms and an emergency telephone (for such events as heart attacks, slips on dangerous rocks).

Now you hike 0.1 mile up to the start of the Mist Trail. ►3 (The 1.1-mile shorter Mist Trail, to the brink of Vernal Fall, past Emerald Pool and across the Silver Apron, certainly is worth taking, but the steep stretch up to the top of Vernal Fall can be wet and slippery and potentially dangerous if

 Stream

 Waterfall

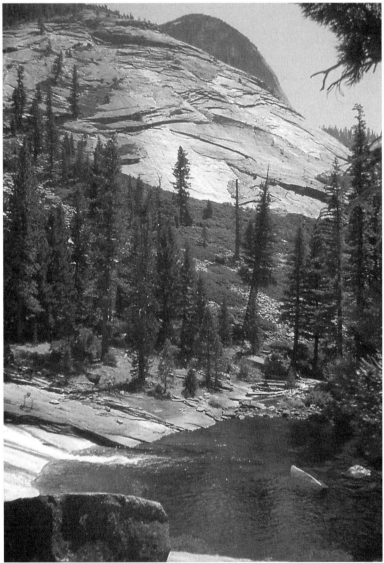

Cascade Cliffs, *east of Little Yosemite Valley*

you're carrying a heavy backpack). Play it safe and take the John Muir Trail 2.7 miles up to the top of the Mist Trail.

This stretch has equal rewards. One is that the first 1.2 miles to Clark Point are along shady, moderately graded switchbacks, which are near ideal for the ascent. From Clark Point ►4 you have less climbing to do, and most of it comes with views across the canyon to Half Dome, Mt. Broderick, and Liberty Cap, the last above Nevada Fall. After 1.1 miles you reach the Glacier Point–Panorama Trail, ►5 then descend 0.2 mile to the bridge over Nevada Fall. ►6 Just a few yards beyond the bridge you can strike northwest to find a short spur trail that drops to a viewpoint beside the fall's brink. This viewpoint's railing is seen from the fall's bridge, thereby giving you an idea where the trail ends. Finally, about 0.2 mile later, you reach the top of the Mist Trail. ►7

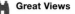 **Waterfall**

 Great Views

From the junction and its adjacent outhouses you begin your 1.0 mile route to Little Yosemite Valley first by ascending a brushy, rocky gully, then quickly descending and reaching both forest shade and the Merced River. Beneath pines, firs, and incense-cedars you continue northeast along the river's azalea-lined bank, then quickly reach a trail fork. ►8 You keep to the main, riverside trail and go a short 0.5 mile to another junction, in the hub of Little Yosemite Valley, ►9 from where the John Muir Trail branches north. Just up it is a large camping area with bear-proof storage boxes, then outhouses, and beyond them a spur trail northeast over to a rangers' camp. Some hikers on their way to Merced Lake spend their first night here, which is about halfway up, measured by total elevation gain and loss.

Stream

You leave the northbound John Muir Trail to embark on a shady 2-mile stroll, following the Merced Lake Trail through the broad, flat valley. The

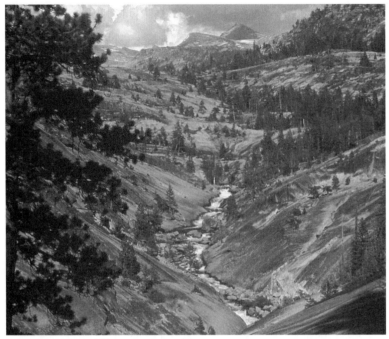

Cascading Merced River, *east of Bunnell Point*

Canyon

Camping

valley's floor has been largely buried by glacial sediments, which, like beach sand, make you work even though the trail is level. Progressing east through Little Yosemite Valley, you stay closer to the base of glacier-polished Moraine Dome than to the Merced River, and along this stretch you can branch off to riverside campsites that are far more peaceful than those near the John Muir Trail junction, which tends to be a "Grand Central Station." The valley's east end is graced by the presence of a beautiful pool—the receptacle of a Merced River cascade. Leaving the camps of the picturesque area, you climb past the cascade and glance back to see the east face of exfoliating Moraine Dome.

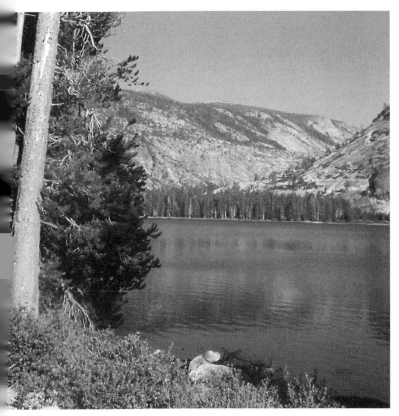

Merced Lake

△ **Camping**

     From this Echo Valley junction near an Echo Creek campsite, there is the start of an alternate route back to the backpackers camp in Little Yosemite Valley, the High Trail. The overall distance is 7.7 miles, versus 7.0 miles along the Merced Lake Trail. When your up-canyon Merced Lake Trail was completed in 1931, the High Trail to Merced Lake fell into disuse, for it is almost a mile longer and climbs 750 feet more. It also has less water, fewer campsites, and fewer views.

Your brief cascade climb heads toward the 1900 foot high Bunnell Point cliff, which is exfoliating at a prodigious rate. Rounding the base of a glacier-smoothed dome, unofficially called the Sugar Loaf, about 1 mile beyond the east end of Little Yosemite Valley you enter Lost Valley, in which no fires are allowed. At the valley's east end, switchback up past Bunnell Cascade, which with the magnificent canyon scenery can easily distract one from the very real danger of this exposed section of trail.

Just beyond the V gorge, the canyon floor widens a bit, and in this area you bridge the Merced River. Your up-canyon walk soon reaches a series of more than a dozen switchbacks that carry you up 400 feet above the river—a bypass route necessitated by another V gorge. Your climb reaches its zenith amid a spring-fed profuse garden, bordered by aspens, which in midsummer supports a colorful array of various wildflowers.

Beyond this glade you soon come out onto a highly polished bedrock surface. Here you can glance west and see Clouds Rest—a long ridge—standing on the horizon. Now you descend back into tree cover, and among the white boles of aspens brush through a forest carpet of bracken ferns and cross several creeklets before emerging on a bedrock bench above the river's inner gorge. From the bench you can study the features of a broad, hulking granitic mass opposite you whose south face is bounded by an immense arch. Traversing the bench, you soon come to a bend in the river and at it bridge the Merced just above the brink of its cascades. Strolling east, you soon reach the west end of spacious Echo Valley, and proceed to a junction at its north edge. ▶10

Caution

Stream

Wildflow

Canyon

In Echo Valley, with Merced Lake your first goal, you immediately bridge Echo Creek, strike southeast through burned-but-boggy Echo Valley, and climb east past the Merced River's largely unseen pools to Merced Lake's west shore. Don't camp here, but rather continue along the north shore for about 0.5 mile and then 0.25 mile east beyond it to Merced Lake High Sierra Camp ▶11 and the adjacent riverside campground, about 9.25 miles beyond the John Muir Trail junction in Little Yosemite Valley. Be sure to use the bear-proof food-storage boxes. Eighty-foot-deep Merced Lake, being a large one at a moderate elevation, supports three species of trout: brook, brown, and rainbow.

≋ **Lake**

▲ **Camping**

🚶	**MILESTONES**
▶1	0.0 Start at shuttle stop 16
▶2	1.0 Vernal Fall bridge
▶3	1.1 Sharp right at Mist Trail
▶4	2.3 Clark Point
▶5	3.4 Glacier Point–Panorama Trail
▶6	3.6 Nevada Fall
▶7	3.8 Straight at top of Mist Trail
▶8	4.4 Right at trail fork
▶9	4.9 Straight in Little Yosemite Valley
▶10	11.9 Straight at Echo Valley junction
▶11	14.2 Merced Lake High Sierra Camp

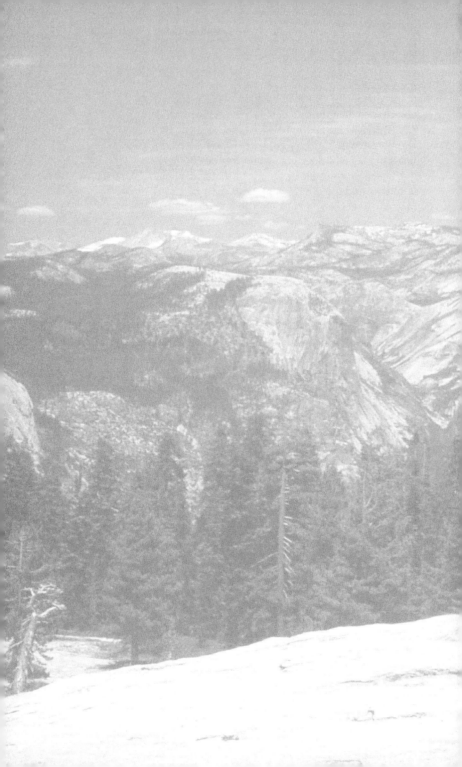

CHAPTER 6

Yosemite Valley's South Rim

Yosemite Valley's South Rim

As was the previous one, this chapter is actually composed of two groups: four trails starting from the end or near the end of the Glacier Point Road and heading to extremely scenic viewpoints, and two trails starting from Glacier Point and descending several thousand feet to the floor of Yosemite Valley.

In the first group, visitor use to each viewpoint is inversely proportionate to its distance from the trailhead. Dewey Point is the farthest and may get one or two dozen visitors on a summer's day, while Glacier Point is easily the closest and may get a thousand visitors. Glacier Point is arguably the best viewpoint in the entire park, if not in the entire Sierra, since more than any other summit it offers an aerial view of the most spectacular part of the valley. I am sure many Sierran hikers have their favorites. (On my list, the views from Mt. Dana and Half Dome compete for first place; Mt. Whitney, the highest peak in the Sierra, is not on my list.) Whereas you can drive almost to Glacier Point (which is a brief walk), and you can drive to Washburn Point (nearly equally spectacular), you'll have to make short hikes (an hour or two, round-trip) to acrophobic Taft Point or to broad-topped Sentinel Dome, both of which offer "Kodak moments."

Of the two trails starting from Glacier Point and descending to Yosemite Valley, the Four Mile Trail is the shortest, half the length of the Glacier Point–Panorama Trail. It also is less spectacular, not passing by three waterfalls or beneath the looming presences of Mt. Broderick and Liberty Cap.

Permits

All of this chapter's described trails are dayhikes, and so no wilderness permit is needed. Still, should you wish to camp in the backcountry, say, near Trail 36's Dewey Point, then try to reserve a permit, rather than get one in person—see the "Fees, Camping, and Permits" section on page 14. If you must get one in person, obtain one either in Yosemite Valley at the Wilderness Center, centrally located in Yosemite Village, or at the Wawona

Overleaf: *Half Dome from Sentinel Dome (Trail 38)*

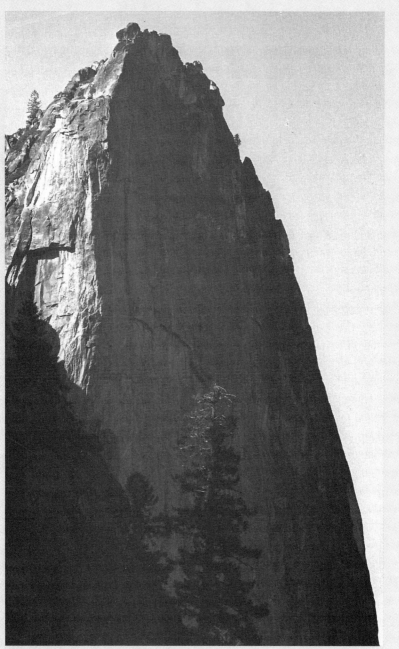

Sentinel Rock *from Four Mile Trail (Trail 40)*

Yosemite Valley's South Rim

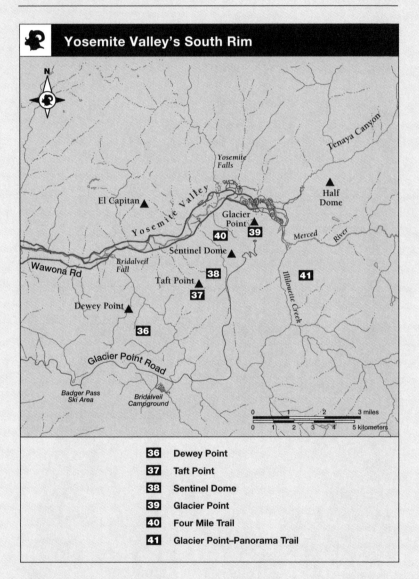

36	Dewey Point
37	Taft Point
38	Sentinel Dome
39	Glacier Point
40	Four Mile Trail
41	Glacier Point–Panorama Trail

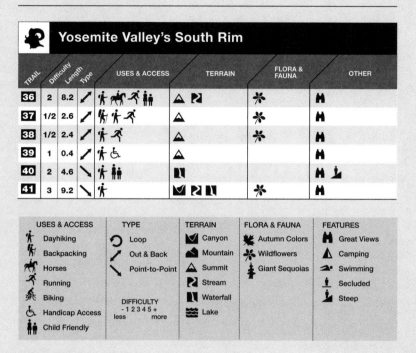

Yosemite Valley's South Rim

TRAIL	Difficulty	Length	Type	USES & ACCESS	TERRAIN	FLORA & FAUNA	OTHER
36	2	8.2	↗	🚶🏇🏃👫	⛰️ ▷	✿	⚔
37	1/2	2.6	↗	🚶🏃	⛰️	✿	⚔
38	1/2	2.4	↗	🚶🏃	⛰️	✿	⚔
39	1	0.4	↗	🚶♿	⛰️		⚔
40	2	4.6	↘	🚶👫	🏔		⚔ 🛁
41	3	9.2	↘	🚶	🏞️ ▷ 🏔	✿	⚔

USES & ACCESS
- 🚶 Dayhiking
- 🎒 Backpacking
- 🏇 Horses
- 🏃 Running
- 🚴 Biking
- ♿ Handicap Access
- 👫 Child Friendly

TYPE
- ↻ Loop
- ↱ Out & Back
- ↘ Point-to-Point

DIFFICULTY
-12345+
less   more

TERRAIN
- 🌊 Canyon
- ⛰️ Mountain
- 🔺 Summit
- ▷ Stream
- 🏔 Waterfall
- 〰️ Lake

FLORA & FAUNA
- 🍁 Autumn Colors
- ✿ Wildflowers
- 🌲 Giant Sequoias

FEATURES
- ⚔ Great Views
- ▲ Camping
- 🏊 Swimming
- 🔱 Secluded
- 🔺 Steep

District Office, on the north side of the South Fork Merced River. From the bridge north across the river, reach this office by starting along the Chilnualna Road and quickly reaching a short spur road, which you take immediately past the Pioneer Yosemite History Center.

Maps

For Yosemite Valley's South Rim, Trails 37 to 41 are on the USGS (1:24,000-scale) Topographic Map of Yosemite Valley, which is readily available in the park. Trail 36 ends on this map, but is shown in its entirety on the USGS El Capitan 7.5-minute (1:24,000-scale) topographic quadrangle.

Yosemite Valley's South Rim

TRAIL 36

Dayhike, Run, Horse
8.2 miles, Out & Back
Difficulty: 1 **2** 3 4 5

Dewey Point 303
This is the easier of two routes to scenic Dewey Point, and it requires less than half the climbing effort of a start up the Pohono Trail. Particularly in the summer, that longer route can be a hot climb. In contrast, yours is a much cooler, rolling traverse confined between 6770 feet and 7385 feet elevation. Because of the relatively gentle nature of the trail, it is suitable for both children and runners.

TRAIL 37

Dayhike, Run, Horse
2.6 miles, Out & Back
Difficulty: **1 2** 3 4 5

Taft Point 307
The views from Taft Point rival those from Glacier Point. However, since Taft Point is reached by trail, it is less visited than mobbed Glacier Point. Generally lacking protective railings, Taft Point and the Fissures are potentially dangerous, so don't bring along children unless you can really keep them under strict control.

TRAIL 38

Dayhike, Run
2.4 miles, Out & Back
Difficulty: **1 2** 3 4 5

Sentinel Dome 311
Sentinel Dome rivals Half Dome as the most-climbed dome in the park. Tuolumne Meadows' Lembert and Pothole domes almost rival them, but neither is a true dome; each is a roche moutonnée—an asymmetrical, glacier-smoothed ridge. Indeed, most of the Sierra's domes, glaciated or unglaciated, are asymmetrical ridges.

Glacier Point 315
From the early 1870s until January 1968, this was the site of the renowned Firefall—an artificial glowing "waterfall" of burning embers. Then, from the early 1970s until mid-1990, people would hang glide here in the early mornings—creating a different spectacle. However, one reason for establishing the park was to protect its natural lands, and you can see a spectacular part of them by making the short pilgrimage out to Glacier Point.

Four Mile Trail 319
This trail provides a very scenic descent to Yosemite Valley—a descent that will acquaint you with the valley's main features. This knee-knocking descent also gives you a feel for the valley's 3000-foot depth. This hike is rated "easy" because not much energy is expended, but if you do a lot of braking on the dozens of switchbacks, you may consider it "moderate."

Glacier Point–Panorama Trail 323
This is the most scenic of all trails descending to the floor of Yosemite Valley, passing three waterfalls and offering spectacular views along the way. Either take a bus up to Glacier Point or have someone drop you there and meet you down at Curry Village.

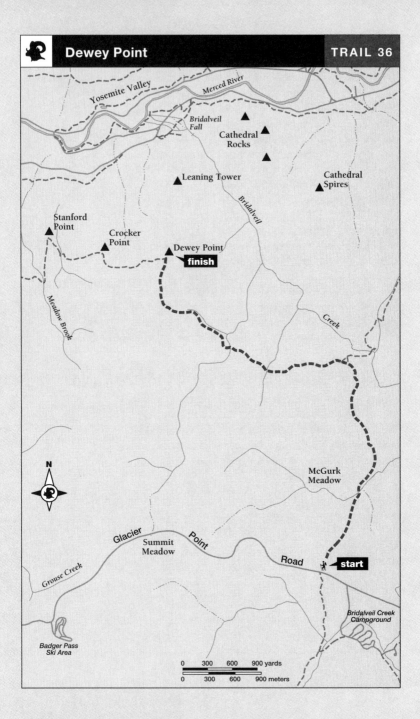

Dewey Point

TRAIL 36

Yosemite Valley

Merced River

Bridalveil
Fall

Cathedral
Rocks

Cathedral
Spires

Leaning Tower

Bridalveil

Stanford
Point

Crocker
Point

Dewey Point

finish

Creek

Meadow Brook

N

McGurk
Meadow

Glacier

Summit
Meadow

Point

Road

start

Grouse Creek

Bridalveil Creek
Campground

Badger Pass
Ski Area

| 0 | 300 | 600 | 900 yards |
| 0 | 300 | 600 | 900 meters |

Dewey Point

This is the easier of two routes to scenic Dewey Point, and it requires less than half the climbing effort of a start up the Pohono Trail, which begins at Discovery View at the east end of Wawona Tunnel, on the Wawona Road 1.5 miles west of the Bridalveil Fall parking lot entrance. Particularly in the summer, that longer route can be a hot climb. In contrast, yours is a much cooler, rolling traverse confined between 6770 feet and 7385 feet elevation. Because of the relatively gentle nature of the trail, it is suitable for both children and runners.

Best Time

Meadow wildflowers are best from about late June to mid-July, when pollinating (and bloodsucking) mosquitoes abound. Therefore, late July onward is best, and because Dewey Point's views do not change much (Ribbon Fall dries up early), the hike is a rewarding one through mid-October.

Finding the Trail

From a signed junction along the Wawona Road, drive 7.4 miles up the Glacier Point Road to the signed trailhead, on your left. This is 0.25 mile before the spur road to the Bridalveil Creek Campground, which is the only campground along the Glacier Point Road.

TRAIL USE
Dayhike, Run, Horse
LENGTH
8.2 miles, 3–4 hours
VERTICAL FEET
+740'/-490'/±2460'
DIFFICULTY
- 1 **2** 3 4 5 +
TRAIL TYPE
Out & Back

FEATURES
Child Friendly
Streams
Summit
Wildflowers
Great Views

FACILITIES
Campground
Water

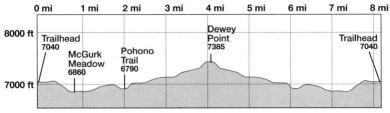

TRAIL 36 Dewey Point Elevation Profile

Trail Description

Of the three Cathedral Rocks seen from Dewey Point, the highest is the only one accessible to competent cross-country hikers–via an exposed walk up its south ridge.

 Wildflowers

▶ **Stream**

Starting from the Glacier Point Road, ▶1 the lodge-pole-shaded trail gently descends almost to the north tip of largely hidden Peregoy Meadow before topping a low divide. Next it drops moderately and reaches the south edge of sedge-filled McGurk Meadow, in which you cross its creek. ▶2 At times, the meadow may have an abundance of wildflowers such as shooting star, paintbrush, cinquefoil, and corn lily. Looking east from the meadow, note the low summits of the Ostrander Rocks. At Peregoy Meadow's north end you first reenter a lodgepole forest, soon crest a shallow, viewless saddle, and then descend at a reasonable gradient to a low-crest trail fork. ▶3 The fork right quickly joins the Pohono Trail and drops to Bridalveil Creek. You could camp in this vicinity, but probably would not want to unless you were doing the entire Pohono Trail from Glacier Point down to Discovery View. If you haven't brought along sufficient water, you can obtain some from this perennial creek.

Pohono Trail

OPTIONS

►4 If you can get someone to meet you at the Wawona Tunnel, then descend 5.5 miles to it along this highly scenic portion of the Pohono Trail, which passes Crocker and Stanford points. The route can be dry, so bring sufficient water.

You fork left, quickly join that trail, and start west on it and cross a broad, low divide. In a fir forest you first cross two Bridalveil Creek tributaries then a smaller third one before you start up a fourth that drains a curving gully. On the gully's upper slopes Jeffrey pine, huckleberry oak, and greenleaf manzanita replace the fir cover. In a few minutes you reach highly scenic 7385-foot Dewey Point, at the end of a short spur trail. ►4 Closer to the Cathedral Rocks than the viewpoints ahead, you look straight down the massive face that supports Leaning Tower. Also intriguing is the back side of Middle Cathedral Rock, with an iron-rich, rust-stained surface. Finally, you see the Cathedral Spires head on so they appear as one. If you are hiking before July, you're also likely to see wispy Ribbon Fall across Yosemite Valley. Bridalveil Fall, however, is blocked by the Leaning Tower.

Great Views

🚶 MILESTONES

►1	0.0	Start at Glacier Point Road trailhead
►2	0.8	McGurk Meadow
►3	2.0	Left on Pohono Trail
►4	4.1	Dewey Point

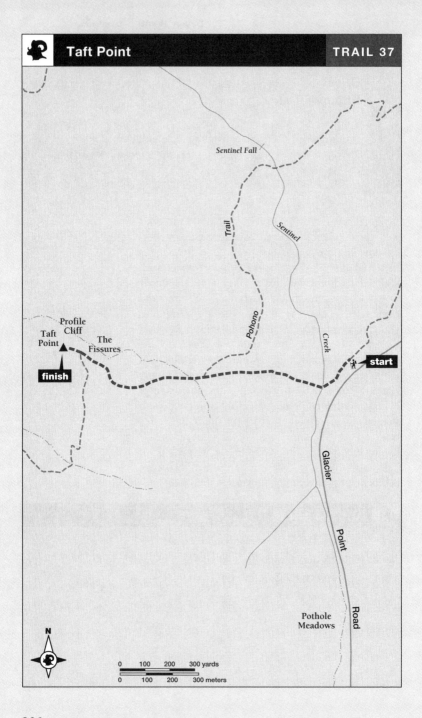

Sentinel Fall

Trail

Sentinel

Pohono

Creek

Profile Cliff

Taft Point

The Fissures

finish

start

Glacier

Point

Road

Pothole Meadows

N

| 0 | 100 | 200 | 300 yards |
| 0 | 100 | 200 | 300 meters |

Taft Point

The views from Taft Point rival those from Glacier Point. However, since Taft Point is reached by trail, it is less visited than mobbed Glacier Point. Generally lacking protective railings, Taft Point and the Fissures are potentially dangerous, so don't bring along children unless you can really keep them under strict control.

Best Time

Because Taft Point provides a good view of Yosemite Falls, you should visit this viewpoint while the falls are still flowing with considerable volume, which is from late June through mid-July. This also is the best time for wildflowers. Before then, the trail is likely to be covered with patches of snow. If you don't mind a wispy to non-existent Yosemite Falls, then you can take the trail through mid-October, when the Glacier Point Road still is likely to be open.

Finding the Trail

From a signed junction along the Wawona Road, drive 13.2 miles up to the Glacier Point Road to a scenic turn out, on your left, which is 2.3 miles before the Glacier Point parking lot entrance. The only campground in the area is Bridalveil Creek Campground, about 7.7 miles up the Glacier Point Road.

TRAIL USE
Dayhike, Run
LENGTH
2.6 miles, 1–2 hours
VERTICAL FEET
+100'/-320'/±840'
DIFFICULTY
- **1 2** 3 4 5 +
TRAIL TYPE
Out & Back

FEATURES
Summit
Wildflowers
Great Views

FACILITIES
Restrooms

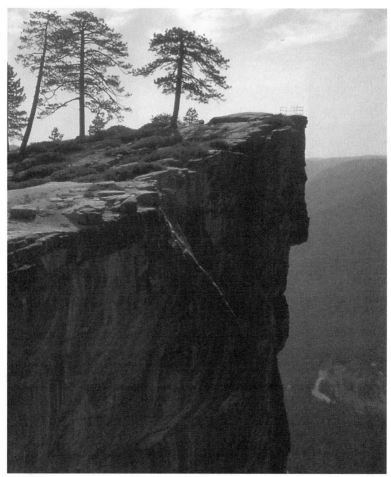

Taft Point

Trail Description

From the road-cut parking area ►1 you descend about 50 yards to a trail, turn left, and start southwest on it. After about 150 yards of easy descent you pass a trailside outcrop that is almost entirely composed of glistening whitish-gray quartz. In a minute you come to seasonal Sentinel Creek, whose limited drainage area keeps Sentinel Fall downstream from being one of Yosemite Valley's prime attractions. After boulder-hopping the creek, your trail undulates west past pines, firs, and brush to a crest junction with the Pohono Trail. ▶2

From the junction you turn left to descend the Pohono Trail to a seeping creeklet that drains through a small field of corn lilies. In this and two other nearby damp areas you may also find bracken fern and an assortment of wildflowers, including green gentian and alpine lily, which can grow to head height. Descending toward the Fissures, you cross drier slopes, which are generally covered with brush drought-tolerant wildflowers. Soon you arrive at the Fissures—five vertical, parallel fractures that cut through overhanging Profile Cliff, just beneath your feet. ▶3 Because the Fissures area, like your entire route, is unglaciated, it is well weathered, and a careless step could result in an easy slip on the loose gravel—dangerous in this area.

Beyond the Fissures, walk briefly up to a small railing at the brink of a conspicuous point and get an acrophobia-inducing view of overhanging Profile Cliff, beneath you. For the best views of Yosemite Valley and the High Sierra walk west to exposed Taft Point. ▶4 From it you see the Cathedral Spires and Rocks, El Capitan, the Three Brothers, Yosemite Falls, and Sentinel Rock. Broad Mt. Hoffmann stands on the skyline just east of Indian Canyon, and east of this peak stands distant Mt. Conness, on the Sierra crest.

Taft Point was named to commemorate President William Howard Taft's October 1909 visit to Yosemite Valley, where he met aged John Muir. Taft jokingly suggested that Yosemite Valley should be dammed, as was proposed for Hetch Hetchy.

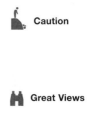 Caution

Great Views

🚶 MILESTONES

▶1 0.0 Start at Glacier Point Road trailhead
▶2 0.7 Left on Pohono Trail
▶3 1.2 The Fissures
▶4 1.3 Taft Point

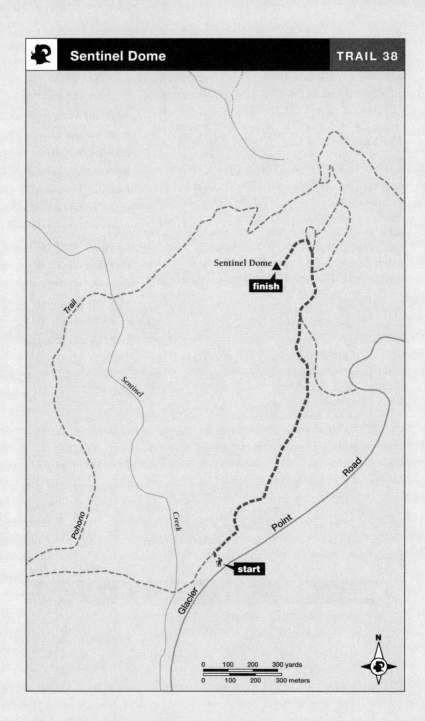

Sentinel Dome ▲
finish

Trail

Sentinel

Pohono

Creek

Road

Point

Glacier

start

0   100   200   300 yards

0   100   200   300 meters

N

Sentinel Dome

Sentinel Dome rivals Half Dome as the most-climbed dome in the park. Tuolumne Meadows' Lembert and Pothole domes almost rival them, but neither is a true dome; each is a roche moutonnée—an asymmetrical, glacier-smoothed ridge. Indeed, most of the Sierra's domes, glaciated or unglaciated, are asymmetrical ridges.

Best Time

Because Sentinel Dome provides a good view of Yosemite Falls, you should visit this viewpoint while the falls are still flowing with considerable volume, which is from late June through mid-July. Before then, the trail is likely to be covered with patches of snow. If you don't mind a wispy to non-existent Yosemite Falls, then you can take the trail through mid-October, when the Glacier Point Road still is likely to be open, and Vernal and Nevada falls, off to the east, are still flowing.

Finding the Trail

From a signed junction along the Wawona Road, drive 13.2 miles up to the Glacier Point Road to a scenic turn out, on your left, which is 2.3 miles before the Glacier Point parking lot entrance. The only campground in the area is Bridalveil Creek Campground, about 7.7 miles up the Glacier Point Road.

TRAIL USE
Dayhike, Run
LENGTH
2.4 miles, 1–2 hours
VERTICAL FEET
+460'/-70'/±1060'
DIFFICULTY
- **1 2** 3 4 5 +
TRAIL TYPE
Out & Back

FEATURES
Waterfalls
Wildflowers
Summit
Great Views

FACILITIES
Restrooms

Trail Description

From the road-cut parking area ▶1 you descend about 50 yards to a trail, turn right and make a curving, generally ascending traverse 0.75 mile north almost to the south base of Sentinel Dome. Here you meet and briefly hike north on a road, and you soon arrive at the dome's north end, where you meet a path ascending from Glacier Point. You now climb southwest up quite safe, unexposed bedrock slopes to the summit. ▶2

At an elevation of 8122 feet, Sentinel Dome is the second highest viewpoint above Yosemite Valley. Only Half Dome—a strenuous hike—is higher. Seen from the summit, El Capitan, Yosemite Falls, and Half Dome stand out as the three most prominent valley landmarks. West of Half Dome are two bald features, North and Basket domes. On the skyline above North Dome stands blocky Mt. Hoffmann, the park's geographic center, while to the east, above Mt. Starr King (an unglaciated, true dome), stands the rugged crest of the Clark Range. In years past almost everyone who climbed Sentinel Dome expected to photograph its windswept, solitary Jeffrey pine, made famous by Ansel Adams. That tree, unfortunately, finally succumbed to vandalism in 1984.

Great Views

MILESTONES

▶1   0.0   Start at Glacier Point Road trailhead
▶2   1.2   Sentinel Dome's summit

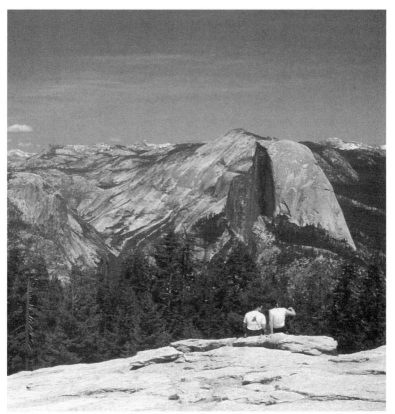

Half Dome *and Tenaya Canyon are just two of the landmarks visible from Sentinel Dome.*

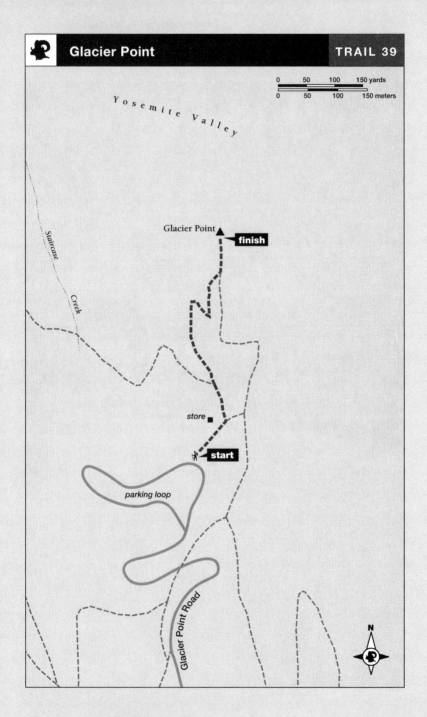

0   50   100   150 yards
0   50   100   150 meters

Y o s e m i t e   V a l l e y

Staircase

Creek

Glacier Point finish

store

start

parking loop

Glacier Point Road

N

Glacier Point

From the early 1870s until January 1968, a large pile of embers was pushed off Glacier Point at evening darkness to create the renowned Firefall—a glowing "waterfall." Quite a spectacle. Then from the early 1970s until June 1990, people in the chilly early morning hours would take running leaps from this vicinity out into space. This hang gliding was also quite a spectacle. However, one reason for establishing the park was to protect its natural lands, and you can see a spectacular part of them by making the short pilgrimage out to nearby Glacier Point, which arguably offers the preeminent view of Yosemite Valley.

Best Time

The best time to visit is when Yosemite Falls are at their greatest, which is about mid-May through June. However, the road to Glacier Point may not be open before mid-June, so late June is best. From early through late July the falls diminish appreciably, are wispy in August, and usually gone in September. However, Vernal and Nevada falls have staying power, and so if Yosemite Falls aren't a high priority, then anytime through late October, when the Glacier Point Road typically closes, is suitable.

Finding the Trail

From a signed junction along the Wawona Road, drive 15.5 miles up the Glacier Point Road to its end. The only campground in the area is Bridalveil Creek Campground, about 7.7 miles up the Glacier Point Road.

TRAIL USE
Dayhike
LENGTH
0.4 mile, 15–30 minutes
VERTICAL FEET
+30'/-10'/±80'
DIFFICULTY
- **1** 2 3 4 5 +
TRAIL TYPE
Out & Back

FEATURES
Child Friendly
Handicap Access
Waterfalls
Great Views

FACILITIES
Restrooms
Bus Stop
Picnic Tables
Phone
Water
Store

Logistics

At their maximum, past glaciers were thick enough to reach the top of Royal Arches but not the level rim just above them.

Rather than drive up to Glacier Point, whose parking lot can be overflowing on summer weekends, consider taking a Yosemite tour bus up to Glacier Point. Check the bus schedule in *Yosemite Today*, a newsletter presented to tourists at all park entrance stations.

Trail Description

The route is short and very obvious, ▶1 so no description is needed. Just follow the throngs of tourists past the restrooms and store out to nearby Glacier Point. ▶2 For a slightly longer route, you can veer right and go out to a small, sheltered viewing room that provides excellent views east.

Great Views

Of more interest to virtually all is the breathtaking panorama visible from the railing at Glacier Point. From west-northwest clockwise you see the following readily identifiable features: Eagle Peak, Yosemite Falls (northwest), Indian Canyon, Royal Arch Cascade (before July), Royal Arches (north), Washington Column with North Dome above, Tenaya Canyon (northeast), Half Dome with Clouds Rest behind it, Mt. Broderick with Vernal Fall below it, higher Liberty Cap with Nevada Fall beside it, Little Yosemite Valley (east) beyond both summits, and Bunnell Point at the end of that valley, Mt. Lyell (the park's highest summit) beyond it clustered with Mt. Florence and Mt. Maclure, and finally, the unglaciated dome, Mt. Starr King (southeast). Best seen from the small, sheltered viewing room is Illilouette Fall, to the south-southeast.

MILESTONES

▶1	0.0	Start from parking lot at end of Glacier Point Road
▶2	0.2	Glacier Point

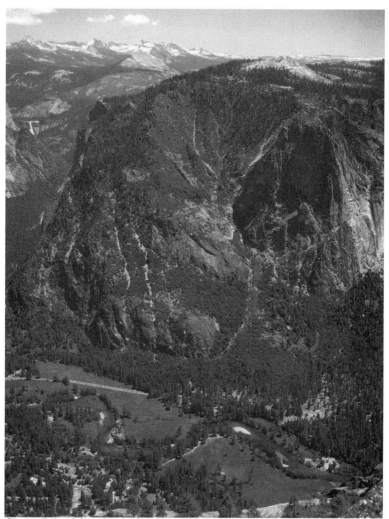

Glacier Point *(left) and Sentinel Rock viewed from Eagle Peak (Trail 30)*

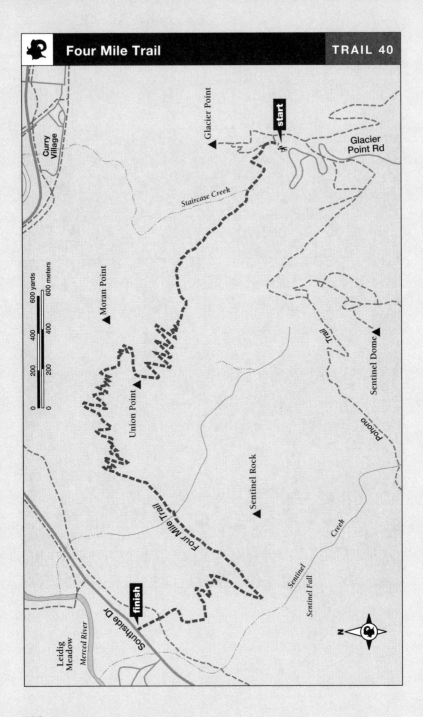

Four Mile Trail

TRAIL 40

Glacier Point

start

Glacier Point Rd

Curry Village

Staircase Creek

Moran Point

600 yards
600 meters

0   200   400

0   200   400

Union Point

Trail

Sentinel Dome

Pohono

Sentinel Rock

Four Mile Trail

Creek

finish

Sentinel Fall

Sentinel

Southside Dr

Merced River

Leidig Meadow

N

Four Mile Trail

This trail provides a very scenic descent to Yosemite Valley—a descent that will acquaint you with the valley's main features. This knee-knocking descent also gives you a feel for the valley's 3000-foot depth. This hike is rated "easy" because not much energy is expended, but if you do a lot of braking on the dozens of switchbacks, you may consider it "moderate."

Best Time

The best time to visit is when Yosemite Falls are at their greatest, which is about mid-May through June. However, the road to Glacier Point may not be open before mid-June, so late June is best. From early through late July the falls diminish appreciably, are wispy in August, and usually gone in September.

Finding the Trail

From a signed junction along the Wawona Road, drive 15.5 miles up the Glacier Point Road to its end. The only campground in the area is Bridalveil Creek Campground, about 7.7 miles up the Glacier Point Road.

Logistics

Rather than drive up to Glacier Point, whose parking lot can be overflowing on summer weekends, consider taking a Yosemite tour bus up to Glacier Point. In the past it has made two morning trips up to the point, giving you ample time to complete

TRAIL USE
Day Hike
LENGTH
4.6 miles, 1–2 hours
VERTICAL FEET
+20'/-3240'/±3260'
DIFFICULTY
- 1 **2** 3 4 5 +
TRAIL TYPE
Point-to-Point

FEATURES
Great Views
Steep

FACILITIES
Restrooms
Bus Stop
Picnic Tables
Phone
Water
Store

Before building the Yosemite Falls Trail (Trail 30) John Conway first worked on this trail, completing it in 1872. Originally about 4.0 miles long, it was rebuilt and lengthened in 1929 but the trail's name stuck.

your hike. Check the bus schedule in *Yosemite Today*, a newsletter presented to tourists at all park entrance stations. This lists schedules, activities, services, etc. available at the time of your visit.

Trail Description

Our trail starts west from the north side of a concessionaire's shop, ▶1 which, along with other minor structures, replaced the grand Glacier Point Hotel. This three-story hotel, together with the adjacent historic Mountain House—built in 1878—burned to the ground in August 1969.

Descending west from the concessionaire's shop, you enter a shady bowl whose white firs and sugar pines usually harbor snow patches well into June. You then contour northwest, eventually emerge from forest shade and, looking east, see unglaciated Glacier Point's two overhanging rocks capping a vertical wall. One of Yosemite's popular geologic myths is that it at least once lay under as much 700 feet of glacier ice. In reality, the glaciers in this vicinity only buried the lower half of Yosemite Valley.

Soon you curve west, veer in and out of a cool gully, then reach a descending ridge. On it you generally exchange views of Royal Arches, Washington Column, and North Dome for those of Yosemite Falls, the Three Brothers, El Capitan and, foremost, Sentinel Rock, which provides a good gauge to mark your downward progress.

Switchbacks begin, and where gravel lies on hard tread, you can easily take a minor spill if you're not

Great Views

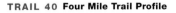

TRAIL 40 Four Mile Trail Profile

Graph axis labels: 0 mi, 1 mi, 2 mi, 3 mi, 4 mi; 7000 ft, 6000 ft, 5000 ft, 4000 ft. Glacier Point 7200. Yosemite Valley floor 3990.

careful. Chinquapin, greenleaf manzanita, and huckleberry oak are shrubs that dominate the first dozen switchback legs, thereby giving you unobstructed panoramas, though making the hike a hot one for anyone ascending from the valley floor on a summer afternoon. However, as you duck east into a gully, shady conifers appear, though they somewhat censor your views.

About midway down the series of switchbacks, canyon live oaks begin to compete with white firs and Douglas-firs, and your view is obstructed even more. After descending two thirds of the vertical distance to the valley floor, the switchbacks temporarily end. A long, steady descent now ensues, mostly past canyon live oaks, whose curved-upward trunks are their response to creeping talus. These talus deposits were erroneously mapped by USGS topographer-turned-geomorphologist François Matthes as glacial deposits. Black oaks and incense cedars also appear, and after 0.25 mile you cross a creeklet that usually flows until early July. Down it you have an excellent view of Leidig Meadow. Your steady descent again enters oak cover and you skirt below the base of imposing but largely hidden Sentinel Rock. At last a final group of switchbacks guide you down to a former parking loop, closed about 1975, and you proceed briefly north, intersecting the valley floor's southside trail just before your end point, Southside Drive.▶2

If you had been on this trail on some early morning, from the 1970s until 1990, when hang gliders were banned, you could have seen pilots land in meadows below you, taking sky trails from Glacier Point to the valley floor.

🚶 MILESTONES

▶1　0.0　Start from parking lot at end of Glacier Point Road
▶2　4.6　Southside Drive in Yosemite Valley

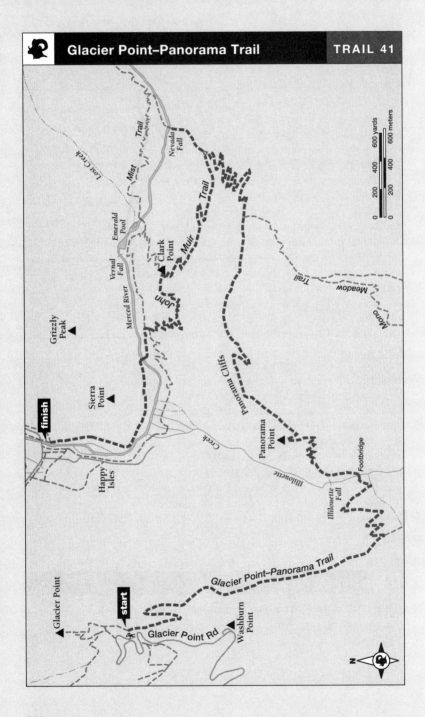

Mist Trail

Lost Creek

Nevada Fall

Emerald Pool

Vernal Fall

Clark Point

Muir Trail

John

Merced River

Grizzly Peak

Sierra Point

finish

Happy Isles

Panorama Cliffs

Meadow

Mono Trail

Creek

Panorama Point

Illilouette

Footbridge

Illilouette Fall

Glacier Point

start

Glacier Point–Panorama Trail

Glacier Point Rd

Washburn Point

0   200   400   600 yards
0   200   400   600 meters

N

Glacier Point–Panorama Trail

This is the most scenic of all trails descending to the floor of Yosemite Valley, passing three waterfalls and offering spectacular views along the way. Either take a bus up to Glacier Point or have someone drop you there and meet you down at Curry Village.

Best Time

All of the trail usually is snow-free by late June, so you can take this hike from then through August. After that Nevada and Vernal falls diminish, so September and early October hikes, done in pleasant weather, may not be as rewarding.

Finding the Trail

From a signed junction along the Wawona Road, drive 15.5 miles up the Glacier Point Road to its end. The only campground in the area is Bridalveil Creek Campground, about 7.7 miles up the Glacier Point Road.

Logistics

Rather than drive up to Glacier Point, whose parking lot can be overflowing on summer weekends, consider taking a Yosemite tour bus up to Glacier Point. In the past it has made two morning trips up to the point, giving you ample time to complete your hike. Check the bus schedule in *Yosemite Today*, a newsletter presented to tourists at all park entrance stations. This lists schedules, activities, services, etc. available at the time of your visit.

TRAIL USE
Dayhike
LENGTH
9.2 miles, 3–5 hours
VERTICAL FEET
+1020'/-4210'/±5230'
DIFFICULTY
- 1 2 **3** 4 5 +
TRAIL TYPE
Point-to-Point

FEATURES
Streams
Waterfalls
Wildflowers
Great Views

FACILITIES
Restrooms
Bus Stop
Picnic Tables
Phone
Water
Store

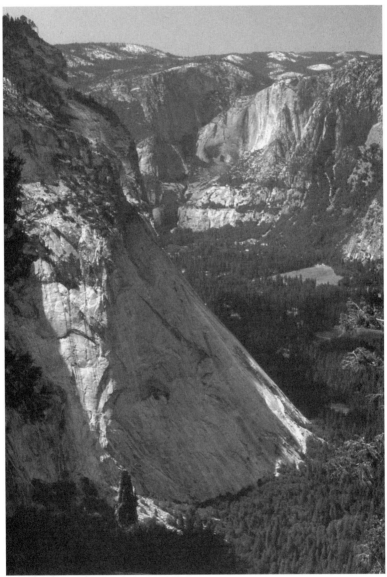

Glacier Point apron *from Panorama Trail*

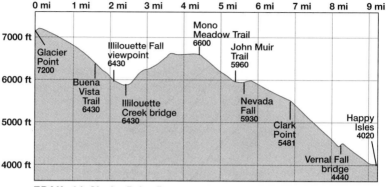

TRAIL 41 Glacier Point–Panorama Trail Elevation Profile

Trail Description

Just east of the entrance to the Glacier Point parking lot ▶1 you take a signed trail that starts south up to a quick fork. ▶2 The Pohono Trail veers right, but you veer left, on the Glacier Point–Panorama Trail, climbing a bit more before starting a moderate descent. A switchback leg helps ease the grade, and then you descend, often with views. A 1987 natural fire blackened most of the forest from near the trailhead to just beyond the upcoming Buena Vista Trail junction, but most trees survived. In open areas, black oaks are thriving, and shrubs have regenerated with a vengeance. Between charred trunks are occasional great views of Half Dome, Mt. Broderick, Liberty Cap, Nevada Fall, and Mt. Starr King. After 1.6 miles and an 800-foot drop, your Glacier Point–Panorama Trail meets the Buena Vista Trail. ▶3 Over 2.2 miles this first heads up-canyon to Illilouette Creek, then leads up along it to intersect the Mono Meadow Trail.

Your trail branches left and switchbacks down to a spur trail that goes a few yards to a railing. ▶4 Here, from your viewpoint atop an overhanging cliff, you have an unobstructed view of 370-foot-high Illilouette Fall, just 200 yards away, which

> **Gravels just above the brink of Illilouette Fall are remnants of a thick accumulation created when the last glacier formed a low ice dam across the creek's mouth.**

🔭 **Great Views**

Waterfall

Stream

Caution

Great Views

splashes down over a low point on the rim of massive Panorama Cliff. Behind it Half Dome rises boldly, while above Illilouette Creek Mt. Starr King rises even higher. In 0.25 mile your trail descends to a wide bridge, wisely placed upstream. ▶5 Illilouette Creek looks tempting for cooling your feet or for wading, but be forewarned that it could carry you swiftly downstream and over the fall.

Your trail soon passes just above the brink of Illilouette Fall, and then starts a major climb along the slopes just above Panorama Cliff. It first climbs briefly along its rim, then switchbacks away, soon returning near Panorama Point. ▶6 The former viewpoint was in part undermined by a monstrous rockfall that broke loose during the winter of 1968–69. The rest of the viewpoint could break loose at any time. About 0.3 mile past this vicinity is a superlative panorama extending from Upper Yosemite Fall east past Royal Arches, Washington Column, and North Dome to Half Dome. Your forested, moderate climb ends after 200 more feet of elevation gain, and then you descend gently to the rim for some more views, contour east, and have even more, these dominated by Half Dome, Mt. Broderick, Liberty Cap, Clouds Rest, and Nevada Fall. Your contour ends at a junction with the Mono Meadow Trail, ▶7 which climbs southwest over a low ridge before descending to Illilouette Creek.

Returning on Mist Trail

OPTIONS

▶8 Rather than descend the John Muir Trail to Happy Isles, you could make an alternate trip down the Mist Trail, a shorter route, which begins a few hundred yards northeast of Nevada Fall. Being 1.1 miles shorter, it is also steeper, and harder on the knees, and it is potentially dangerous for those who try to descend it too rapidly. This wet route down the aptly named Mist Trail is described in the opposite direction in the first part of Trail 33.

Beyond the trail junction you make a mile-long, switchbacking, generally viewless descent to a trail split, each branch descending a few yards to the John Muir Trail. ▶8 You'll descend along it, but first walk over to the nearby brink of roaring Nevada Fall and back, a round-trip distance of about 0.4 mile. ▶9 (This option is described in Trail 33, page 270)

▮▮ Waterfall

The recommended route is to take the John Muir Trail down to Happy Isles. In brief, from the junction with the Glacier Point–Panorama Trail, which you have descended, you start along the John Muir Trail, having grand views of Nevada Fall, Liberty Cap, Mt. Broderick, and Half Dome before you reach Clark Point. ▶10 Ahead the John Muir Trail is largely viewless, and on its well-graded switchbacks you descend to the bottom of the Mist Trail ▶11 and walk but a minute to the Vernal Fall bridge, ▶12 from which you hike your last mile down to the shuttle stop at Happy Isles. ▶13 From it you can take a shuttle bus over to Curry Village or any other eastern Yosemite Valley destination.

ᴴ Great Views

⯑ Stream

⚡ MILESTONES

▶1	0.0	Start from parking lot at end of Glacier Point Road
▶2	0.1	Left at Pohono Trail
▶3	1.6	Left at Buena Vista Trail
▶4	2.1	Illilouette Fall viewpoint
▶5	2.4	Bridge Illilouette Creek
▶6	3.0	Trail nears Panorama Point
▶7	4.4	Straight at Mono Meadow Trail
▶8	5.4	Straight at John Muir Trail
▶9	5.8	To Nevada Fall and back to JMT
▶10	6.9	Clark Point
▶11	8.1	Left at Mist Trail
▶12	8.2	Vernal Fall bridge
▶13	9.2	Happy Isles

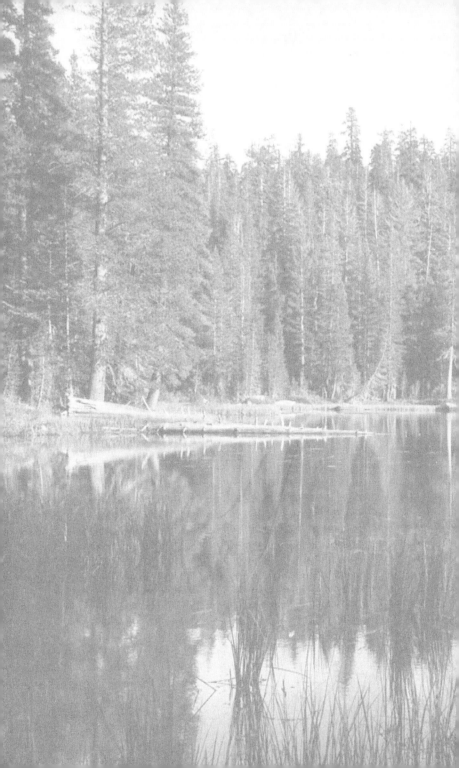

CHAPTER 7

South Yosemite

South Yosemite

S outh Yosemite mirrors Chapter 4's Northwest Yosemite, its lands having a smattering of lakes, some falls, and a grove of giant sequoias (also known as Big Trees). Like in that area, this one's backcountry lakes are not as heavily visited as are those of Chapter 2's Tuolumne Meadows. On summer weekends, Ostrander Lake, which requires a relatively modest effort to reach it, will get considerable use. The lakes along the Vandeberg–Lillian Lakes loop, just outside the park in a western part of Ansel Adams Wilderness, also require only a relatively modest effort to reach them. However, the long drive up lengthy Forest Service roads to the trailhead diminishes their popularity.

Between Ostrander Lake and the South Fork Merced River stands unimposing, subalpine Buena Vista Peak, the westernmost and most accessible (but not highest) summit of the Buena Vista Crest. Relatively small glaciers flowing north, west, and south from the peak once excavated the relatively small and generally shallow lakes that encircle it. The most inspiring is Royal Arch Lake, and Trail 43 visits this one and several others that are perched on relatively gentle uplands above the deep South Fork Merced River canyon. From the Wawona area you can gain an appreciation of the canyon's depth by ascending a trail to the highest of the Chilnualna Falls, its brink on the lip of the canyon. Unlike the park's other falls, these falls descend unglaciated slopes. A common geologic myth is that waterfalls owe their existence to deep erosion of trunk canyons by glaciers, but the Chilnualna Falls stand as evidence against this myth, as do the world's greatest waterfalls, which are located in unglaciated, tropical lands.

But the falls are not the prime attraction. That lies south of the South Fork Merced River canyon: the Mariposa Grove of Big Trees. This grove is unique in that it has a network of trails among the giant sequoias; no such trail system exists at the park's two other groves, the Tuolumne and Merced. Although thousands of persons visit this chapter's Mariposa Grove each week during summer, the vast majority ride trams. The few who explore the grove on foot are richly rewarded.

Overleaf: *Grouse Lake (Trail 45)*

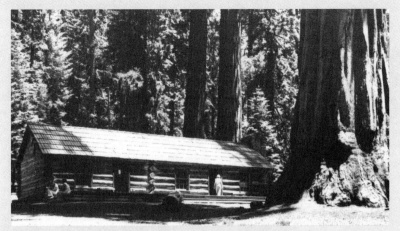

Mariposa Grove Museum *(Trail 44)*

Because the South Fork's uplands are lower than those of the Merced River proper through Yosemite Valley, there is less snowmelt, and the South Fork warms considerably by the time it reaches the Wawona area. By mid-afternoon in July and August, the river can reach into the low 70s, which is about 10 degrees warmer than the Merced River through Yosemite Valley. A string of swimming holes that vary in quality from year to year (floods can remove or deposit sediments and debris) are popular attractions for visitors and local residents. These extend from the Swinging Bridge down to the Covered Bridge to the Wawona Picnic Area and to the Wawona Campground and below it.

Permits

If you want to reserve a permit, rather than get one in person, see the "Fees, Camping, and Permits" section on page 14. However, within the park only Ostrander Lake (Trail 42) is likely to reach its quota of backpackers, and then only on summer weekends. Therefore, most backpackers will probably get their permits in person at the Wawona District Office, on the north side of the South Fork Merced River. From the bridge north across the river, reach this office by starting along the Chilnualna Road and quickly reaching a short spur road, which you take immediately past the Pioneer Yosemite History Center.

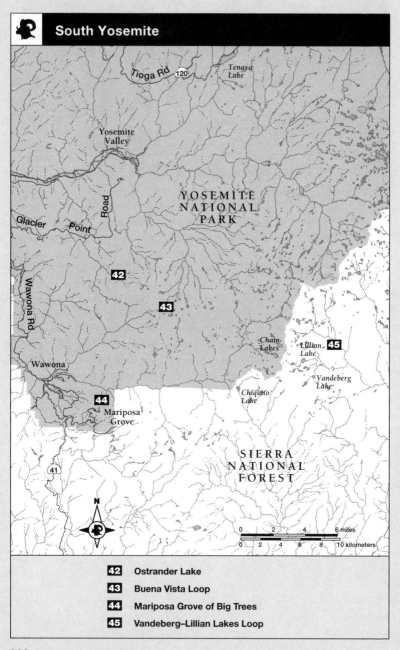

South Yosemite

42 Ostrander Lake

43 Buena Vista Loop

44 Mariposa Grove of Big Trees

45 Vandeberg–Lillian Lakes Loop

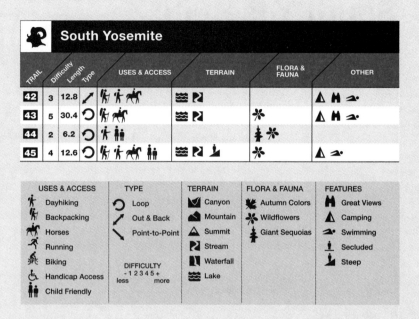

South Yosemite

TRAIL	Difficulty	Length	Type	USES & ACCESS	TERRAIN	FLORA & FAUNA	OTHER
42	3	12.8	Out & Back	Backpacking, Dayhiking, Biking	Lake, Stream		Camping, Great Views, Swimming
43	5	30.4	Loop	Backpacking, Horses	Lake, Stream	Wildflowers	Camping, Great Views, Swimming
44	2	6.2	Loop	Dayhiking, Child Friendly		Giant Sequoias, Wildflowers	
45	4	12.6	Loop	Backpacking, Dayhiking, Horses, Child Friendly	Lake, Stream, Waterfall	Wildflowers	Camping, Swimming

USES & ACCESS	TYPE	TERRAIN	FLORA & FAUNA	FEATURES
Dayhiking	Loop	Canyon	Autumn Colors	Great Views
Backpacking	Out & Back	Mountain	Wildflowers	Camping
Horses	Point-to-Point	Summit	Giant Sequoias	Swimming
Running		Stream		Secluded
Biking	DIFFICULTY	Waterfall		Steep
Handicap Access	- 1 2 3 4 5 + less more	Lake		
Child Friendly				

Trail 45 starts on lands of the Sierra National Forest, and so you must get a permit at a Forest Service office. It probably is best to get one at the office in the Yosemite–Sierra Visitors Center (559-658-7588), located in downtown Oakhurst. Also, you can get one at the Clover Meadow Ranger Station, which you'll find near Trail 45's trailhead. (When the station is not staffed, there may be permits that have been left outside for you to complete.) Permits are also available at the Mariposa–Minarets Ranger District Office (559-877-2218), in the tiny settlement of North Fork, but for most people this is out of the way.

Maps

For South Yosemite, here are the USGS 7.5-minute (1:24,000 scale) topographic quadrangles that you will need, listed in the order that you will need them as you hike along your route.

Trail 42: Half Dome
Trail 43: Half Dome, Mariposa Grove
Trail 44: Mariposa Grove
Trail 45: Timber Knob

South Yosemite

TRAIL 42

Dayhike, Backpack,
Horse
12.8 miles
Out & Back
Difficulty: 1 2 **3** 4 5

Ostrander Lake 337

Ostrander Lake, being the closest lake to the Glacier Point Road, is the objective of many summertime weekend backpackers. It is also popular in winter and spring with cross-country skiers. You might consider dayhiking to it, since with a day pack it is only a two- to three-hour hike to the lake, and day-hiking lessens human impact on the lake's environment.

TRAIL 43

Backpack, Horse
30.4 miles, Loop
Difficulty: 1 2 3 4 **5**

Buena Vista Loop 341

The subalpine lakes nestled around Buena Vista Peak can be reached from the Chilnualna Falls trail-head in North Wawona or from three trailheads along the Glacier Point Road. This hike starts from one of these trailheads and visits five of the peak's lakes. While it can be done at a moderate pace in three days, I recommend a more-relaxed pace in four or more days so that you can savor the lakes you meet along this relatively easy route.

TRAIL 44

Dayhike
6.2 miles, Loop
Difficulty: 1 **2** 3 4 5

Mariposa Grove of Big Trees 349

Near the southwest end of the parking lot is an information kiosk where visitors can get introduced to the Mariposa Grove while waiting to take the tram. The tram ride gives you an instructive, guided tour of the grove's salient features and, at its stops, you can step off, explore the immediate area, and then get on the next tram. However, by hiking you get a more intimate experience with the giant sequoia, or Wawona, as the Indians called them.

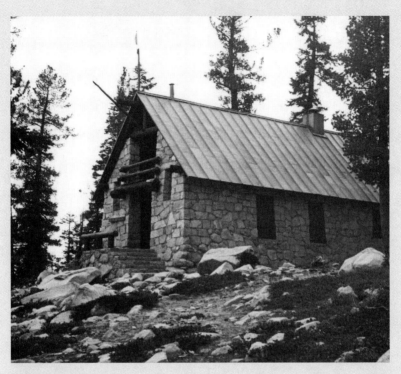

Ostrander Hut (*Trail 42*)

Vandeberg–Lillian Lakes Loop 355

If you are in shape, you could hike this entire circuit in one day without overexerting yourself. However, it is so scenic that three days are recommended—sufficient time to visit Lady, Chittenden, Staniford, and Rainbow lakes. Visiting all four of these desirable lakes lengthens your route to about 21 miles, adds about 2400 feet of ascent and descent, and changes its classification to a moderate three-day hike.

TRAIL 45

Dayhike, Backpack, Horse
12.6 miles
Loop
Difficulty: 1 2 3 **4** 5

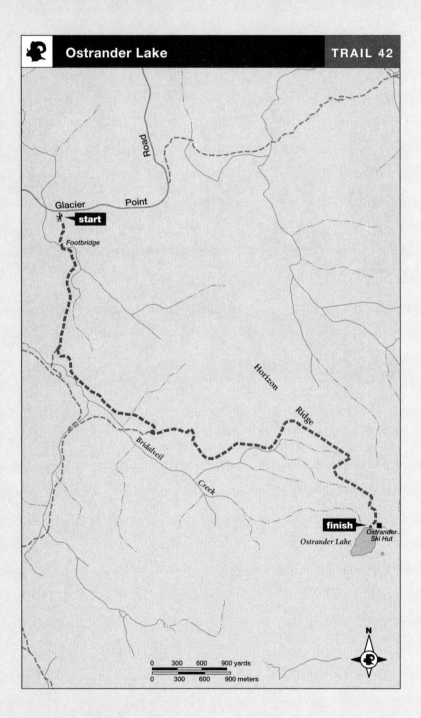

Ostrander Lake

TRAIL 42

Road

Glacier Point

start

Footbridge

Horizon

Ridge

Bridalveil

Creek

finish

Ostrander Lake

Ostrander
Ski Hut

| 0 | 300 | 600 | 900 yards |
| 0 | 300 | 600 | 900 meters |

N

Ostrander Lake

Ostrander Lake, being the closest lake to the Glacier Point Road, is the objective of many summertime weekend backpackers. It is also popular in winter and spring with cross-country skiers. You might consider dayhiking to it, since with a day pack it is only a two- to three-hour hike to the lake, and dayhiking lessens human impact on the lake's environment.

Best Time

All of the trail is usually snow-free by early July, but mosquitoes linger in the meadowy flats along the first half of the hike well into July, so the optimal time is from about late July through August. By September, Ostrander Lake is too cool for pleasant swimming, but it still is a very desirable destination through early October. Major storms aren't likely in this period, but if one hit, you could get out in two or three hours, especially since the upper half of the route is an easily followable old road.

Finding the Trail

From a signed junction with the Wawona Road drive 8.9 miles up the Glacier Point Road to a turnoff on your right. This parking area is 1.2 miles past the spur road to Bridalveil Creek Campground, which is the only one along the Glacier Point Road.

TRAIL USE
Dayhike, Backpack, Horse

LENGTH
12.8 miles,
6 hours–2 days

VERTICAL FEET
+1720'/-210'/±3860'

DIFFICULTY
- 1 2 **3** 4 5 +

TRAIL TYPE
Out & Back

FEATURES
Streams
Lake
Wildflowers
Great Views
Swimming

FACILITIES
Campground

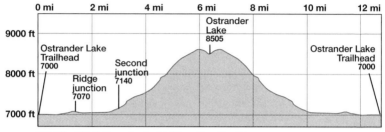

TRAIL 42 Ostrander Lake Elevation Profile

Trail Description

**Ostrander Lake is at
the headwaters of
Bridalveil Creek,
which produces
Bridalveil Fall. In early
days, the fall was
known as Pohono,
and its source,
Pohono Lake.**

Stream

The first half of your hike is easy—a gentle ascent
through a forest that is interspersed with an assortment of meadows. From Glacier Point Road ►1 you
start along a former jeep road and soon encounter
the first of several areas of lodgepole forest badly
burned in a 1987 fire. Farther up, on Horizon
Ridge, you'll see a forest burned in a 1994 fire. Just
0.33 mile from the trailhead you cross a sluggish
creek, then amble an easy mile to a ridge junction.
►2 From it a short lateral right drops to Bridalveil
Creek—possibly a difficult June crossing—then
climbs equally briefly to the Bridalveil Creek Trail.

From the junction, your route contours southeast past unseen Lost Bear Meadow, and after a mile
makes a short ascent east up along a trickling creek
to its crossing. Just beyond the ford your route
curves west to a nearby junction ►3 with a second
lateral that branches right to Bridalveil Creek and
then to the Bridalveil Creek Trail. Though you are
now about halfway to Ostrander Lake, you've
climbed very little, and from this junction you face
1500 feet of vertical gain, mostly through burned
forests. Nevertheless, some trees survived.

The steepening road climbs east through a forest, then climbs more gently, south across an open
slab that provides the first views of the Bridalveil
Creek basin. You then curve southeast into a Jeffrey

pine stand, before climbing east through a white-fir forest. These firs are largely supplanted by red firs by the time you top a saddle that bisects Horizon Ridge. Climbing southeast up that ridge, your road passes through a generally open stretch that surprisingly has sagebrush. About 400 feet above your first saddle the road switchbacks at a second one, then curves up to a third. From it the road makes a momentary descent southeast before bending to start a short, final ascent south into unburned forest surrounding Ostrander Lake. Near this bend you get far-ranging views across the Illilouette Creek basin. You can see the tops of Royal Arches and Washington Column and, above and east of them, North, Basket and Half domes. Behind Half Dome stands the park's geographic center, broad-topped Mt. Hoffmann. Reigning over the Illilouette Creek basin is Mt. Starr King and its entourage of lesser domes. To the east and northeast the jagged crest of the Clark Range cuts the sky.

Beyond the short, final ascent south you drop in several minutes to Ostrander Hut, on the north shore of Ostrander Lake. ▶4 When it is snowbound, cross-country skiers can stay in it if they've first obtained reservations from the valley's Wilderness Center. The hut is on a rocky glacial moraine left by a glacier that retreated perhaps 16,000 years ago. Behind it, lying in a bedrock basin, is 25-acre, trout-populated Ostrander Lake. Here, camping is good along the west shore.

M Great Views

R Stream

 Lake

A Camping

🚶 **MILESTONES**		
▶1	0.0	Start at Ostrander Lake trailhead
▶2	1.4	Left at ridge junction
▶3	3.0	Left at second junction
▶4	6.4	Ostrander Lake

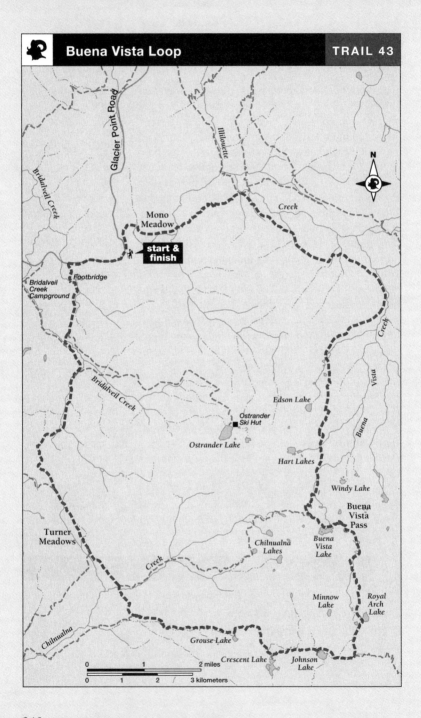

Glacier Point Road

Illilouette

N

Bridalveil Creek

Creek

Mono Meadow

start & finish

Footbridge

Bridalveil Creek Campground

Bridalveil Creek

Edson Lake

Ostrander Ski Hut

Ostrander Lake

Hart Lakes

Windy Lake

Buena Vista Creek

Buena Vista Pass

Turner Meadows

Creek

Chilnualna Lakes

Buena Vista Lake

Minnow Lake

Royal Arch Lake

Chilnualna

Grouse Lake

Crescent Lake

Johnson Lake

0   1   2 miles
0   1   2   3 kilometers

Buena Vista Loop

The subalpine lakes nestled around Buena Vista Peak can be reached from North Wawona or from three trailheads along the Glacier Point Road. This hike starts from one of these trailheads and visits five of the peak's lakes. Although this route is slightly longer than a start from Wawona's Chilnualna Falls trailhead, it requires 20 percent less climbing effort. While it can be done at a moderate pace in three days, I recommend a more-relaxed pace in four or more days so that you can savor the lakes you meet along this relatively easy route.

Best Time

Mosquitoes and snow patches can linger well into July, so the optimal time is in August. By September, the lakes are too cool for pleasant swimming, but are still very desirable destinations. Because you can get about 15 miles from the trailhead, I don't recommend this route in early or mid-October unless you are prepared for a major, if rare, storm. The advantage of late-season hiking, of course, is that you have the wilderness virtually to yourself.

Finding the Trail

From a signed junction on the Wawona Road, drive 10.1 miles up Glacier Point Road to a forested saddle with a parking area on your right. The only campground in the area is Bridalveil Creek Campground, about 7.7 miles up the Glacier Point Road.

TRAIL USE
Backpack, Horse
LENGTH
30.4 miles, 3–5 days
VERTICAL FEET
+5240'/-5240'/±10,480'
DIFFICULTY
- 1 2 3 4 **5** +
TRAIL TYPE
Loop

FEATURES
Backcountry Permit
Lakes
Streams
Wildflowers
Camping
Great Views
Swimming

FACILITIES
Restrooms
Campground
Patrol Cabin

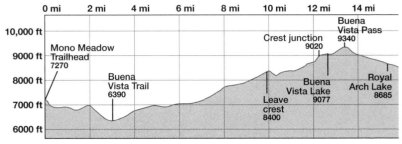

TRAIL 43 Buena Vista Loop Elevation Profile

Trail Description

You start your trail at the Mono Meadow Trailhead ▶1 with a steady, moderate descent north, followed by an easing gradient east to lodgepole-fringed Mono Meadow. Should the route be vague in early season, know that the trail crosses the meadow on a 120-degree bearing, and it becomes obvious once you're within the forest's edge. Beyond the meadow your Mono Meadow Trail crosses a low divide, then makes a generally viewless, easy descent to a major tributary of Illilouette Creek. Here, 1.5 miles from your trailhead, is your first possible campsite. You ford the tributary at the brink of some rapids, and in early season this ford could be a dangerous one. From the tributary you gain 200 feet on a short ascent to a crest, and on your descent east from it you're rewarded with views of North, Basket, and Half domes, Clouds Rest, and Mt. Starr King.

After a descent through a fir forest you emerge on an open slope with a thin veneer of grus, or granitic gravel. On the slope you descend straight toward Mt. Starr King, the highest of the Illilouette Creek domes, and immediately after the view disappears, you reach a junction with the Buena Vista Trail, which links Glacier Point with the Buena Vista Peak area. ▶2

⚠ **Camping**

👤 **Caution**

🏛 **Great Views**

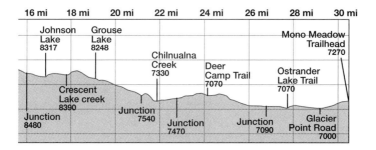

Stream

Camping

Camping

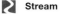
Stream

You turn right and go just 40 yards up-canyon to a second junction, from where the Mono Meadow Trail goes 300 yards east past campsites to ford broad Illilouette Creek. From it the trail climbs a slope veneered with glacial outwash—stream deposits from the last glaciers that existed up-canyon—then it crosses a spacious bedrock bench that is suitable for camping.

From the junction before the creek crossing your route heads southeast up the Buena Vista Trail. Over much of the route up toward Buena Vista Peak the vegetation has been burned by several large, natural fires. Usually a burn is quite unsightly for a year or two, but wildflowers often abound there, and after several years brush and young trees soften the visual effect. In 1.25 miles you come to a creeklet with a fair camp on its west bank. The trail's gradient gradually eases, then you cross a broad divide and in 0.25 mile angle sharply left to descend along the edge of a sloping meadow. Beyond are aspens that hide a step-across creek. Just a few minutes' walk east of it you cross a slightly larger creek, then make a gentle ascent southeast across sandy soils to steep slopes above Buena Vista Creek. Camping is poor along the west bank, but good—and isolated—above the east bank. Fallen trees may provide access across the bouldery creek to these sites.

From Buena Vista Pass, Buena Vista Peak is easily reached and, true to its name "good view," provides an unrestricted panorama of the park's southern lands.

 Camping

Caution

Lake

 Camping

Soon your trail leaves Buena Vista Creek, curves southwest, and climbs moderately in that direction for 1.5 miles to a ford, between two meadows, of diminutive Edson Lake creek. From a poor campsite the trail ascends along a moraine crest, then in 1.0 mile leaves it ►3 to angle southeast up to a higher crest. Your trail follows this crest southwest for more than 300 yards, finally leaves the burned area, and then makes a 0.25-mile, view-blessed descent to Hart Lakes creek. Now you make a short contour over to Buena Vista Creek, which has a small campsite on its east bank. After 0.5 mile of moderate ascent you cross a creek that bends northeast, then continue south up a slightly shorter ascent to a recrossing of that creek. Immediately beyond you cross its western tributary, then follow this stream south briefly up to two ponds, from which you switchback up a cirque wall with ice-shattered blocks to a crest junction.►4

The first lake you encounter, about 0.33 mile southeast from the junction, is rather bleak Buena Vista Lake, which has rainbow and brook trout.►5 Nestled on a broad bench at the base of the cool north slope of Buena Vista Peak, this lake is the highest and coldest one you'll see. It does, however, have at least two good, if somewhat exposed camps. In threatening weather, camp lower down. Starting at the lake's outlet, take short switchbacks up to a nearby, broad, viewless Buena Vista Pass, which at 9340 feet is your trip's highest elevation.►6

From the pass you descend 2.0 easy, winding trail miles to a favorite lake on this loop, Royal Arch Lake, which lies below a broad, granitic arch.►7 This lake, like Buena Vista Lake, has rainbow and brook trout. Just past the outlet is an excellent, popular campsite. Leaving Royal Arch Lake, you parallel its outlet creek for 0.5 mile, then angle south across slabs to a junction with an east-climbing trail.►8 Here you meet the route from

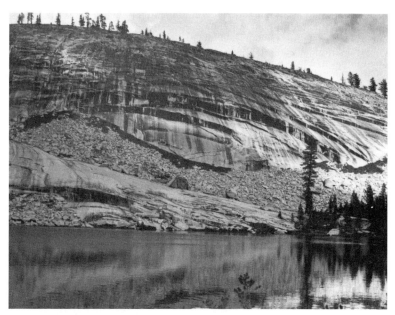

Royal Arch Lake

Chiquito Pass, which crosses the South Fork
Merced River and climbs to Buck Camp, a ranger
station about 1.5 miles from your junction.

Turning right, you descend west toward
Johnson Lake,▶9 reaching good campsites along its
northwest shore in just 0.75 mile—with hordes of
mosquitoes in early season. You don't see large
Crescent Lake, but on meeting its inlet creek, ▶10
about 0.33 mile beyond a meadowy divide, you can
walk 150 yards downstream, passing a fair camp
before reaching the lake's shallow, trout-filled
waters. You might visit or camp near the lake's
south end, for from its outlet you can peer into the
2800 foot deep South Fork Merced River canyon.

Beyond Crescent Lake's inlet creek your trail
quickly turns north, passes a small creekside
meadow, and then climbs more than 150 feet to a

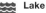 **Lake**

 Camping

Chilnualna Lakes

▶13 Should you want to visit the mediocre Chilnualna Lakes, take the 5.3 mile trail east up past them to the crest junction, then back-track 13.1 miles to your trailhead. This route is 10.0 miles longer than the following route, including its 1.2 mile walk along the Glacier Point Road back to the trailhead.

Lake

▲ **Camping**

Stream

second broad divide. From it you descend into the headwaters of a Chilnualna Creek tributary. Your moderate-to-steep gradient ends when you approach easily missed Grouse Lake. ▶11 Look for a trail that descends about 100 yards to a fair camp-site on the north shore of this shallow, reedy lakelet.

Lodgepoles and red firs monopolize the slopes along your 2-mile descent from this lake down to a hillside junction. ▶12 Now you first top a nearby divide, then descend more than 400 feet to Chilnualna Creek. ▶13 Just above its north bank is a good, medium-sized campsite, and just beyond that is another trail junction.

Spurning the longer option, head northwest from Chilnualna Creek. During midsummer, your gently ascending traverse is brightened by the orange sunbursts of alpine lilies, growing chest-high along the wetter parts of your trail. You encounter a junction before Turner Meadows, ▶14 from which a trail departs southwest to a junction near the brink of upper Chilnualna Fall, from which a steep trail descends to the Wawona area.

You now ascend past and through a series of "Turner Meadows," then top a forest pass to quickly meet a trail ▶15 descending to Deer Camp. You, however, keep right, traverse to a crest, and descend to a tributary of Bridalveil Creek. Before reaching Bridalveil Creek, you meet a junction, ▶16 turn left, and then cross the tributary creek. Along it you momentarily pass a moderate-sized campsite and then in 0.5 mile reach another junction. ►17 The main trail continues 1.6 miles northwest to Bridalveil Creek Campground, but you veer right and over the next 0.3-mile trail segment you first drop to nearby Bridalveil Creek, ford it, and then make an equally short climb up to the Ostrander Lake Trail—a former Jeep road. ►18 In 1.4 miles this northbound route ends at the Glacier Point Road, ►19 beside which you walk 1.2 miles east to your Mono Meadow trailhead. ►20

▟ **Stream**

▲ **Camping**

🚶 MILESTONES

- ►1   0.0 Start at Mono Meadow trailhead
- ►2   3.0 Right on Buena Vista Trail
- ►3   9.9 Trail leaves moraine crest
- ►4   12.2 Left at crest junction
- ►5   12.6 Buena Vista Lake
- ►6   13.3 Buena Vista Pass
- ►7   15.3 Royal Arch Lake
- ►8   16.0 Right at east-climbing trail
- ►9   16.8 Johnson Lake
- ►10 17.8 Crescent Lake's inlet creek
- ►11 19.1 Grouse Lake
- ►12 21.2 Right at hillside junction
- ►13 21.9 Chilnualna Creek
- ►14 22.8 Straight at junction before Turner Meadows
- ►15 24.2 Trail descending to Deer Camp
- ►16 26.8 Left at junction by tributary creek
- ►17 27.5 Right at junction above Bridalveil Creek
- ►18 27.8 Left at Ostrander Lake Trail
- ►19 29.2 Right at Glacier Point Road
- ►20 30.4 Mono Meadow trailhead

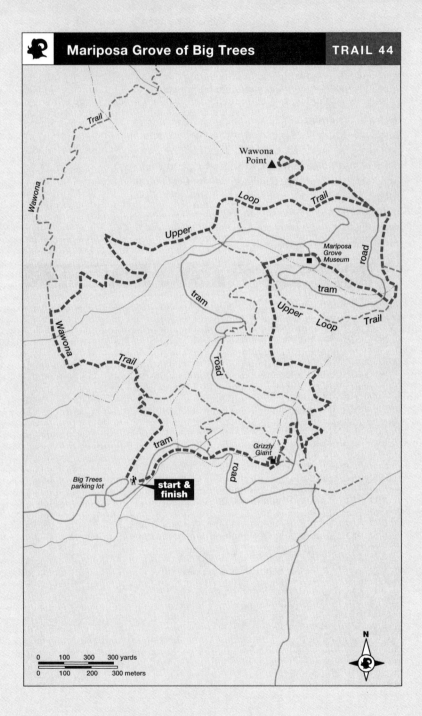

Wawona
Point ▲

Loop   Trail

Upper

Trail

road

Wawona

Mariposa
Grove
Museum

tram

tram

Upper   Loop   Trail

Wawona   Trail

road

tram

Grizzly
Giant

Big Trees
parking lot

road

**start &
finish**

| 0 | 100 | 300 | 300 yards |
| 0 | 100 | 200 | 300 meters |

N

Mariposa Grove of Big Trees

Near the southwest end of the parking lot is an information kiosk where visitors can get introduced to the Mariposa Grove while waiting to take the tram. The tram ride gives you an instructive, guided tour of the grove's salient features and, at its stops, you can step off, explore the immediate area, and then get on the next tram. However, by hiking you get a more intimate experience with the giant sequoia, or Wawona, as the Indians called them.

Best Time

The Mariposa Grove is best visited no sooner than late May, when the snow has melted and grasses, wildflowers, and deciduous trees and shrubs have awoken from their long winter's slumber. Because the grove is shady, it is not a botanist's paradise, but if you do like wildflowers, then visit the grove by early July. The modest seasonal wildflower display will be gone by September, but so too will be the summer's hordes of tourists. If possible, visit on a weekday, preferably from mid-September through early November.

Finding the Trail

From the park's south entrance station drive east 2.1 miles up to road's end at the Big Trees parking lot. Be forewarned that by mid-morning the lot can be full, since the grove is very popular, receiving up to 2 million visitors a year. The only campground in the Wawona area is the Wawona Campground, which is 0.8 mile past the bridge across the South Fork Merced River as you travel north along the Wawona Road.

TRAIL USE
Dayhike

LENGTH
6.2 miles, 2–3 hours

VERTICAL FEET
+1530'/-1530'/±3060'

DIFFICULTY
- 1 **2** 3 4 5 +

TRAIL TYPE
Loop

FEATURES
Child Friendly
Giant Sequoias
Wildflowers

FACILITIES
Restrooms
Bus Stop
Picnic Tables
Phone
Water

Logistics

During summer and early fall, take the free shuttle bus that leaves from the Wawona Store, just northwest of the Wawona Hotel, since parking space is not always available at the grove.

Trail Description

Two trails, a northern and a southern one, leave from the eastern, upper end of the parking lot. The northern one is the Outer Loop Trail, which makes a switchbacking climb 0.6 mile north to a junction with a trail east, then a winding traverse 0.6 mile northwest to a junction with a trail 5 miles down to Wawona.

Your route from the eastern, upper end of the Mariposa Grove's parking lot ▶1 is the southern trail, which actually starts at the kiosk and runs along the edge of the parking lot. On this nature trail you momentarily parallel the tram road east before crossing a creeklet and the road. The signs along this trail not only identify the notable sequoias, but also educate you on their natural history, including such items as bark, cones, fire, reproduction, and associated plants and animals.

At the tram-road crossing lies the Fallen Monarch, largely intact, including its roots. From the south side of the road your nature trail climbs 0.25 mile east before crossing the road. At this spot stand the Bachelor and the Three Graces. In a similar distance your trail reaches the Grizzly Giant. ▶2 Like the Leaning Tower of Pisa, this still-growing giant seems ready to fall any second, and one wonders how such a top-heavy, shallow-rooted specimen could have survived as long as it has. Though it's the largest tree in the park—and probably the oldest at almost 3000 years—there are at least 25 specimens elsewhere larger than it is. It has a trunk volume of about 34,000 cubic feet, compared to about 52,500 cubic feet for the largest, the General Sherman, in Sequoia National Park's Giant Forest Grove.

Heading north from the east end of the enclosure circling the Grizzly Giant, you reach in 50 yards the California Tree, also enclosed, but with a path through it. It once had a deep burn, which was cut away in 1895 so that tourists could ride a stage through it. Beyond this tree a trail traverses 0.5 mile west to the Outer Loop Trail. You, however, take an ascending trail that parallels the tram road north for 250 yards before crossing it. Your trail then climbs to a nearby switchback from where a lightly used trail winds southeast down to an old road. You start north and quickly reach a lackluster trail that traverses northwest to the tram road, from where another trail, equally lackluster, descends southwest to the Outer Loop Trail. Additionally a switchbacking one climbs northeastward to a loop in the upper part of the tram road.

Your trail gains 400 feet elevation climbing to the same spot, starting north and then going briefly east before switchbacking to wind northwest to the upper end of the switchbacking trail, the junction being about 15 yards from the tram road. Here too is the Upper Loop Trail, which parallels the tram road counterclockwise as both circle the upper grove. (Although this area is called the Mariposa Grove, it is really two groves, a lower one, which includes the Grizzly Giant and trees below it, and an upper one, which is mostly encircled by the Upper Loop Trail.)

This guide's suggested route from the junction is to start on a trail a few paces away, which descends north about 90 yards to a junction with an east-west trail. This winds about 250 yards eastward, skirting below restrooms and then passing a west-heading nature trail before reaching the Mariposa Grove Museum, ▶3 which has an adjacent water fountain.

> **The Grizzly Giant has enough timber to build about 20 homes, but fortunately sequoia wood is very brittle, shattering when a tree falls—a feature that saved it from being logged into oblivion.**

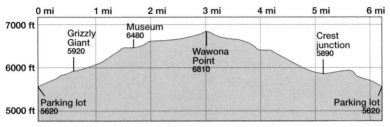

TRAIL 44 Mariposa Grove Elevation Profile

The 2200-year-old Wawona Tree, like many others, had a fire-scarred base, and it was enlarged in 1881 for first stagecoaches and much later automobiles to pass through it. Today, the fallen tree is not much to look at.

In the museum you will find information and displays on the giant sequoia, its related plants and animals, and the area's history. From just east of it you could take a trail 0.33 mile east up to the tram road, beside which you'd spy the lower end of the Fallen Wawona (Tunnel) Tree, which toppled during the late winter or spring of 1969.

The suggested route, however, continues from the museum momentarily east along the tram road to a bend. Here is the amazing Telescope Tree, ▶4 which has been hollowed out by fire. Inside it you can look straight up to the heavens. Despite its great internal loss, this tree is still very much alive, for its vital fluids—as in all trees—are conducted in the sapwood, immediately beneath the thick bark. The heartwood is just dead sapwood whose function is support.

From the back side of the tree you take a trail that climbs 50 yards to the Upper Loop Trail, mentioned earlier. On it you hike 0.33 mile counterclockwise to pass just above the Fallen Wawona Tree, then continue about 250 yards to a crest saddle. Just 40 yards east of it is the Galen Clark Tree, ▶5 a fine specimen named for the man who first publicized this grove and later became its first guardian. From the saddle a road branches from the tram-road loop, and on it you make an easy climb 0.5 mile to Wawona Point. ▶6 No sequoias grow along this route, probably because of insufficient groundwater. From the point you see the large, partly human-constructed meadow at Wawona, to the northwest, and the long, curving cliff of Wawona Dome, breaking a sea of green, to the north.

After returning 0.5 mile to the crest saddle, ►7 descend west along the Outer Loop Trail, which takes you down almost three essentially viewless, sequoia-less miles to the parking lot. The descending trail winds westward about 0.7 mile to a junction. From here a connecting trail goes about 270 yards southeast down to the tram road and the adjacent west end of the nature trail. Onward the Outer Loop Trail descends about 200 yards to a second connecting trail, descending about 150 yards southeast to cross the grove's tram road. You continue 0.8 mile southwest on the Outer Loop Trail down to the broad-crest junction, ►8 from where you could head 5.0 miles down to Wawona. Instead, you start south, left, on the Outer Loop Trail, which soon begins a winding, rolling traverse 0.5 mile southwest over to a junction with a northeast-climbing trail, then walk 0.1 mile farther to another junction, the eastbound trail from it leading to the California Tree and the Grizzly Giant. Unless you want to make another visit to them (and add about 0.5 mile to your hike) continue southward 0.5 mile down to the parking lot. ►9

A giant sequoia can live to 2000-plus years in age, producing over a half-billion seeds in this time. Only one seed is required to replace the parent.

🚶	**MILESTONES**

►1	0.0	Mariposa Grove parking lot
►2	0.6	Grizzly Giant
►3	1.7	Mariposa Grove Museum
►4	2.0	Telescope Tree
►5	2.5	Galen Clark Tree
►6	3.0	Wawona Point
►7	3.5	Return to crest saddle
►8	5.1	Left at broad-crest junction
►9	6.2	Mariposa Grove parking lot

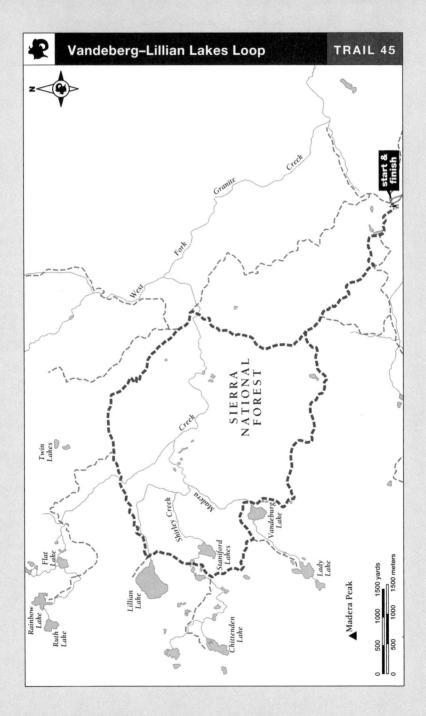

N

Granite   Creek

West   Fork

start & finish

SIERRA
NATIONAL
FOREST

Twin
Lakes

Shirley Creek

Madera

Creek

Vandeburg
Lake

Stanford
Lakes

Flat
Lake

Lillian
Lake

Lady
Lake

Rainbow
Lake

Ruth
Lake

Chittenden
Lake

▲ Madera Peak

0   500   1000   1500 yards

0   500   1000   1500 meters

Vandeberg–Lillian Lakes Loop

If you are in shape, you could hike this entire circuit in one day without overexerting yourself. However, it is so scenic that three days are recommended—sufficient time to visit Lady, Chittenden, Staniford, and Rainbow lakes. Visiting all four of these desirable lakes lengthens your route to about 21 miles, adds about 2400 feet of ascent and descent, and changes its classification to a moderate three-day hike.

Best Time

This is classic subalpine Sierran country, and as elsewhere, the trails are mostly snow-free by early July, but mosquitoes keep most away until late July. From then through mid-August, the lakes are optimal for swimming. To avoid crowds and find wilderness solitude, try hiking from mid-September through mid-October.

Finding the Trail

From the Highway 49 junction in Oakhurst, drive north on Highway 41 for 3.5 miles up to a junction with Road 222. Follow this east 3.5 miles to a fork, veer left and continue east 2.4 miles on Malum Ridge Road 274 to a junction with north-climbing Forest Route 7, or Beasore Road. (South, Beasore Road descends briefly to Pines Village, just above the north shore of Bass Lake.) Paved Forest Route 7 climbs north 4.0 miles to Chilkoot Campground, then it climbs to an intersection at Cold Springs Summit, 7.4 miles beyond the campground. Road 6S10 (an alternate, 0.2-mile-longer route to Cold

TRAIL USE
Dayhike, Backpack,
Horse
LENGTH
12.6 miles,
6 hours–3 days
VERTICAL FEET
+2650'/-2650'/±5300'
DIFFICULTY
- 1 2 3 **4** 5 +
TRAIL TYPE
Loop

FEATURES
Backcountry Permit
Child Friendly
Lakes
Streams
Wildflowers
Camping
Steep
Swimming

FACILITIES
Ranger Station
Restrooms
Campgrounds
Horse Staging
Ranger Station

Springs Summit) heads west from this intersection, winding 5.5 miles over to a junction near Kelty Meadow. From the summit, Forest Route 7 winds 8.6 miles, going past Beasore Meadows, Jones Store, Muglers Meadows, and Long Meadow before coming to a junction with Road 5S04, opposite Globe Rock, 20.0 miles from the start of Forest Route 7.

Continue along your road, an obvious route, 7.5 miles to a junction with Road 5S86. This junction is 0.4 mile past the Bowler Group Camp entrance and 100 yards before Forest Route 7 crosses Ethelfreda Creek. This alternate trailhead lies at a road's end parking area above Norris Creek, 1.9 miles up this road. Be aware that there may be a rough creek bed crossing about 0.5 mile before the parking area. This trailhead provides the shortest mileage for any hike along the Lillian Loop Trail. The second trailhead—the one from which this trip's trail mileages are based—is at the end of Road 5S05. This forks left only 100 yards after Forest Route 7 crosses Ethelfreda Creek. Take Road 5S05 2.3 miles to the trailhead and its large turnaround/parking area.

Should you need a wilderness permit or a campground, then continue east on Forest Route 7 drive east from the Road 5S05 fork, passing Road 5S88, which branches south 0.4 mile to Minarets Pack Station and then in 250 yards reaches a junction. Here, 30 miles from the start of Forest Route 7, you meet the end of Forest Route 81, a.k.a. Minarets Road, ascending 52 paved miles north from community of North Fork. From this junction, drive northeast 1.8 miles on Road 5S30 to a junction at the Clover Meadow Ranger Station. The entrance to the Clover Meadow Campground is just beyond it, and it is the closest campground for those taking Trail 45.

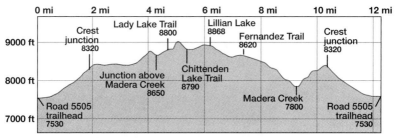

TRAIL 45 Vandeberg–Lillian Lakes Loop Elevation Profile

Trail Description

From the second trailhead at the end of Road 5S05, ▶1 you start west up the Fernandez Trail, passing through a typical mid-elevation Sierran forest: white fir, Jeffrey pine, lodgepole pine, and scrubby huckleberry oak. After 0.3 mile of gentle ascent across morainal slopes, you reach the lower end of a small meadow and meet a junction at its west side. ▶2 From it an easily missed old trail meanders almost a mile to the vicinity of the first trailhead.

Beyond the junction your trail's gradient becomes a moderate one, and red firs quickly begin to replace white firs. The forest temporarily yields to brush as you struggle up short, steep switchbacks below a small, exfoliating "dome." Now entering Ansel Adams Wilderness, you have a steady 0.5-mile pull up to a near-crest junction ▶3 with a steep, mile-long trail from the first trailhead. If you come up this short, exhausting route, remember this junction, for if it is not properly signed it can be easy to miss as you later descend the Fernandez Trail. You continue a moderate ascent up the Fernandez Trail for only a few more minutes, then reach a crest junction. ▶4

⚑ Steep

The Fernandez Trail continues right, but you branch left, along the start of the Lillian Loop Trail. While you could go either way, branching left, clockwise, is more desirable in that you'll reach a

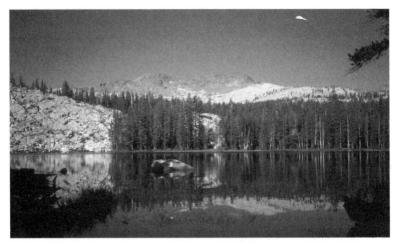

Vandeberg Lake

lake sooner than you'd reach a lake if you went
counterclockwise. For some folks, Vandeberg Lake,
the first one you'll encounter, is a worthy goal in
itself, ideal for novice backpackers, dayhikers, or
those with children.

Heading west toward peaks and lakes, you veer
left and start up the Lillian Loop Trail. This trail's
first 2 miles are generally easy. Conifers shade your
way first past a waist-deep pond, on your right, then
later past two often wet, moraine-dammed meadows; then the trail climbs to a bedrock notch in a
granitic crest. On the crest you arc around a stagnant
pond, then make a short descent to a junction above
Madera Creek. ►5 If you plan to camp at very popular Vandeberg Lake, at 8650 feet elevation, you
could leave the trail here and descend southwest to
find some campsites along its east shore.

⚑ Stream

From the junction the right branch—for horses—descends north to Madera Creek, then circles counterclockwise 0.3 mile to rejoin the left branch above the lake's west shore. You take the left branch, curving above good-to-excellent campsites along the lake's north shore. From them, steep, granitic Peak 9852, on Madera Peak's northeast ridge, is reflected in the lake's placid early morning waters. Where the two trail branches of the loop trail reunite, you start a 250-yard climb up bedrock to the edge of a lodgepole flat that has a junction with a trail to Lady Lake. ▶6

 Lake

▲ **Camping**

Lady Lake

OPTIONS

▶6 Here a spur trail takes off south and climbs gently to moderately 0.5 mile up to a large campsite on the north shore of granite-rimmed, 8908-foot-high **Lady Lake**. On the east-shore moraine that juts into the lake, you'll find an even better campsite, though not quite as large. This lake's irregular form, speckled with several boulder islands, makes it a particularly attractive lake to camp at or to visit, especially since it is backdropped by hulking, metamorphic Madera Peak. Like all the lakes you might visit along this hike, Lady Lake has trout. Because it is shallow, it is a good lake for swimming from late July through mid-August.

Beyond the Lady Lake Trail junction your Lillian Loop Trail crosses the lodgepole flat, then climbs a couple of hundred feet up fairly open granitic slabs. On them you can stop and appreciate the skyline panorama from the Minarets south to the Mt. Goddard area in Kings Canyon National Park. Descending northwest from a ridge on a moderate-to-steep gradient, you reach, in 0.2 mile, an easily missed junction—if it is not well signed—with a trail to Chittenden Lake. ▶7

Chittenden Lake

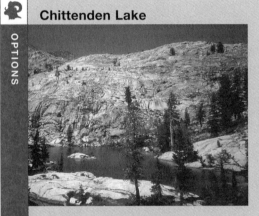

▶7 Here, close to a Staniford Lakes creek, you can start a mile-long climb up to cliff-bound 9182-foot-high Chittenden Lake. (If you miss this junction, then you probably wouldn't be able to follow the obscure trail to that lake anyway.)

Chittenden may be the most beautiful of all the lakes in this part of Ansel Adams Wilderness, though Lady and Rainbow lakes offer competition. Although Chittenden's water temperature does not usually rise above the low 60s, the lake's three bedrock islands will certainly tempt some swimmers. If there are more than two back-packers in your group, don't plan to camp at this fairly deep lake, for flat space is really at a premium.

On the Lillian Loop Trail, you go north only about 200 yards past the Chittenden Lake Trail junction before you see a Staniford lake. A waist-deep, grass-lined lakelet, this water body, like Shirley Lake, is best avoided. After a similar distance you'll come to a trailside pond atop a broad granitic crest. ▶8

Stream

More ponds are seen along the northbound Lillian Loop Trail before it dips into a usually dry gully. It then diagonals up along a ridge with many glacier-polished slabs. You soon cross the ridge, then quickly descend to Lillian Lake's outlet creek. A short walk upstream ends at the a low dam on Lillian Lake ▶9 and an adjacent, lodgepole-shaded area that once comprised the largest campsite in this

Staniford Lakes

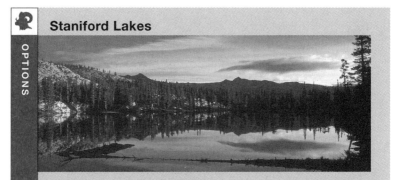

▶8 In this vicinity you can leave the trail, and on your third optional excursion descend southeast briefly cross-country on low-angle slabs to the largest of the **Staniford Lakes**, lying at 8708 feet. This is certainly the best lake to swim in, and if any sizable lake along this route will warm up to the low 70s in early August, it will be this one. The great bulk of the lake is less than 5 feet deep, its only deep spot being at a diving area along the west shore. Among the slabs you can find camp spots.

Rainbow Lake

▶10 Your fourth optional side trip ascends the Fernandez Trail 1.0 mile northwest up to a junction, from which the Rainbow Lake Trail first wanders 0.9 mile southwest up a ridge that is just north of Lillian Lake. On the ridge the trail may become vague on bedrock slabs where it bends from southwest to northwest, and unsuspecting hikers may continue southwest down toward Lillian Lake, 400 feet below, before realizing their error. If you are good at cross-country hiking, you can start from the northeast shore of Lillian Lake and hike up this "erroneous" route, and just beyond its ridge's crest locate the trail, saving about 2 miles of hiking. From the ridge the Rainbow Lake Trail then roller-coasters northwest 0.7 mile to prized **Rainbow Lake**, where camping is prohibited within 0.25 mile of the lakeshore. One can cross this multi-lobed lake by swimming from island to island.

part of the wilderness. Since camping is prohibited within 400 feet of the northeast shore, be inventive and try elsewhere. Being the largest and deepest lake you'll see along this hike, Lillian Lake is also the coldest, and its large population of trout does attract anglers.

With your basic hike now half over, you leave the lake's outlet and descend a forested mile east to a two-branched creek with easy fords. The Lillian Loop Trail ends in 0.3 mile, after a short, stiff climb over a gravelly knoll. Here, at a junction on a fairly open slope, you rejoin the Fernandez Trail, ►10 which you'll take back to the crest junction on which you started your loop. First, you might consider the side trip to Rainbow Lake (above).

From the Lillian Loop–Fernandez trails junction, you descend 0.3 mile east on the Fernandez Trail to a linear gully, follow it a bit, then drift over to the crest of a moraine, about 0.5 mile from the previous junction. From here a now abandoned, former route of the Fernandez Trail once ascended this ridge for about 0.7 mile northwest to the Twin Lakes, then a similar distance and bearing up to a minor saddle now crossed by the current route. Your route, which has been eastward, now turns southeast and follows the crest to its end, from where you soon engage a few short switchbacks near some junipers, and here get a good view of much of your basin's landscape.

Below the switchbacks the Fernandez Trail descends 0.5 mile to a junction. ►11 If you were to follow the trail north 70 yards to a crest saddle, you would see that it forks into the Post Creek Trail (left) and the Timber Creek Trail (right). The Post Creek Trail ends after a 1.9-mile climb to a packer camp on the West Fork of Granite Creek. The Timber Creek Trail climbs about 5.8 miles up to the Joe Crane Lake Trail.

From the junction the Fernandez Trail descends briefly past lodgepoles and junipers to a gravelly flat along the north bank of Madera Creek. ▶12 This spacious flat is well suited for camping, and from it you can inspect the dark plug of olivine basalt above you, which was once part of the throat of a cinder cone. On the flat you may see an old trail heading east, the former Walton Trail, which crossed Madera Creek about 250 yards below the Fernandez Trail ford, which once provided an alternate route to your trailhead. With that goal in mind, cross the creek and gain about 500 feet on the Fernandez Trail, your ridge ascent ending after a brief contour southeast to the crest junction with the start of your loop. ▶13 From it retrace your steps back to the parking area at the end of Road 5S05. ▶14

 Stream

 Camping

🚶	MILESTONES	
▶1	0.0	Start at parking area at end of Road 5S05
▶2	0.4	Straight at old-trail junction
▶3	1.7	Straight at near-crest junction
▶4	1.9	Left at crest junction
▶5	4.3	Left at junction above Madera Creek
▶6	4.7	Right at trail to Lady Lake
▶7	5.4	Right at trail to Chittenden Lake
▶8	5.6	Trailside pond atop a broad granitic crest
▶9	6.2	Lillian Lake
▶10	7.4	Right on Fernandez Trail
▶11	9.0	Straight at junction
▶12	9.3	Madera Creek
▶13	10.4	Left at crest junction
▶14	12.3	End at parking area at end of Road 5S05

Top Rated Trails

Appendix I

Campgrounds and RV Parks

Yosemite National Park Campgrounds

Hetch Hetchy

Hetch Hetchy Backpacker

Big Oak Flat Road, eastward

Hodgdon Meadow
Crane Flat

Tioga Road, eastward

Tamarack Flat
White Wolf
Yosemite Creek
Porcupine Flat
Tuolumne Meadows

Yosemite Valley

North Pines
Upper Pines
Lower Pines
Sunnyside Walk-in
Backpackers Walk-in

Glacier Point Road

Bridalveil Creek

Wawona

Wawona

National Forest Campgrounds

For each chapter on hiking trips, campgrounds close to the trailheads are listed. However, these are often full, so you may have to stay in a campground that is a considerable way from your trailhead. Below is a list of campgrounds for each national forest, and these are listed in the order you will encounter them as you drive toward the park or its adjacent Forest Service lands. For the east-side (Highway 395) campgrounds in the Humboldt–Toiyabe and Inyo National Forests, the campgrounds are listed from north to south. Campgrounds located miles away from routes to the trailheads are not listed. "R" means you can reserve.

Highway 41—
Sierra National Forest

West of Fish Camp

Summit Campground

East of Fish Camp

Big Sandy Campground
Little Sandy Campground
Fresno Dome Campground–R

North of Fish Camp

Summerdale Campground

Bass Lake

Crane Valley Campground
Forks Campground
Lupine/Cedar Campground
Spring Cove Campground
Wishon Point Campground

**Forest Route 7
(North from Bass Lake)**

Chilkoot Campground–R
Upper Chiquito Campground
Bowler Campground
Clover Meadow Campground
Granite Creek Campground

**Forest Route 81
(North from North Fork)**

Fish Creek Campground
Rock Creek Campground
Soda Springs Campground

Highway 108—
Stanislaus National Forest

West of Sonora Pass

Meadowview & Pinecrest
Cascade Creek
Mill Creek
Niagara Creek
Boulder Flat
Dardanelle
Pigeon Flat
Eureka Valley
Baker

Highway 108—
Humboldt–Toiyabe National Forest

East of Sonora Pass

Sonora Bridge
Leavitt Meadow

Highway 120—
Stanislaus National Forest

West of Yosemite National Park

The Pines
Lost Claim
Sweetwater

Cherry Road

Cherry Valley

Evergreen Road

Dimond O

Highway 120—
Inyo National Forest

East of Yosemite National Park

Lower Lee Vining
Cattleguard
Boulder
Moraine
Aspen Grove
Big Bend
Ellery
Junction & Sawmill Walk-In
Tioga Lake
Saddlebag Lake

Highway 395—Humboldt–
Toiyabe National Forest

South of Highways 108/395 junction

Obsidian

FS Road 017 (West of Bridgeport)

Buckeye

**Twin Lakes Road
(South from Bridgeport)**

Honeymoon Flat
Robinson Creek
Paha
Crags
Lower Twin Lakes

**Green Creek Road 142
(South of Bridgeport)**

Green Creek

**Virginia Lakes Road 021
(South from Conway Summit)**

Trumbull Lake

Highway 395—
Inyo National Forest

North of Lee Vining

Lundy Canyon

South of Lee Vining

June Lake Loop

Oh! Ridge
June Lake
Reversed Creek
Gull Lake
Silver Lake

Obsidian Dome Road

Hartley Springs

Glass Creek Road

Glass Creek

Deadman Creek Road

Deadman

Mammoth Lakes

Shady Rest
Pine Glen

Devils Postpile

Agnew Meadows
Upper Soda Springs
Pumice Flat
Minaret Falls
Devils Postpile
Reds Meadow

Private Campgrounds and RV Parks Outside Yosemite National Park

The following is a list of private facilities for camping. Most of these are RV parks, which cater more to those with motor homes, fifth wheels, and trailers than to those with tents, who are more likely to camp in one of the Forest Service campgrounds near the park. For each of the western Sierra highways below, the facilities are listed by their distance to the park, starting with those in the closest sites or towns. For east-side Highway 395, the facilities are listed from north to south.

Highway 41

Bass Lake

Bass Lake Recreational Resort, (559) 642-3145

Oakhurst

Elks Lodge, (559) 683-2717
High Sierra RV & Mobile Park, (559) 683-7662
Oakhurst RV Park, (559) 642-4488

Highway 120

East of Buck Meadows

Yosemite Lakes RV Park, (209) 962-0121

Groveland

Pine Mountain Lake Campground, Groveland, (209) 962-8615, -8625
Yosemite Pines RV Resort, just east of Groveland, (877) 962-7690

Midpines

KOA Yosemite–Mariposa, (209) 966-2201
Yosemite Trail Camp, (209) 966-6444

Highway 140

Mariposa

Mariposa Fairgrounds (s. on Hwy. 49), (209) 966-3686

Highway 395

Bridgeport

Annett's Mono Village (at Upper Twin Lake), (760) 932-7071

Between Bridgeport and Lee Vining
Lundy Lake Resort, (626) 309-0415

Lee Vining

Mono Vista RV Park, Lee Vining, (760) 647-6401

June Lake & Silver Lake

June Lake RV & Lodge, (760) 648-7967
Pine Cliff RV Resort, (760) 648-7558
Silver Lake Resort & RV Park, (760) 648-7525

APPENDIX II

Hotels, Lodges, Motels, and Resorts

I've tried to list all reputable facilities other than B&Bs, since B&Bs have a tendency to come and go. My apologies to the owners and managers of good facilities that I have failed to mention. On the Internet you can access most of these. For additional facilities, you might start by visiting www.yosemite.com for accommodations and services outside the park. For each of the western Sierra highways below, the facilities are listed by their distance to the park, starting with those in the closest sites or towns. For the eastside Highway 395, the facilities are listed from north to south.

Yosemite National Park—Concessionaire
Delaware North, (559) 252-4848, www.yosemitepark.com

Yosemite Valley
Ahwahnee Hotel

Camp Curry
Housekeeping Camp
Yosemite Lodge

Wawona

Wawona Hotel

Tioga Road

Tuolumne Meadows High Sierra Camp
White Wolf

Private—Yosemite National Park

The Redwoods in Yosemite, (559) 375-6666,
www.redwoodsinyosemite.com
Yosemite West, (559) 642-2211, www.yosemitewest.com

Private—Outside the Park

Only phone numbers are given.

Highway 41

Fish Camp

Apple Tree Inn, (559) 683-5111
Narrow Gauge Inn, (559) 683-7720
Tenaya Lodge at Yosemite, (559) 683-6555

Bass Lake

Forks Resort, (559) 642-3737
Pines Resort, (559) 642-3121

Oakhurst

America's Best Value Inn, (800) 658-2888
Best Western Yosemite Gateway Inn, (800) 545-5462
Comfort Inn–Oakhurst, (800) 321-5261
Days Inn, (800) DAYSINN
Oakhurst Lodge, (800) OKLODGE
Ramada Limited Yosemite, (559) 658-5500
Shilo Inn, (800) 222-2244
Sierra Sky Ranch Resort, (559) 683-8040

Highway 120

Buck Meadows

Yosemite Westgate Lodge, (800) 253-9673

Groveland

Groveland Hotel, (209) 962-4000, -7865
Pine Mountain Lake Realty (vacation home rentals), (209) 962-7156

El Portal

Cedar Lodge, (209) 379-2612
Yosemite View Lodge, (209) 379-2681

Highway 140

Midpines

Bear Creek Cabins, 209-966-5253
KOA Yosemite-Mariposa, (209) 966-2201
Muir Lodge Motel, (209) 966-2468
Whispering Pines Motel, (209) 966-5253
Yosemite Bug Lodge & Hostel, (209) 966-6666

Mariposa

Best Value Mariposa Lodge, (209) 966-3607
Best Western Yosemite Way Station Motel, (209) 996-7545
Comfort Inn–Mariposa, (209) 966-4344
E C Lodge Yosemite, (209) 742-6800
Mariposa Lodge, (209) 966-3607
Miners Inn, (209) 742-7777
Mother Lode Lodge, (209) 966-2521
Super 8 Motel, (209) 966-4288

Highway 395

Bridgeport

Annett's Mono Village (at Upper Twin Lake), (760) 932-7071
Best Western Ruby Inn, (760) 932-7241
Big Meadow Lodge, (760) 932-9801

Bodie Motel, (760) 932-7020
Bridgeport Inn, (760) 932-7380
Redwood Motel, (760) 932-7060
Silver Maple Inn, (760) 932-7383
Walker River Lodge, (760) 932-7021

Lee Vining

Best Western Lake View Lodge, (760) 647-6543
El Mono Motel, (760) 647-6310
Heidelbert Inn, (760) 648-7718
Lee Vining Motel, (760) 647-6440
Murphey's Motel, (760) 647-6316
Tioga Lodge (w. of Hwy. 395, near Tioga Pass), (760) 647-6423

June Lake & Silver Lake

Boulder Lodge, (760) 648-7533
Double Eagle Resort, (760) 648-7004
Fern Creek Lodge, (760) 648-7722, -7741
Four Seasons, (760) 648-7476
Gull Lake Lodge, (760) 648-7516
The Haven, (800) 648-7524
June Lake Motel & Cabins, (760) 648-7547
June Lake Pines Cottages, (760) 648-7522
June Lake Villager, (760) 648-7712
Lake Front Cabins, (760) 648-7527
Reverse Creek Lodge, (760) 648-7535
Silver Pines Chalet, (760) 648-2403
Whispering Pines Motel, (760) 648-7762

Mammoth Lakes

There are dozens of lodging opportunities in the small city of
Mammoth Lakes. Online, you might start by visiting
www.mammothweb.com.

APPENDIX III

Useful Books and Maps

Backpacking and Mountaineering

Beck, Steve. *Yosemite Trout Fishing Guide*. Portland, OR: Amato Publications, 1995, 158 p.

Beffort, Brian. *Joy of Backpacking*. Berkeley, CA: Wilderness Press, 2007, 320 p.

Berger, Karen. *Hiking Light Handbook*. Seattle, WA: The Mountaineers Books, 2004, 171 p.

Darvill, Fred, Jr. *Mountaineering Medicine*. Berkeley, CA: Wilderness Press, 1998, 110 p.

Ladigin, Don. *Lighten Up! A Complete Handbook for Light & Ultralight Backpacking*. Guilford, CT: The Globe Pequot Press, 2005, 100 p.

Guidebooks

Medley, Steven P. *The Complete Guidebook to Yosemite National Park*. El Portal, CA: Yosemite Association, 2002, 120 p. [Not a complete guidebook, but packed with information.]

Schaffer, Jeffrey P. *Hiker's Guide to the High Sierra: Tuolumne Meadows*. Berkeley, CA: Wilderness Press, 2006, 135 p.

Schaffer, Jeffrey P. *Hiker's Guide to the High Sierra: Yosemite*. Berkeley, CA: Wilderness Press, 2006, 126 p.

Schaffer, Jeffrey P. *Yosemite National Park: A Complete Hiker's Guide*. Berkeley, CA: Wilderness Press, 2006, 393 p.

History and Literature

Brewer, William H. *Up and Down California in 1860–64*. Berkeley, CA: University of California Press, 1930 (1974), 583 p.

Bunnell, Lafayette H. *Discovery of the Yosemite in 1851*. El Portal, CA: Yosemite Association, 1880 (1990), 314 p.

Farquhar, Francis P. *History of the Sierra Nevada*. Berkeley, CA: University of California Press, 1965, 262 p.

King, Clarence. *Mountaineering in the Sierra Nevada*. Lincoln, NB: University of Nebraska Press, 1972 (1997), 320 p.

Muir, John. *The Mountains of California*. Berkeley, CA: Ten Speed Press, 1894 (1977), 400 p.

Muir, John. *My First Summer in the Sierra*. San Francisco, CA: Sierra Club, 1911 (1990), 208 p.

Muir, John, and Galen Rowell. *The Yosemite*. San Francisco, CA: Sierra Club, 1989, 223 p.

Righter, Robert W., *The Battle Over Hetch Hetchy*. New York, NY: Oxford University Press, 2005, 303 p.

Russell, Carl P. *100 Years in Yosemite*. El Portal, CA: Yosemite Association, 1968 (1992), 267 p.

Sanborn, Margaret. *Yosemite: Its Discovery, its Wonders and its People*. El Portal, CA: Yosemite Association, 1989, 289 p.

Geology

Huber, N. King. *The geologic story of Yosemite National Park*. US Geological Survey Bulletin 1595, 1987, 64 p. [Good bedrock geology; poor uplift and glacial geology.]

Matthes, François E. *Geologic History of the Yosemite Valley*. US Geological Survey Professional Paper 160, 1930, 137 p. [The widely acclaimed classic on Yosemite Valley, but in reality an artificial construct at odds with the geologic evidence.]

Matthes, François E. *The Incomparable Valley*. Berkeley, CA: University of California Press, 1950, 160 p. [Popular account of the above, and equally flawed.]

Schaffer, Jeffrey P. *The Geomorphic Evolution of the Yosemite Valley and Sierra Nevada Landscapes: Solving the Riddles in the Rocks*. Berkeley: Wilderness Press, CA, 1997, 388 p. [The only comprehensive source on Sierran uplift and glaciation based solely on field evidence.]

Schaffer, Jeffrey P. *Seeing the Elephant: How Perceived Evidence in the Sierra Nevada Biased Global Geomorphology*. (unpub. ms. completed in 2006). [Volume 2 of the previous entry.]

Geologic Maps

Alpha, Tau Rho, Clyde Wahrhaftig, and N. King Huber. *Oblique map showing maximum extent of 20,000-year-old (Tioga) glaciers, Yosemite National Park, central Nevada, California.* US Geological Survey Map I-1885, 1987. [Considerably underestimates the lengths and thicknesses of these glaciers.]

Bateman, Paul C., and Konrad B. Krauskopf. *Geologic map of the El Portal quadrangle, west-central Sierra Nevada, California.* US Geological Survey Map MF-1998, 1987.

Bateman, Paul C., and others. *Geologic map of the Tuolumne Meadows quadrangle, Yosemite National Park, California.* US Geological Survey Map GQ-1570, 1983.

Calkins, Frank C., and others. *Bedrock geologic map of Yosemite Valley, Yosemite National Park, California.* US Geological Survey Map I-1639, 1930 (1985).

Chesterman, Charles W. *Geology of the Matterhorn Peak Quadrangle, Mono and Tuolumne Counties, California.* California Division of Mines and Geology Map Sheet 22, 1975.

Dodge, F.C.W., and L.C. Calk. *Geologic map of the Lake Eleanor quadrangle, central Sierra Nevada, California.* US Geological Survey Map GQ-1639, 1987.

Huber, N. King, and C. Dean Rinehart. *Geologic map of the Devils Postpile quadrangle, Sierra Nevada, California.* US Geological Survey Map GQ-437, 1965.

Huber, N. King, Paul C. Bateman, and Clyde Wahrhaftig. *Geologic map of Yosemite National Park and vicinity, California.* US Geological Survey Map I-1874, 1989. [Dates on metamorphic rocks are poor; glacial deposits are inaccurate.]

Kistler, Ronald W. *Geologic map of the Mono Craters quadrangle, Mono and Tuolumne Counties, California.* US Geological Survey Map GQ-462, 1966.

Kistler, Ronald W. *Geologic map of the Hetch Hetchy Reservoir quadrangle, Yosemite National Park, California.* US Geological Survey Map GQ-1112, 1973.

Peck, Dallas L. *Geologic map of the Merced Peak quadrangle, central Sierra Nevada, California.* US Geological Survey Map GQ-1531, 1980.

Peck, Dallas L. *Geologic map of the Yosemite quadrangle, central Sierra Nevada, California.* US Geological Survey Map I-2751, 2002.

Wahrhaftig, Clyde. *Geologic map of the Tower Peak quadrangle, central Sierra Nevada, California.* US Geological Survey Map I-2697, 2000. [Dates and interpretations of metamorphic rocks are poor.]

Biology

Botti, Stephen J., and Walter Sydoriak. *An Illustrated Flora of Yosemite National Park.* El Portal, CA: Yosemite Association, 2001, 484 p.

Gaines, David. *Birds of Yosemite and the East Slope.* Lee Vining: Artemisia Press, 1992, 352 p.

Horn, Elizabeth L. *Sierra Nevada Wildflowers.* Missoula, MT: Mountain Press, 1998, 215 p. [This contains over 220 photographs of common shrubs and wildflowers. It is a good introduction for those who prefer plant identification by photos rather than by keys.]

Storer, Tracy I., Robert L. Usinger, and David Lukas. *Sierra Nevada Natural History.* Berkeley: University of California Press, 2004, 439 p. [An updated classic, but erroneous, century-old glaciation and uplift geology.]

Weeden, Norman F. *A Sierra Nevada Flora.* Berkeley: Wilderness Press, 1996, 259 p.

Willard, Dwight. *A Guide to the Sequoia Groves of California.* El Portal: Yosemite Association, 2000, 124 p.

Index

Author

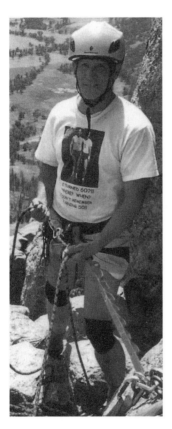

Jeffrey P. Schaffer

Jeffrey P. Schaffer has been hiking and climbing in Yosemite National Park since 1964. He's logged thousands of miles on trail in the Park, and has completed some 70 different roped ascents, including several first ascents. In 1972 he began work on his first book for Wilderness Press, *The Pacific Crest Trail*. Since then he has written and contributed to more than a dozen Wilderness Press guidebooks, including *Yosemite National Park: A Complete Hiker's Guide*. Today he teaches a variety of natural sciences courses at San Francisco Bay Area community colleges, does Sierran geomorphic research, lead-climbs both outdoors and in climbing gyms, and lives with his wife in the Napa Valley.

Series Creator
Joe Walowski

Joe Walowski conceived of the Top Trails series in 2003, and was series editor of the first three titles: *Top Trails Los Angeles*, *Top Trails San Francisco Bay Area*, and *Top Trails Lake Tahoe*. He currently lives in Seattle.

Also available from
WILDERNESS PRESS

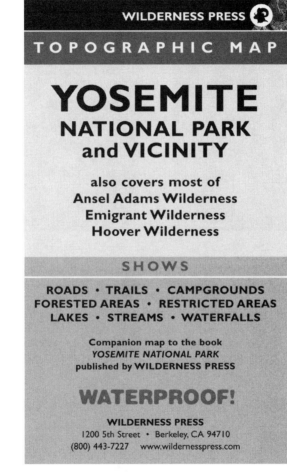

WILDERNESS PRESS

TOPOGRAPHIC MAP

YOSEMITE
NATIONAL PARK
and VICINITY

also covers most of
**Ansel Adams Wilderness
Emigrant Wilderness
Hoover Wilderness**

SHOWS

**ROADS • TRAILS • CAMPGROUNDS
FORESTED AREAS • RESTRICTED AREAS
LAKES • STREAMS • WATERFALLS**

Companion map to the book
YOSEMITE NATIONAL PARK
published by WILDERNESS PRESS

WATERPROOF!

WILDERNESS PRESS
1200 5th Street • Berkeley, CA 94710
(800) 443-7227   www.wildernesspress.com

ISBN 0-89997-370-1

More TOP TRAILS™ from WILDERNESS PRESS

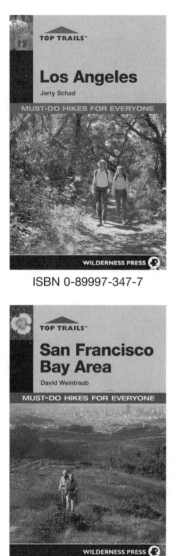

ISBN 0-89997-347-7

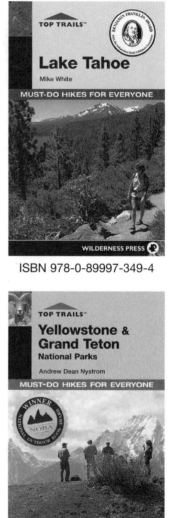

ISBN 978-0-89997-349-4

ISBN 0-89997-348-5

ISBN 0-89997-368-X

For ordering information, contact your local bookseller
or Wilderness Press, www.wildernesspress.com